Replication and Evidence Factors in Observational Studies

MONOGRAPHS ON STATISTICS AND APPLIED PROBABILITY

Editors: F. Bunea, R. Henderson, N. Keiding, L. Levina, R. Smith, W. Wong

Recently Published Titles

Multistate Models for the Analysis of Life History Data
Richard J. Cook and Jerald F. Lawless 158

Nonparametric Models for Longitudinal Data
with Implementation in R
Colin O. Wu and Xin Tian 159

Multivariate Kernel Smoothing and Its Applications
José E. Chacón and Tarn Duong 160

Sufficient Dimension Reduction
Methods and Applications with R
Bing Li 161

Large Covariance and Autocovariance Matrices
Arup Bose and Monika Bhattacharjee 162

The Statistical Analysis of Multivariate Failure Time Data: A Marginal Modeling Approach
Ross L. Prentice and Shanshan Zhao 163

Dynamic Treatment Regimes
Statistical Methods for Precision Medicine
Anastasios A. Tsiatis, Marie Davidian, Shannon T. Holloway, and Eric B. Laber 164

Sequential Change Detection and Hypothesis Testing
General Non-i.i.d. Stochastic Models and Asymptotically Optimal Rules
Alexander Tartakovsky 165

Introduction to Time Series Modeling
Genshiro Kitigawa 166

Replication and Evidence Factors in Observational Studies
Paul R. Rosenbaum 167

For more information about this series please visit: https://www.crcpress.com/
Chapman--HallCRC-Monographs-on-Statistics--Applied-Probability/book-series/
CHMONSTAAPP

Replication and Evidence Factors in Observational Studies

Paul R. Rosenbaum

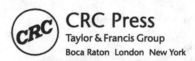

CRC Press
Taylor & Francis Group
Boca Raton London New York

CRC Press is an imprint of the
Taylor & Francis Group, an **informa** business

A CHAPMAN & HALL BOOK

First edition published 2021
by CRC Press
6000 Broken Sound Parkway NW, Suite 300, Boca Raton, FL 33487-2742

and by CRC Press
2 Park Square, Milton Park, Abingdon, Oxon, OX14 4RN

CRC Press is an imprint of Taylor & Francis Group, LLC

Library of Congress Control Number: 2021930860

ISBN: 978-0-367-48388-3 (hbk)
ISBN: 978-0-367-75170-8 (pbk)
ISBN: 978-1-003-03964-8 (ebk)

Typeset in Computer Modern font
by Cenveo Publisher Services

For Paul, Noah, and Sara

With a true view all the facts harmonize, but with a false one they soon clash.

Aristotle [2, p. 372, 1098b10]

A conclusion cannot be more certain than that some one of the facts that support it is true, but it may easily be more certain than any one of those facts. ... We have ... a variety of facts .... Some arbitrary hypothesis may otherwise explain any one of these facts; this is the only theory which brings them to support one another.

Charles Sanders Peirce [171, pp. 18, 20]

No genuine science is formed by isolated conclusions .... Science does not emerge until these various findings are linked up together to form a coherent system—that is, until they reciprocally confirm and illuminate one another.

John Dewey [55, pp. 21–22]

It must, however, be stressed that the harmonization of knowledge is nowadays to be seen in fundamentally pragmatic terms. It is not a matter of discovery—of finding at the end of a long course of inquiry that we have discovered a harmonious reality. Instead, it is the other way round: The standard of acceptability that we ourselves endorse with respect to the distinction between conjecture and fact views the harmony of fact as a pivotal validating factor in our entitlement to certain contentions as true rather than merely problematic or conjectural.

Nicholas Rescher [180, p. 27]

Contents

Preface

Two Facts and a Question about Them

Let us begin with two facts and a question about them.

The first fact is that association does not imply causation. The treatments that individuals receive may be associated with the outcomes they exhibit, yet that association may or may not reflect effects caused by the treatments. In formal statistical terms, taken alone, the observable distributions—the distributions of the data that we can see—do not identify the effects caused by the treatments. The same observable distributions are compatible with an effect caused by the treatment or with an unobserved bias in the way treatments are allocated to individuals. This ambiguity would persist even if we collected an infinite quantity of data from these observable distributions: more data isn't the solution. In a slightly idealized randomized trial, treatments are allocated to individuals on the basis of random numbers generated by a computer; then, association does imply causation, as biased treatment assignment has been prevented. But in a study of treatment effects without random assignment of treatments—in an observational study—association does not imply causation: the causal effects are not identified by the observable distributions. A short survey of these issues is given in Part I: Aspects of Causal Inference.

The second fact is that cigarette smoking causes lung cancer in human beings, and we know this; indeed, we know this as well as we know anything. True, scientists would listen, perhaps briefly, to a critic who claimed the second fact is mistaken, not a fact after all; however, unless that critic quickly delivered substantial new evidence or reasons for doubting this second fact, scientists would stop listening, dismissing the critic as a paid lobbyist, a quack, or someone who likes to argue for the enjoyment of arguing. Moreover, we know the second fact in the absence of randomized trials forcing individuals to smoke or not smoke. The direct evidence that smoking causes lung cancer in people comes from observational studies of the kind described in the first fact, studies in which association does not imply causation.

The question is: How can the first fact and the second fact both be true?

A Neglected Aspect of Causal Inference

This book is about a neglected aspect of formal causal inference, an aspect that is commonly present and often decisive in informal discussions of the evidence of cause and effect. A common answer to the question at the end of the previous section is to hand over several massive summary reports about smoking and health prepared by the US Surgeon General [249, 250, 251]. That is an answer of a certain kind, perhaps adequate in its way, yet it leaves us puzzled in another way: How can a large quantity of ambiguous evidence become unambiguous? If more data isn't the solution, how can more data ever become decisive?

If one sought an answer in a brief slogan, it would be this: Fallible comparisons all fallible in the same way, no matter how numerous, are never decisive, but fallible comparisons fallible in very different ways may ultimately be decisive. This brief, nontechnical answer is known and has been advocated when thinking about replication of observational studies. A series of observational studies that all suffer from the same ambiguity may not be much more convincing than the first study in the series, particularly if all of the investigators are competent and sample sizes are large. If three witnesses testify to the innocence of the defendant, but they are all siblings of the defendant, then the evidence they supply shares a single ambiguity, an ambiguity not resolved by seeking the testimony of the defendant's other siblings. In contrast, a series of ambiguous observational studies not inconsistent with a treatment effect may be much more convincing than any one of those studies if the ambiguities in different studies are very different. Could the stars align with such malice that each study has a different ambiguity, unrelated to the ambiguities of earlier studies, yet each study gives the false appearance of treatment effect? In his *Meditations Concerning First Philosophy*, Descartes entertained the possibility that "a certain malign spirit, maximally powerful and clever, has employed all his industry so that I am deceived"; however, if only that could explain why a series of observational studies concur, then we fall short of logical proof but may have more than we need to formulate policy.

It is a mistake to conflate "doing a new study" and "facing a different ambiguity." A series of studies may share one ambiguity. Conversely, one study may permit several comparisons, each ambiguous, yet ambiguous in very different ways. The central task of this book is to bring this informal aspect of causal reasoning into formal causal inference, introducing new statistical analyses for a single observational study that can quantitatively demonstrate stronger evidence of cause and effect when ambiguous comparisons concur.

Two or more comparisons suffer from different ambiguities. In what sense may they combine to provide stronger evidence together than they provide on their own? First, the combined analysis may be insensitive to larger unmeasured biases than each comparison is by itself. Second, evidence may be demarcated: each part of the evidence may be set aside in turn, to see if the conclusion stands without it. View any one part with total skepticism, as facing infinite bias, the victim of Descartes' "malign spirit": Would the conclusion about treatment effects remain in place without that part? It may happen that there is strong evidence for a conclusion no matter which part of the evidence is omitted.

Organization of the Book

This is a second book about causal inference, a book about a topic. The book is self-contained—there is no need to read something else first—but the book is not comprehensive—many important topics in causal inference are mentioned only briefly and others are not mentioned at all.

The book has four parts. Part I is background, intended to make the book self-contained. Chapters 1 and 2 discuss selected aspects of causal inference in randomized experiments and observational studies. Topics appear or not in these chapters precisely to the extent that the topics are needed later in the book. These chapters introduce some notation and terminology that will be used later. Chapter 3 discusses replication in observational studies—how biases can replicate along with treatment effects, how successful replication is not repetition but rather disrupts the most plausible sources of bias. Given that replication is not repetition—not more data of the same kind—Chapter 3 is a prelude to the book's central question: Can a single observational study replicate itself? Are there evidence factors?

Part II discusses evidence factors in terms of examples, concepts, and practical methods, delaying theoretical justification of these methods to Part III. My hope is that a reader will be able to use evidence factors in a standard way having read Part II, and will be able to develop new evidence factors having read Part III. Part IV is brief: it discusses the algorithmic aspects of designing observational studies to contain evidence factors.

How to Read This Book

As I mentioned, this is a second book about causal inference, a book about a specific topic. How should a second book begin? How should you read it?

Chapters 1–3 of Part I are background. They start at the beginning, but move quickly, focusing on aspects of causal inference that arise in later chapters. The material in Chapters 1–3 may be entirely familiar, entirely unfamiliar, or familiar in part. No matter: read what seems helpful or interesting in these chapters; then, move along. You can always come back if you omitted something you find you need later.

The book begins in earnest with the motivating examples in Chapter 4. It is reasonable to begin the book by reading Chapter 4, returning to Part I, if needed, with a clearer sense of purpose. It is equally reasonable to begin reading with Chapter 1.

Between Chapter 4 and Chapter 12, the book develops in a straight line, one thing following another. Even here, there are many options to skip material and move on, as discussed below. Chapter 13 is different: it may be read immediately after Chapter 4, or not at all. Chapter 14 is a brief look back at the earlier chapters.

A technically minded reader who skips the motivation, applications, and examples may miss more than a practically minded reader who skips the mathematics.

Certain topics may be skipped. Chapter 1 spends some time combatting the mistaken notion that randomization inference is limited to tests of no effect; so, confidence intervals for various measures of the magnitude of effect are discussed in some detail in Chapter 1. If this mistaken notion is not your notion, then you might limit your time with this material.

A general concept is often illustrated with two or more examples. One example is the simplest nontrivial instance of the general concept. A second example may be more complex, intended to provide a sense of the scope of the general concept. For instance, in Chapter 2, there are two examples of sensitivity analysis in observational studies. The example in §2.2 involves 11 pairs of two people matched for two covariates, and the mathematics involves 11 independent coin flips. The example in §2.3 involves 2475 people in 104 strata defined by observed covariates, with additional robust covariance adjustment for these covariates, with reference to the journal literature and R packages for technical details and implementation. At a certain level of abstraction, the two examples are entirely parallel, but there is definitely more stuff in the second example. The point I am making by including both examples is that the material in this book is applicable to general concepts, both simple instances and complex instances of these concepts. The simple instance is included as an aid to understanding. The complex instance is an aid to an investigator who would like to incorporate the general concept in a study that has various unavoidable complexities. You can skip the second, more complex example, yet understand the general concept and its role in subsequent discussion.

Some chapters have additional sections, called "Complements," that appear after the chapter summaries. These sections complete the chapter: they might have been sections of the chapter, but their placement at the end is intended to emphasize that they are not needed if the goal is to see the big picture quickly. A "Complement" explores a potentially useful variation on a theme, where earlier sections of the chapter have adequately explored the theme. When you reach the chapter summary: If you want more, read the "Complement"; otherwise, move on.

Some chapters have an optional section entitled "Using R." Such a section shows how to perform a few statistical analyses that were done earlier in the chapter.

In contrast, a chapter or section with an asterisk (*) is a bit more technical than other material in the same part of the book. The second example mentioned in a previous paragraph is in §2.3, and this section has an asterisk. Sometimes, a section with an asterisk contains material that is fussy, as in §10.3. At other times, this technical material refers to concepts that are interesting, not difficult, but possibly unfamiliar and also not essential. For instance, it is often enlightening, but not essential, to note that a particular set of permutation matrices is a subgroup, or a coset, or a system of distinct representatives of the cosets of a subgroup. Sections that make use of elementary group theory have asterisks: you can skip them without loss of continuity, but you may be skipping material that offers an organized perspective on evidence factors as a whole. In a subsection of §2.4, an asterisk indicates a concise survey of material that plays a role when deciding to use one test statistic rather than another. A reader who is content to trust my choices of test statistics could omit §2.4, or return to it later if the need arises. This book has nothing new to say about the choice of a test statistic for use in a sensitivity analysis—see Ref. [223, Chapter 19] for discussion of this topic—but it is necessary to choose a statistic when an analysis is done, and §2.4 concisely discusses this choice. Nonetheless, design sensitivity—the topic of §2.4 as a whole—does make repeated brief appearances throughout the book.

Finding What You Need

In the index, a **bold** page number signifies a definition. The index contains an entry for notation, where mathematical symbols are listed. The index contains an entry for examples—empirical studies with evidence factors—many of which are discussed repeatedly in different parts of the book. There are a few technical glosses intended to simplify the book; these may be located using the index, under the entry "without further mention."

R Package

A companion R package, `evident`, is available from CRAN. The package contains data sets used in the book. The help-files for these data sets reproduce some analyses from the book. Some exercises ask you to perform additional analyses using data from `evident`.

Terminology

Terms used in this book come from standard English, from experimental design, from statistical theory, and from abstract algebra. As in English, one word may have several meanings. There are treatment "groups," control "groups," and algebraic "groups" of permutation matrices. Worse than this, the word "block" has a meaning in experimental design and a different meaning in group theory, still another meaning in "block diagonal matrices," even though the theory of experimental design employs group theory, and there are groups of block diagonal matrices. As in English, I try to avoid introducing strange new terminology merely to avoid familiar multiple meanings; instead, I let the context indicate the relevant meaning. If I suggest that you go to the bank to get some cash, then you know I mean the bank in town, not the river bank. In parallel, I let the context distinguish treatment groups from matrix groups. I try to be alert to possible ambiguity of expression, but I belabor it only when there is a cash machine at the river bank.

Notation in Part III

The slightly technical discussion in Part III uses the following notation. Notation is defined as it is introduced. For convenient quick reference later as you read, a few aspects of the notation are collected here.

The indicator $\chi(E)$ of an event E is $\chi(E) = 1$ if E occurs and $\chi(E) = 0$ if E does not occur. If $\mathscr{A}$ is a finite set, then $|\mathscr{A}|$ denotes the number of elements in $\mathscr{A}$.

Logical notation is used to combine two null hypotheses to produce a new hypothesis, $\wedge$ for "and," $\vee$ for "or." The conjunction hypothesis is the hypothesis that asserts that hypotheses H and H' are both true, and it is denoted by $H \wedge H'$. The disjunction hypothesis asserts that either hypothesis H or hypothesis H' or both are true, and it is denoted by $H \vee H'$.

Lower-case bold **a** signifies a fixed matrix or column vector, while $\mathbf{a}^T$ is its transpose. In contrast, $\mathbf{a}'$ does not signify transpose, but rather a close relative—a sibling or cousin—of **a**, whose exact meaning will be clear from the context. Upper-case bold **A** is a random matrix or vector. A treatment assignment for N individuals is represented by an $N \times N$ permutation matrix **a**; see Chapter 8. A set of fixed permutation matrices of the same size is denoted A, and some of these sets happen to be groups of permutation matrices; see Chapter 9. The number of elements **a** of A is $|A|$, so if the permutation matrices **a** in A are $N \times N$, then $|A| \leq N!$. Two $N \times N$ permutation matrices, **a** and **b**, can be multiplied, but so can two sets, A and B, of such matrices; see §9.2. A probability distribution **p** on A is a vector of dimension $|A|$ with nonnegative coordinates summing to one, so **p** gives the distribution of a random permutation matrix **A** taking values in A; see §10.1. A set $\mathscr{P}$ of distributions on A is simply a set of such vectors **p**; see §10.2. A sensitivity analysis in an observational study considers a growing or nested family of sets $\mathscr{P}_\Gamma$ of distributions on A indexed by a parameter Γ; see §10.4. The knit product of two sets of probability distributions, $\mathscr{P}' \oslash \mathscr{P}''$, is defined in Definition 9 in Chapter 11.

The Greek letter upsilon, $\Upsilon(\bullet)$, signifies either an upper tail probability of a test statistic with a single known distribution **p** in (10.2), or the upper bound on such a tail probability over a set $\mathscr{P}$ of distributions **p** in (10.6).

Subscripts occur throughout the book, but their use is contextual: the same subscript may have a different meaning in different parts of the book. Subscripts, such as i, j, k, ℓ, s, are used to distinguish individuals, treatment assignments, strata, treatment groups, doses, and so on. If the meaning of a subscript is unclear, look nearby, earlier in the same chapter; do not jump to another chapter where the meaning may be different.

Exercises

Some chapters end with exercises. In this book, exercises are optional, not required reading. Proofs in the text are complete as they stand; they do not depend upon doing the exercises.

Exercises provide optional practice with data, R, concepts, and notation. Some exercises ask you to do an easy simulation to check some claim about design sensitivity. Exercises develop some topics in greater detail than is needed for the text. For instance, there is more about groups of permutation matrices in the exercises than in the text. An exercise may ask you to examine an issue more closely than was needed in the text itself. An exercise may ask: Where does a particular proof in the text go wrong if a needed premise is dropped?

Acknowledgments

I am grateful to Bikram Karmakar, Bo Lu, Mark Neuman, Jeffrey H. Silber, Dylan S. Small, and José R. Zubizarreta for collaborations that are discussed in this book. I am grateful to Colin Fogarty, Bikram Karmakar, Judith A. McDonald, Samuel Pimentel, José R. Zubizarreta, and three anonymous reviewers for comments on a draft of this book.

Part I

Background: Aspects of Causal Inference

Chapter 1

Causal Inference in Randomized Experiments

Abstract

Causal inference in randomized experiments is briefly reviewed in notation that will be used throughout the book. Treatment assignments permute N individuals into N positions in an experimental design, and a randomized experiment selects the treatment assignment at random, using random numbers generated by the computer, so that no pretreatment attribute of an individual predicts their assigned treatment. Causal effects are comparisons of potential outcomes under different treatment assignments, and they are radically simplified if only the treatment an individual receives affects the outcomes of that individual, a condition known as "no interference between individuals." Randomization provides a basis for testing Fisher's null hypothesis of no causal effect, and various devices invert this test to provide confidence sets for the magnitude of effect.

1.1 A Randomized Experiment

1.1.1 Treatment of Hypertension

In 2002, the *Journal of the American Medical Association* published the results of a randomized trial [75] called ALLHAT, the short form of "Antihypertensive and Lipid Lowering Treatment to Prevent Heart Attack Trial." Appropriately, the design of the trial and plans for its analysis had been published six years earlier [53]. The trial compared three drugs, of different types, used to treat hypertension with a view to reducing heart attack and cardiovascular mortality. The drugs were: (i) amlodipine, a calcium channel blocker, (ii) lisinopril, an ACE inhibitor, and (iii) chlorthalidone, a diuretic, a relatively standard treatment approved in 1960 by the Food and Drug Administration. To increase power when compared to the standard, about 1.7 times as many patients were allocated to chlorthalidone.[1]

---

[1] The ALLHAT experiment will be used to illustrate and anchor certain concepts of causal inference in randomized experiments. The actual trial is more complex than my description of it: I will ignore certain issues discussed in Ref. [75] that are unrelated to the concepts this example is intended to exemplify. Some of the issues I ignore are consequential in the trial, but peripheral to the current discussion; for instance, as in any prolonged trial, there is some loss to follow up as the years passed. Other issues I ignore are largely inconsequential technical variations on how randomization is implemented. Finally, I

The ALLHAT trial was essentially an equitable lottery: $N = 33,357$ individuals—patients—were assigned to three treatments at random. Treatment assignment favored no individual above another. In ALLHAT, individuals were assigned to the three drugs using random numbers generated by the computer. Because more patients were assigned to chlorthalidone, every patient was more likely to receive chlorthalidone than, say, amlodipine; however, this was true in the same way for every patient. For every individual, there was a $0.46 = 1.7/(1 + 1 + 1.7)$ probability of receiving chlorthalidone, a $0.27 = 1/(1 + 1 + 1.7)$ probability of amlodipine, and a 0.27 probability of lisinopril. Think of this as $N = 33,357$ lottery tickets, 46% marked chlorthalidone, 27% marked amlodipine, 27% marked lisinopril, with either tickets or individuals randomly permuted to allocate each individual to one ticket.

1.1.2   Equitable Treatment Assignment

There are an enormous number of possible ways to permute 33,357 individuals to 33,357 treatment positions, with 46% of positions marked chlorthalidone, 27% marked amlodipine, 27% marked lisinopril. Each of these possible permutations was given the same probability, and one permutation was selected at random.

Because the lottery was fair, was randomized, and the sample size was large, the winners and losers looked quite similar in terms of covariates, that is, in terms of variables measured prior to treatment. The average age was 66.9 years in all three treatment groups, 32% of patients were non-hispanic blacks in all three groups, and 22% of patients were cigarette smokers in all three groups [75, Table 1]. Luck did produce some small imbalances: 47% of patients were women in both the chlorthalidone and amlodipine groups, but 46% of patients were women in the lisinopril group.

It is important to observe that luck—a fair lottery—produced similar treatment groups: age, race, and gender were not used to decide treatments. This is important because there are covariates that were not measured, possibly important ones—there are unobserved covariates—and yet a fair lottery should tend to balance these as well. Perhaps a decade from now, a genetic variant of great importance to cardiovascular risk will be discovered; however, that discovery will not invalidate the ALLHAT experiment, because randomization should make that variant occur with almost equal relative frequency in the three groups, as it did with age, race, smoking, and gender. More precisely and more importantly, individuals with and without that genetic variant received lottery tickets in exactly—not approximately—the same way, with exactly the same probabilities. The sample proportions are approximately the same, but the true underlying probabilities are exactly the same, with and without the genetic variant. Using those treatment assignment probabilities, appropriate statistical analysis of a properly conducted randomized trial takes full account of baseline covariate differences that randomization could produce by chance. Yes, there is a tiny probability that a fair lottery will end up looking very unfair. Yes, there is, in a fair lottery, a tiny probability of a giant imbalance in an unmeasured covariate; however,

---

will focus on a secondary outcome—achieved blood pressure control at year one—rather than the primary cardiovascular outcome, for which no effect was demonstrated. This secondary outcome is better as an illustration of certain issues; however, it is of less clinical importance.

the randomization inference is telling us precisely how improbable it is that we are being misled by this highly improbable event. Randomization and its theoretical properties were developed by Sir Ronald A. Fisher [68].

1.1.3 Randomized Trials Contain Simpler Randomized Trials

Randomized trials often contain other simpler randomized trials. Two randomized trials inside the ALLHAT experiment will be mentioned. One trial compares two of the three treatment groups. The other trial compares the third treatment group to a peculiar treatment formed as a type of lottery. The lottery treatment group is exposed to a lottery that assigns individuals to one of the first two treatments.

Imagine that we set aside the individuals who received amlodipine. It is fairly clear that what remains is a fair lottery between chlorthalidone and lisinopril for the people who have not been set aside. Said more precisely, conditionally given who received amlodipine, the distribution of treatment assignments for the remaining individuals is randomized between chlorthalidone and lisinopril. So, conditioning on who received amlodipine creates a smaller randomized trial inside the ALLHAT experiment, namely a trial that compares chlorthalidone and lisinopril.

We could merge the chlorthalidone and lisinopril treatment groups. The single merged group is the cl-lottery, namely the peculiar treatment consisting of a lottery between chlorthalidone and lisinopril in ratio 1.7-to-1. It is fairly clear that the ALLHAT experiment contains a randomized experiment comparing amlodipine to the cl-lottery: it is just luck whether a patient is assigned to amlodipine or to the cl-lottery. Of course, there was nothing special in our choice of amlodipine: the same reasoning applies to each drug.

In randomized trials, the issues just described are simple enough that we use them without noticing them. Parallel issues will arise in a more noticeable form in observational studies in Parts II and III.

1.2   Structure and Notation

1.2.1   One Treatment Position for Each Individual

An experimental design begins with N treatment positions. In some designs, the N treatment positions involve N distinct treatments,[2] but in clinical trials, there are usually only a few distinct treatments, with many individuals allocated to the same treatment. In the ALLHAT experiment, there was one treatment position for each patient—$N = 33,357$ treatment positions for $N = 33,357$ patients—but there were only three distinct treatments. That is, there were $N = 33,357$ lottery tickets to be assigned to the $N = 33,357$ patients, but there were only three kinds of tickets, and many tickets of each kind. In ALLHAT, think of the first 46% of positions as labeled chlorthalidone, the next 27% as labeled amlodipine, and the final 27% as labeled lisinopril.

---

[2]The N treatment positions are typically distinct in fractional factorial designs; see, for instance Ref. [160].

1.2.2   Treatment Assignments Permute Individuals to Treatment Positions

A treatment assignment g permutes the N individuals into the N treatment positions. Let us index the individuals by j, so we have individuals $j = 1, \dots, N$. Let us index the treatment positions by ℓ, so we have individuals $\ell = 1, \dots, N$. A treatment assignment is a permutation g, sending individuals to treatment positions. If g assigns individual j to treatment position ℓ, then write $g(j) = \ell$ or more concisely $gj = \ell$. Every treatment position is filled by a different individual.[3] Of course, in ALLHAT, positions $\ell = 1$ and $\ell = 2$ are different positions, but the different patients in those different positions both receive chlorthalidone.

> **Treatment Assignment** The experiment has N treatment positions, which may or may not represent N distinct treatments. There are N individuals. A treatment assignment is a permutation: it places the N individuals into the N treatment positions.

For any finite set S, write $|S|$ for the number of elements of S.

There are $N!$ permutations g of N individuals, far more than we need to represent the ALLHAT experiment. The ALLHAT experiment does not change if we switch two distinct people, j and j', between two distinct treatment positions, ℓ and ℓ', that both received chlorthalidone. The simplest approach to avoiding redundancy is to pick one representative permutation among many equivalent permutations. Consider the set of all of the permutations g that are the same in the sense of assigning the same people to the chlorthalidone, amlodipine, and lisinopril treatment groups. Some of those permutations assign individual j to the first position in the chlorthalidone group, others assign j to the second position, and so on, but j is always assigned to chlorthalidone, with an analogous pattern for every individual. The permutations in this set differ only in how they order the individuals inside each treatment group, and we do not care about that. So, let us pick one g to represent the entire set. The one representative is picked arbitrarily, just to avoid redundancy. A simple way to do this is to always use the one permutation g that preserves the original order inside each treatment group.[4] Collect these distinct representatives g in a set G. If $g \neq g'$ with $g \in G$ and $g' \in G$, then g and g' are meaningfully different: there is at least one person j who receives a different drug under treatment assignment g than under treatment assignment g'.[5] So, we have represented the $N!$ permutations, many of which

---

[3] In other words, a permutation $g(\cdot)$ is a 1-1 function. That is, if j and j' both get assigned to the same position ℓ, then j and j' must be the same person; $gj = \ell$ and $gj' = \ell$ implies $j = j'$. In Chapter 8, the function $g(j) = \ell$ or $gj = \ell$ is replaced by an $N \times N$ permutation matrix $\mathbf{g}$ that sends individuals $\mathbf{n} = (1, \dots, N)^T$ to N treatment positions as $\mathbf{gn}$. Where the function $g(j)$ acts on individual j, the matrix $\mathbf{g}$ acts on all N individuals at once.

[4] If $j < j'$ are assigned to different positions in the same treatment group, say amlodipine, then $gj = \ell < \ell' = gj'$, so the people in the amlodipine group are in increasing order in terms of their original indices j. These single representatives are the pick matrices in Chapter 8.

[5] If C people receive chlorthalidone, A people receive amlodipine, and L people receive lisinopril, where $N = C + A + L$, then the set G contains $|G| = N! / (C! \times A! \times L!)$ permutations g that are meaningfully

assign the same drugs to the same people, by a smaller set G, with $|G| < N!$, where different $g \in G$ represent meaningfully different treatment assignments.

The Set of Treatment Assignments The set, G, of possible treatment assignments contains $N!$ treatment assignments *only if* all N treatment positions represent distinct treatments and there are no restrictions on treatment assignment. More commonly, $|G| < N!$.

If the goal were to describe the ALLHAT experiment alone, then a simpler notation would be possible. Instead, the goal is to have a single notation that describes a wide variety of studies.

In brief, under treatment assignment g, individual j receives treatment gj. Distinct $g \in G$ change the drugs received by at least two of the $N = 33,357$ individuals, perhaps swapping person j who received chlorthalidone for person j' who received lisinopril.

1.2.3   What Is a Randomized Experiment?

In the current book, a randomized experiment entails picking a treatment assignment, a permutation $g \in G$ of individuals to treatment positions, at random, so each $g \in G$ has probability $1/|G|$. Write G for the resulting treatment assignment, so the chance that $G = g$ is $1/|G|$ for each $g \in G$. In this case, individual j is randomly assigned to treatment Gj. More complex forms of randomization are sometimes used in clinical trials [235], but they do not arise in this book.

If we listed the elements of G in some definite order, $g_1, g_2, \ldots, g_{|G|}$, then there is a corresponding vector

$$\mathbf{p}^T = \left(p_{g_1}, p_{g_2}, \ldots, p_{g_{|G|}} \right) \text{ with } p_{g_k} \geq 0, \, k = 1, \ldots, |G| \text{ and } 1 = \sum_{k=1}^{|G|} p_{g_k}. \quad (1.1)$$

In a randomized experiment,

$$\mathbf{p}^T = \left(p_{g_1}, p_{g_2}, \ldots, p_{g_{|G|}} \right) = \left(\frac{1}{|G|}, \ldots, \frac{1}{|G|} \right). \quad (1.2)$$

As the book proceeds, there will be other sets G of treatment assignments g in randomized experiments, but (1.2) will be the distribution of treatment assignments in these randomized experiments. Other distributions besides (1.2) will arise in non-randomized or observational studies, where treatment assignment may be inequitable or biased. Uncertainty about the true distribution of treatment assignments in an observational study will be represented by a set $\mathscr{P}$ of distributions of the form (1.2). But let us deal with that in due course.

---

different, and each $g \in G$ represents $C! \times A! \times L!$ permutations that assign the same people to the same drugs.

Table 1.1 *Achievement of blood pressure goal* $< 140/90$ *mm Hg in ALLHAT for individuals at risk at one year after the start of treatment*

	Chlorthalidone	Amlodipine	Lisinopril
Achieved	7434	4200	3806
Not achieved	5428	3409	3715
Total	12862	7609	7521
Percent achieved	57.8%	55.2%	50.6%

1.3 Covariates and Outcomes

1.3.1 Covariates

A covariate is a variable measured or measurable prior to treatment assignment, hence unaffected by the treatment an individual will later receive. A covariate is observed if its value is measured and recorded. A covariate is unobserved if its value was not measured and recorded. The observed covariate for individual j is $\mathbf{x}_j$. An unobserved covariate for individual j is $\mathbf{u}_j$. Either $\mathbf{x}_j$ or $\mathbf{u}_j$ may be a vector representing several variables. As an individual j is permuted among treatment positions, that individual's covariates, $\mathbf{x}_j$ and $\mathbf{u}_j$, move with him or her, but they do not change. If a woman is 60 years old at baseline, before treatment assignment, then she remains a woman who was 60 years old at baseline whether she is assigned to chlorthalidone or lisinopril. Write $\mathbf{x}$ for the matrix with N rows whose jth row is $\mathbf{x}_j^T$, and $\mathbf{u}$ for the matrix with N rows whose jth row is $\mathbf{u}_j^T$,

There are borderline cases, and these are classified as follows: If a covariate is measured with error, the fallible recorded value is part of $\mathbf{x}_j$, and the difference between the fallible recorded value and the true unrecorded value is part of $\mathbf{u}_j$. If a covariate is sometimes observed, sometimes missing, then: (i) place in $\mathbf{x}_j$ either its observed value or an asterisk (*) signifying that its value is missing; (ii) place in $\mathbf{u}_j$ an asterisk (*) if the covariate is observed, and its missing value if the value is missing. In other words, in all cases, what is observed is in $\mathbf{x}_j$ and what is not observed is in $\mathbf{u}_j$. For instance, we can adjust for the observed covariates plus the pattern of missing covariates [229, Appendix], as all of this is recorded in $\mathbf{x}_j$, but we cannot adjust for the missing values themselves as they are in $\mathbf{u}_j$.

1.3.2 The Complete Array of Potential Outcomes

A secondary outcome in the ALLHAT experiment was a binary indicator of whether the blood pressure goal had been achieved at one year after the start of treatment. The goal was 140/90 mm Hg. Table 1.1 summarizes the results for individuals in the trial at one year.

To say that treatment with lisinopril caused person j to have lower systolic blood pressure than person j would have had under chlorthalidone is to compare two potential outcomes for person j under different treatment assignments. The formal expression of causal effects as comparisons of potential outcomes under alternative treatments is due to Jerzy Neyman [164] and Donald Rubin [237]. See also

Refs. [48, 93, 129, 285, 289] and Ref. [245, Chapter 9]. Potential outcomes are described in a more general notation in the current subsection, with the next subsection describing the Neyman-Rubin notation.

In principle, individual j has a different potential outcome or response under each treatment assignment $g \in G$, or $|G|$ possible outcomes,

$$\mathbf{r}_j^T = \left(r_{jg_1}, r_{jg_2}, \ldots, r_{jg_{|G|}} \right). \tag{1.3}$$

This says that individual j would exhibit response r_{jg_k} if treatments were assigned according to permutation $g_k \in G$. For the binary outcome in Table 1.1, $r_{jg_k} = 1$ if individual j would achieve the blood pressure goal if randomization picked treatment assignment $g_k \in G$, and $r_{jg_k} = 0$ otherwise.

Write $\mathbf{r}$ for the $N \times |G|$ matrix of $|G|$ potential outcomes for N individuals. The rows of $\mathbf{r}$ refer to distinct individuals, the columns to distinct ways of assigning individuals to treatment positions. Keep in mind that $\mathbf{r}$ is a large matrix, with many columns. If $N = 10$ individuals were permuted into two treatment groups each containing 5 individuals, then there are $|G| = 10!/(5! \times 5!) = 252$ possible treatment assignments $g \in G$, so $\mathbf{r}$ is 10×252. In the ALLHAT trial, $\mathbf{r}$ is unthinkably large, but quite simple in concept. The matrix $\mathbf{r}$ simply indicates which of the N specific individuals j would achieve the blood pressure goal under every possible random assignment $g_k \in G$.

We see a single column, $\mathbf{R}$, of $\mathbf{r}$, the column that corresponds to the treatment assignment $g \in G$ that was actually selected by randomization. That is, we see one column $\mathbf{R}$ of $\mathbf{r}$ picked at random from the $|G|$ columns, where each column $g \in G$ has the same probability $1/|G|$. Taken together, $g \in G$ and $\mathbf{R}$ tell us who received which treatment, and what outcomes were observed under the treatments individuals received, so that, from $g \in G$ and $\mathbf{R}$, we could produce, for instance, Table 1.1.

When we speak of the probability of a treatment assignment $g \in G$, we mean the conditional probability given $\mathbf{r}$, $\mathbf{x}$, and $\mathbf{u}$, or $p_{g_k} = \Pr(G = g_k \mid \mathbf{r}, \mathbf{x}, \mathbf{u})$. Randomization means $p_{g_k} = \Pr(G = g_k \mid \mathbf{r}, \mathbf{x}, \mathbf{u}) = 1/|G|$ for all $g_k \in G$, or (1.2). What is key about randomization is that treatment assignment is a fair lottery in which $(\mathbf{r}, \mathbf{u})$ plays no role: if someone told us the (mostly unobserved) potential outcomes $\mathbf{r}$, or the unobserved covariates, $\mathbf{u}$, that would not help us guess which treatment assignment $g_k \in G$ will occur.[6]

In What Sense Is Randomization Equitable? A randomized experiment is equitable in the sense that there is equality of the $|G|$ conditional probabilities given potential outcomes $\mathbf{r}$ and covariates $(\mathbf{x}, \mathbf{u})$ of each treatment assignment $g \in G$. Treatment assignment does not favor some individuals over others based on potential outcomes or covariates.

---

[6]If $\Pr(G = g_k \mid \mathbf{r}, \mathbf{x}, \mathbf{u})$ were not constant but depended only on the observed covariate, $\mathbf{x}$, then the required analysis would be a little more complex, but inferences could be drawn about treatment effects [238]. The condition $\Pr(G = g_k \mid \mathbf{r}, \mathbf{x}, \mathbf{u}) = \Pr(G = g_k \mid \mathbf{x})$ is called ignorable treatment assignment [228].

A nonrandomized or observational study is similar, except randomization is not used, so we do not know the treatment assignment probabilities $p_{g_k} = \Pr(G = g_k \mid \mathbf{r}, \mathbf{x}, \mathbf{u})$ and quite possibly (1.2) does not hold.

1.3.3 Fisher's Hypothesis of No Effect

If changing the drugs individuals receive changes whether their blood pressure goal is achieved, then the drugs have different effects on this outcome; otherwise, the drugs do no differ in their effects on this outcome. Randomization moves individuals at random from one column of Table 1.1 to another, but if that is all it does—if it does not change whether individuals achieve the blood pressure goal—then the treatments do not differ in their effects on this outcome.

Expressed in terms of (1.3) and the matrix $\mathbf{r}$, the treatments do not differ in their effects if the $|G|$ columns of $\mathbf{r}$ are all the same, and this is what Fisher's [68, §2] "hypothesis of no effect" asserts. Perhaps it would be better to speak of "Fisher's hypothesis that the treatments do not differ in their effects"—that is mathematically what the hypothesis asserts—rather than speak of the "hypothesis of no effect," but the short, slightly inaccurate form of expression is traditional and concise. If Fisher's hypothesis H_0 were true, then the one random column $\mathbf{R}$ of $\mathbf{r}$ that the randomized experiment allowed us to see is the only column there is: all the other columns are the same.

1.3.4 No Effect Means No Effect

No effect means no effect. Suppose the trial had two drugs, amlodipine and chlorthalidone, and $N = 2$ people, you, $j = 1$, and me, $j = 2$. There are two treatment assignments: g_1 gives you amlodipine and me chlorthalidone, while g_2 gives you chlorthalidone and me amlodipine. So, $\mathbf{r}$ is a $N \times |G| = 2 \times 2$ matrix whose first row describes you and whose second row describes me. The first column of $\mathbf{r}$ refers to treatment assignment g_1 and the second column refers to treatment assignment g_2, so in each column, half the population receives amlodipine. As it happens, you would achieve the blood pressure goal if you took amlodipine under g_1, so $r_{11} = 1$, but not if you took chlorthalidone under g_2, so $r_{12} = 0$. The opposite is true for me: I would achieve the blood pressure goal if I took chlorthalidone under g_1, so, $r_{21} = 1$, but not if I took amlodipine under g_2, so $r_{22} = 0$. In fact, we are both better off under g_1, both worse off under g_2. Fisher's hypothesis of no effect is false: the two columns of $\mathbf{r}$ are different. When Fisher's hypothesis is false, it makes a difference how treatments are assigned: we are both better off under g_1. In this situation, we would like, if possible, to reject the null hypothesis of no effect, because that hypothesis is false in a consequential way.

Notice, however, that on average, amlodipine and chlorthalidone are equally effective. Half the population—you and not me—benefits from amlodipine but not from chlorthalidone, and half the population—me and not you—benefits from chlorthalidone and not from amlodipine. So, on average, the benefit of amlodipine for you and the benefit of chlorthalidone for me cancel. In the population consisting of the two of us, the two drugs are equally effective, on average. Moreover, in a randomized experiment that picks treatment assignments g_1 or g_2 each with probability $1/2$, the expectation of the amlodipine-minus-chlorthalidone difference in mean responses is also zero, $0 = 0 \times 0.5 + 0 \times .5$. The average treatment effect can fail to capture what is important when Fisher's hypothesis of no effect is false.

Consider a larger population. If half the population benefits from amlodipine but not from chlorthalidone, and half the population benefits from chlorthalidone but not from amlodipine, then the entire population could benefit if each person received the appropriate medication. In practical terms, rejecting Fisher's hypothesis of no effect in this situation would be greatly aided by identifying some pretreatment quantity—some observed covariate—that distinguishes people like you, who benefit from amlodipine, from people like me, who benefit from chlorthalidone. With such a covariate in a large study, we could see effect modification, that is, a different treatment effect at different levels of the covariate [112, 113, 137]. Without such a covariate, we might make the serious mistake of thinking that amlodipine and chlorthalidone are equally effective, because, in expectation, half of the patients randomly assigned to each treatment achieve the blood pressure goal under that treatment.

Admittedly, we might not be able to find this covariate that distinguishes the subpopulation that benefits from amlodipine and the subpopulation that benefits from chlorthalidone; so, we might make the serious mistake of thinking that there is no difference between the two medications, when in fact there is a substantial difference. Thinking that there is no effect when there is merely no effect on average is clearly a grave mistake in this context: it would be immediately recognized as a mistake when some other investigator discovered the covariate and improved the health of the population by using it to appropriately allocate medications to patients.

If Fisher's hypothesis of no effect is false, then we must do our best to understand the manner in which it is false, and to determine whether the manner in which it is false can be put to constructive use.

In a parallel fashion, a small effect on average may be important if it is composed of a large effect for a small subpopulation and no effect for everyone else [45, 202, 243].

1.3.5 No Interference between Individuals

There is "interference between individuals" if the treatment given to one individual can affect the response of another individual [51, 240]. If you are vaccinated against flu, then perhaps I do not catch the flu because I do not catch it from you; whereas, if you are not vaccinated, then I do catch the flu from you. In this case, my response, whether or not I develop flu, is affected by the treatment you received. In studies of vaccination, interference between individuals, or herd immunity, is a central concern: vaccinate enough people and many unvaccinated people will also benefit [116].

Interference is common, often important, when the individuals under study are people who talk to one another, listen to one another, observe or react to one another [260]. In a classroom, a teacher who praises a student for asking a good question may elicit questions from other students. This is, again, interference: what was done to one student affects other students.

Interference There is interference between individuals if changing the treatment given to one person can cause a change in the outcome of someone else.

The vector $\mathbf{r}_j$ for individual j in (1.3) and the matrix $\mathbf{r}$ both record interference. Suppose that $g_1, g_2 \in G$ are two treatment assignments that assign individual j to the same treatment group, but assign other individuals differently. If $r_{jg_1} \neq r_{jg_2}$, then there is interference: by assumption, g_1 and g_2 gave the same treatment to individual j, yet the response of individual j is different under g_1 and g_2, so there is interference.

We often speak of one person's behavior as causing a rise in the blood pressure of another person, but perhaps that way of speaking is more common as a metaphor than clinical observation. It seems much less likely that the choice of blood pressure medication in ALLHAT for person j affects the blood pressure of another person, $j' \neq j$ in ALLHAT. It is not entirely inconceivable that because j received amlodipine instead of chlorthalidone, j's blood pressure remained high, causing j to experience stress and anxiety that j would not have experienced under chlorthalidone, and j's stress was shared with j's employee j' whose blood pressure rose as a result. That would constitute interference. However, this possibility seems sufficiently remote and limited in scope that we might ignore it to focus on other more pressing concerns in the interpretation of an experiment like ALLHAT. We might make a different judgment in a vaccine trial, or in an agricultural experiment in which adjacent fields of a farm are treated with different insecticides.

There is "no interference between individuals" if each person j may be affected by the treatment given to j but is unaffected by the treatment given to other people [51]. When we speak, as we often do, of the effect of a treatment on person j without mentioning other people, there is a tacit assumption that interference is either absent or negligible. No interference between individuals places an enormous number of restrictions on the matrix $\mathbf{r}$, namely $r_{jg_1} = r_{jg_2}$ whenever g_1 and g_2 gave the same treatment to individual j.

In randomized experiments, interference introduces some complexities and occasional ambiguities, but it does not preclude straightforward inference about treatment effects [11, 36, 203, 270]. For instance, in a randomized experiment, Wilcoxon's rank sum test may be used to draw inferences about the magnitude of the effect of amlodipine versus chlorthalidone on systolic blood pressure, with no assumptions about interference [203]. Inference is further facilitated if interference is limited in scope or form [116].

Fisher's hypothesis of no effect entails no interference between individuals. As a consequence, interference does not affect those properties of a test that presume the null hypothesis to be true, such as the level of the test and the size of the test. In contrast, the power of a test is computed assuming the null hypothesis is false, so interference does affect power. Indeed, there are often some rather extreme alterna-

Table 1.2 *Achievement of blood pressure goal* $< 140/90$ *mm Hg under chlorthalidone and lisinopril in ALLHAT for individuals at risk at one year after the start of treatment*

	Chlorthalidone $Z_j = 1$	Lisinopril $Z_j = 0$
Achieved $R_j = 1$	7434	3806
Not achieved $R_j = 0$	5428	3715
Total	12862	7521
Percent achieved	57.8%	50.6%

tives with interference that cannot be distinguished from no effect so that a test has power equal to its size against such alternatives [203].

Although interference is an interesting topic, it has no special connection to replication and evidence factors. As a consequence, without further mention, the assumption of no interference between individuals is made in this book.

1.4 Causal Effects with Two Treatment Groups

1.4.1 Treatment versus Control

In the simplest case, there are just two treatment groups, as in Table 1.2, comparing chlorthalidone and lisinopril. Table 1.2 is a smaller randomized trial contained within the ALLHAT experiment, and the discussion that follows shifts to this smaller, notationally simpler experiment, setting aside individuals assigned to amlodipine.[7] The sample size, N, now refers to this smaller trial, and j distinguishes the individuals in this smaller trial, $j = 1, \ldots, N$. If there is no interference between individuals in this smaller trial, then each individual j in Table 1.2 has two potential outcomes, say r_{Tj} under chlorthalidone or r_{Cj} under lisinopril. Because there is no interference, whenever a treatment assignment $g \in G$ assigns individual j to chlorthalidone, the response for j is r_{Tj}, and whenever $g \in G$ assigns individual j to lisinopril, the response is r_{Cj} for individual j.

In the Neyman-Rubin [164, 237] notation, a treatment effect or a causal effect is a comparison of two potential responses an individual might exhibit under alternative treatment assignments. The effect on individual j of assigning individual j to chlorthalidone rather than lisinopril is $r_{Tj} - r_{Cj}$. For instance, for the binary outcome in Table 1.2, $r_{Tj} - r_{Cj} = 1 - 0 = 1$ signifies that individual j would have achieved the blood pressure goal under chlorthalidone, but not under lisinopril, so giving chlorthalidone rather than lisinopril would cause individual j to achieve the goal. Of course, we cannot see $r_{Tj} - r_{Cj}$ because individual j receives only one treatment, so we see r_{Tj} or r_{Cj} but not both, so we cannot calculate $r_{Tj} - r_{Cj}$ for one person j. Causal inference is difficult because it is about something that we cannot see.

Let $Z_j = 1$ signify that individual j did receive chlorthalidone rather than lisinopril. In a randomized trial like ALLHAT, Z_j is a random variable with a known

---

[7]Formally, Table 1.2 is the trial formed by conditioning on the identities of the individuals assigned to amlodipine.

distribution: it is a function of the randomly selected treatment assignment $G \in \mathbf{G}$ whose known distribution is (1.2). In what follows, the number of people assigned to chlorthalidone, $m = \sum Z_j$, is regarded as fixed.[8]

The outcome individual j actually exhibits is $R_j = Z_j r_{Tj} + (1 - Z_j) r_{Cj}$. That is, R_j is the outcome for individual j observed under the treatment ℓ that individual j actually received, either chlorthalidone if $Z_j = 1$ or lisinopril if $Z_j = 0$. A causal inference proceeds from what we see, namely (R_j, Z_j), to an inference about we cannot see, namely a causal effect such as $r_{Tj} - r_{Cj}$. Write $\delta_j = r_{Tj} - r_{Cj}$ for the causal effect on individual j so that $R_j = Z_j r_{Tj} + (1 - Z_j) r_{Cj} = r_{Cj} + Z_j \delta_j$ and $R_j - Z_j \delta_j = r_{Cj}$.

1.4.2   Hypotheses Concerning Causal Effects

Under Fisher's hypothesis H_0 of no effect, $r_{Tj} = r_{Cj}$ for each j. Were H_0 true, each causal effect would be zero, $\delta_j = r_{Tj} - r_{Cj} = 0$ for each j.

With no additional assumptions beyond the absence of interference, a general hypothesis about the causal effects is of the form $H_{\delta_0} : \delta = \delta_0$, where

$$\delta^T = (\delta_1, \ldots, \delta_N) = (r_{T1} - r_{C1}, \ldots, r_{TN} - r_{CN}), \quad \delta_0^T = (\delta_{01}, \ldots, \delta_{0N}), \quad (1.4)$$

so that δ is the unknown N-dimensional vector of causal effects, and δ_0 specifies a hypothesized value for each causal effect. Fisher's hypothesis of no effect is the special case in which $\delta_0 = (0, \ldots, 0)^T = \mathbf{0}$.

When there are logical constraints on the outcome, there may be logical constraints on δ, and hence logical constraints on the hypotheses $H_{\delta_0} : \delta = \delta_0$ that merit attention. In Table 1.2, R_j, r_{Tj}, and r_{Cj} are binary, 1 or 0, so $\delta_j = r_{Tj} - r_{Cj}$ must be -1, 0 or 1; hence, if hypothesis $H_{\delta_0} : \delta = \delta_0$ asserts otherwise, then H_{δ_0} is impossible and may be rejected with no possibility of error. In parallel, in Table 1.2, because $R_j = r_{Cj} + Z_j \delta_j$, having seen R_j and Z_j, there are always two possible values for δ_j: (i) if $Z_j = 0$ and $R_j = 1$, then δ_j must be either 0 or -1, (ii) if $Z_j = 0$ and $R_j = 0$ then δ_j must be either 0 or 1, (iii) if $Z_j = 1$ and $R_j = 1$, then δ_j must be either 0 or 1, and (iv) if $Z_j = 1$ and $R_j = 0$, then δ_j must be either 0 or -1; so, any hypothesis $H_{\delta_0} : \delta = \delta_0$ that asserts otherwise is logically false, and may be rejected with no possibility of error. In Table 1.2, there are 2^N hypotheses $H_{\delta_0} : \delta = \delta_0$ that are logically possible, of which one is true and $2^N - 1$ are false.

> **General Hypotheses about Causal Effects**   Every specific hypothesis about causal effects may be reduced to Fisher's hypothesis of no effect for an adjusted outcome.

---

[8]The group size, $\sum Z_j$, would be fixed by design if each g were a permutation to a fixed number of group labels. Alternatively, $\sum Z_j$ could be fixed by conditioning on its realized value, having determined Z_j by flipping one coin independently. The reduced sample size at risk at one year in Tables 1.1 and 1.2 is a practical issue that is being ignored in the current conceptual discussion.

Table 1.3 *Table of observed counts*

	Chlorthalidone, $Z_j = 1$	Lisinopril, $Z_j = 0$
Achieved, $R_j = 1$	$\sum Z_j R_j$	$\sum (1 - Z_j) R_j$
Not achieved, $R_j = 0$	$\sum Z_j (1 - R_j)$	$\sum (1 - Z_j)(1 - R_j)$

Every logically possible hypothesis, $H_{\delta_0} : \delta = \delta_0$, is Fisher's hypothesis of no effect for an adjusted response, so that, if we know how to test Fisher's hypothesis, we also know how to test every hypothesis, $H_{\delta_0} : \delta = \delta_0$, about causal effects. Specifically, if $H_{\delta_0} : \delta = \delta_0$ is logically impossible, reject it with no possibility of error. Otherwise, define $A_{j,\delta_0} = R_j - Z_j \delta_{0j}$, where A_{j,δ_0} can be computed from the observed data, (R_j, Z_j), for any specific hypothesis, $H_{\delta_0} : \delta = \delta_0$. If $H_{\delta_0} : \delta = \delta_0$ is the one true hypothesis, then $A_{j,\delta_0} = R_j - Z_j \delta_{0j} = R_j - Z_j \delta_j = r_{Cj}$ for $j = 1,\ldots,N$, and Fisher's hypothesis of no effect is true for $A_{j,\delta_0} = r_{Cj}$.

1.4.3 Attributable Effects with Binary Outcomes

The quantity $A = \sum Z_j (r_{Tj} - r_{Cj}) = \sum Z_j \delta_j$ is a random variable that cannot be observed. It is a random variable because it depends upon the randomized treatment assignment, $G \in \mathsf{G}$, which determines the value of the random variable Z_j, so the distribution of A is governed by the distribution of treatment assignments $p_{g_k} = \Pr(G = g_k \mid \mathbf{r}, \mathbf{x}, \mathbf{u})$. Here, $\delta_j = r_{Tj} - r_{Cj}$ is determined by $\mathbf{r}$ so that given $\mathbf{r}$ the attributable effect A is a random variable only because Z_j is a random variable. The random variable $A = \sum Z_j (r_{Tj} - r_{Cj})$ cannot be observed because $\delta_j = r_{Tj} - r_{Cj}$ is never observed. The quantity $A = \sum Z_j (r_{Tj} - r_{Cj})$ is called the attributable effect [192]: among people who received chlorthalidone with $Z_j = 1$, the attributable effect A is the net increase in the number of individuals who achieved the blood pressure goal because of effects, $r_{Tj} - r_{Cj}$, caused by giving chlorthalidone in place of lisinopril. If Fisher's hypothesis of no effect were true, then $r_{Tj} - r_{Cj} = 0$ for each j, and consequently $A = 0$.[9]

A logically possible hypothesis $H_{\delta_0} : \delta = \delta_0$ yields a corresponding hypothesized value $A_0 = \sum Z_j \delta_{0j}$ of the attributable effect. If $H_{\delta_0} : \delta = \delta_0$ were true, then $A = A_0$. For any logically possible hypothesis, $H_{\delta_0} : \delta = \delta_0$, it is straightforward to compute $A_0 = \sum Z_j \delta_{0j}$, as Z_j is observed and the hypothesis specifies δ_0.

Table 1.4 *Table of counts that would have been observed had all individuals in both groups actually received lisinopril*

	Chlorthalidone, $Z_j = 1$	Lisinopril, $Z_j = 0$
Achieved, $r_{Cj} = 1$	$\sum Z_j r_{Cj}$	$\sum (1 - Z_j) r_{Cj}$
Not achieved, $r_{Cj} = 0$	$\sum Z_j (1 - r_{Cj})$	$\sum (1 - Z_j)(1 - r_{Cj})$

---

[9]Dividing A by the fixed number of people, $\sum Z_j$, who received chlorthalidone yields a proportion, $A / \sum Z_j$, rather than a count. A confidence set for the count immediately yields a confidence set for the proportion, if that is preferred.

Table 1.5 *Adjustment of Table 1.3 by the hypothesized value A_0 of an attributable effect A.*

	Chlorthalidone, $Z_j = 1$	Lisinopril, $Z_j = 0$
Achieved, $R_j = 1$	$\sum Z_j R_j - A_0$	$\sum (1 - Z_j) R_j$
Not achieved, $R_j = 0$	$\sum Z_j (1 - R_j) + A_0$	$\sum (1 - Z_j)(1 - R_j)$

Tables 1.3–1.5 examine the relationship between an observed table like Table 1.2 and a table adjusted for A_0. Table 1.3 is the general form of the observed table, of which Table 1.2 is a particular case. Table 1.4 is not observed: it imagines that we determined Z_j at random behind closed doors, as in the actual trial, but we gave everyone Lisinopril observing r_{Cj} for all N individuals. Fisher's hypothesis of no effect is true in the unobservable Table 1.4, because everyone received Lisinopril, whether $Z_j = 1$ or $Z_j = 0$, and there is no difference in effect between giving Lisinopril with $Z_j = 1$ behind closed doors, and giving Lisinopril with $Z_j = 0$ behind closed doors.

If Fisher's hypothesis H_0 of no effect were true about Chlorthalidone and Lisinopril, then Tables 1.3 and 1.4 would be equal.

Suppose the logically possible hypothesis $H_{\delta_0} : \delta = \delta_0$ is the one true hypothesis of the 2^N logically possible hypotheses. Then, $A = \sum Z_j (r_{Tj} - r_{Cj}) = \sum Z_j \delta_j = \sum Z_j \delta_{0j} = A_0$ so that

$$\sum Z_j R_j - A_0 = \sum Z_j (r_{Cj} + \delta_j) - \sum Z_j \delta_j = \sum Z_j r_{Cj}$$

and

$$\sum Z_j (1 - R_j) + A_0 = \sum Z_j (1 - r_{Cj}),$$

so that Tables 1.4 and 1.5 are equal. In brief, if the logically possible hypothesis $H_{\delta_0} : \delta = \delta_0$ is true, then Fisher's hypothesis of no effect is true of Table 1.5, and we can calculate Table 1.5 from the observed Table 1.3 and the specified hypothesis, $H_{\delta_0} : \delta = \delta_0$. In a moment, this simple piece of algebra will allow us to invert a test of Fisher's hypothesis of no effect to yield a confidence set for the attributable effect, A.

1.5 Inference with Random Assignment

1.5.1 Testing the Hypothesis of No Effect

With two treatments in a randomized experiment, a fixed number $m = \sum Z_j$ of individuals are picked at random from N individuals for the treatment, say Chlorthalidone, with the remaining $N - m$ individuals receiving the control, say Lisinopril. With a binary outcome, such as achieving the blood pressure goal, an observed table results, here Table 1.2 in ALLHAT or Table 1.3 in general. If Fisher's hypothesis H_0 of no effect were true in such a randomized trial, then Table 1.3 would equal Table 1.4, whose conditional distribution given $\mathbf{r}, \mathbf{x}, \mathbf{u}$ is the hypergeometric distribution. That is to say, the distribution of Table 1.3 under H_0 is a known distribution in a randomized experiment, with no assumptions at all. Randomization creates the null distribution required for testing the hypothesis that giving the treatment rather than the control has no causal effect. This is Fisher's [68, Chapter 2] celebrated result: randomized treatment assignment makes causal inference straightforward with no assumptions of any kind.

In Table 1.2, a one-sided test of Fisher's hypothesis of no effect H_0 asks whether the count 7434 is too large to plausibly be produced by the hypergeometric distribution, yielding a P-value of 2.2×10^{-16}. Were H_0 true, a count of 7434 or more would be exceedingly improbable. A two-sided P-value is obtained by doubling this one-sided P-value.[10]

1.5.2 A Confidence Set for the Magnitude of the Effect

A $1 - \alpha$ confidence set for the attributable effect, $A = \sum Z_j \left(r_{Tj} - r_{Cj} \right) = \sum Z_j \delta_j$, is obtained by testing each of the 2^N logically possible hypotheses $H_{\delta_0} : \delta = \delta_0$ and retaining those values of δ_0 in (1.4) and the corresponding values of $A_0 = \sum Z_j \delta_{0j}$ that are not rejected by a level α test [192]. Of the 2^N logically possible hypotheses, $H_{\delta_0} : \delta = \delta_0$, one is true and $2^N - 1$ are false. When the one true hypothesis is tested at level α, it is falsely rejected with probability at most α, so the random set of values of δ_0 and $A_0 = \sum Z_j \delta_{0j}$ that are not rejected includes these true values with probability at least $1 - \alpha$.

The computations are straightforward. In principle, we apply Fisher's test of no effect to Table 1.5: if $H_{\delta_0} : \delta = \delta_0$ were true in a randomized experiment, then Table 1.5 would have the hypergeometric distribution, so each δ_0 could be tested by comparison with the hypergeometric distribution. In practice, we need not test the 2^N logically possible hypotheses $H_{\delta_0} : \delta = \delta_0$ one at a time; instead, we accept or reject these hypotheses in large collections based on the value of $A_0 = \sum Z_j \delta_{0j}$.

For Table 1.2, the hypothesis of no effect is rejected in Table 1.5 in a one-sided, 0.05 level test for all logically possible $H_{\delta_0} : \delta = \delta_0$ such that $A_0 \leq 770$ and accepted for all logically possible $H_{\delta_0} : \delta = \delta_0$ such that $A_0 \geq 771$, so the one-sided 95% confidence set for A is $A \geq 771$. In words, we estimate a net increase of $A \geq 771$ in the number of Chlorthalidone-treated patients who achieved the blood pressure goal because of effects caused by receiving Chlorthalidone rather than Lisinopril, or an increase of at least $771/(7434 + 5428) = 6\%$.

The important aspect of the confidence interval $A \geq 771$ is that it is derived from the random assignment of treatments, with no assumed model for treatment effects. Unlike Fisher's test of no effect in Table 1.2, this inference depends upon the assump-

---

[10] In general, the hypergeometric distribution is skewed. For skewed null distributions, there are several ways to construct a two-sided test. The method here takes the smaller of two one-sided P-values and doubles it, as suggested by Cox [49] and Shaffer [252]. This approach views a two-sided test as two one-sided tests with a Bonferroni correction for testing twice. It has the virtue, not shared by some other approaches, of controlling the probability of misstating the direction of the treatment effect, and not just the truth or falsity of the null hypothesis H_0 of no effect. Here, rejecting at level $\alpha/2$ in two one-sided tests allows us to be $1 - \alpha$ confident that Chlorthalidone increased the number of people who achieved the blood pressure goal, compared to Lisinopril. People often take this property for granted, but it is not assured by some methods for constructing a two-sided test from a test statistic with a skewed null distribution. Without further mention, throughout this book, a level α two-sided test is constructed from two one-sided tests conducted at level $\alpha/2$.

tion of no interference between individuals; however, like Fisher's test, it requires no further assumption beyond the actual use of randomization in the ALLHAT experiment.

The half-line $A \geq 771$ is a confidence set for a random variable, $A = \sum Z_j \delta_j$, that we cannot observe. Although confidence sets for random variables are less commonly seen than confidence sets for fixed parameters, they have been known for quite some time [69, 284].

1.6 Randomization Tests for Continuous Outcomes

1.6.1 Randomization Tests in General

If Fisher's hypothesis, H_0, of no effect is true, then assignment to one treatment or another does not alter an individual's outcomes; rather, it merely moves the individual from one part of the experimental design to another. If $t(\cdot)$ is a test statistic computed from observed outcomes, observed covariates, and the treatment assignment, $g \in G$, then under H_0, we may write $t(\cdot)$ simply as a function of the treatment assignment, $t(g)$, because nothing else about individuals is changing as g changes. If H_0 is true, then the observed outcome is the only outcome for each individual, and that observed outcome and the individual's observed covariate $\mathbf{x}_j$ are simply permuted about the experimental design by switching from one treatment assignment to another.

Suppose the test rejects for large values of $t(\cdot)$. If H_0 were true in a randomized experiment, what is the probability that $t(G) \geq c$? Recall that G is the random treatment assignment picked from G, where each $g_k \in G$ has the same probability, $p_{g_k} = \Pr(G = g_k \mid \mathbf{r}, \mathbf{x}, \mathbf{u}) = 1/|G|$. Clearly, under H_0, the desired probability is simply the proportion of treatment assignments g_k that have $t(g_k) \geq c$, or, more precisely,

$$\Pr\{t(G) \geq c \mid \mathbf{r}, \mathbf{x}, \mathbf{u}\} =$$

$$\sum_{g_k \in G:\, t(g_k) \geq c} p_{g_k} = \sum_{g_k \in G:\, t(g_k) \geq c} \frac{1}{|G|} = \frac{|\{g_k \in G : t(g_k) \geq c\}|}{|G|}. \quad (1.5)$$

Setting c equal to the observed value, $t(G)$, in (1.5) yields the P-value. In the case of random assignment to treatment or control, G contains $N!/\{m!\,(N-m)!\}$ permutations that pick m individuals for treatment and these have equal probability.[11]

The hypergeometric P-value in §1.5 is a special case of (1.5) in which $t(G)$ is the count in the first row and column of Table 1.3, where Tables 1.3 and 1.4 are equal if H_0 is true. If H_0 is true, then an individual never moves from one row of Table 1.3 to the other row, but changing the treatment assignment, $g \in G$, may move an individual from one column, Chlorthalidone, to the other, Lisinopril. We saw in §1.5 that a value as large or larger than the observed $t(G)$ in Table 1.2 would be highly improbable were H_0 true.

---

[11]These are the pick matrices in Definition 4 of §8.3 in Chapter 8.

With continuous outcomes—say, systolic blood pressure in the ALLHAT experiment—one of the many familiar randomization tests of H_0 comparing treated and control groups is based on Wilcoxon's rank sum statistic [140, 288]. Wilcoxon's statistic $t(G)$ ranks the N outcomes from 1 to N, with average ranks for ties, and $t(G)$ is the sum of the ranks of the m treated individuals. Under H_0, an individual's outcomes are the same under all treatment assignments, so the ranks of outcomes also remain the same. Under H_0, the randomization distribution of $t(G)$ in (1.5) is simply the distribution of $m = \sum Z_j$ ranks picked at random without replacement from the N ranks [140].

If $t(G)$ is the treated-minus-control difference in mean outcomes, then (1.5) is the distribution for Pitman's permutational t-test [175].

1.6.2 Randomization Tests and Permutation Tests

Randomization tests and permutation tests often coincide, but are logically distinct. A randomization test is based on the randomized assignment of treatments in an experiment. A permutation test is derived from certain symmetries possessed by a probability distribution when a certain null hypothesis is true [142]. A randomization test may coincide with a permutation test when the experimental design possesses certain symmetries.

Set aside randomized experiments, and consider independent samples from two continuous distributions, one sample of size m, the other of size $N - m$. Consider testing the null hypothesis that the two distributions are equal. If that null hypothesis were true, then swapping individuals in the two samples would not alter the distribution of responses. A permutation test of the form (1.5) may be used to test this null hypothesis.

The phrase "may be used" is too weak; more can be said. If the null hypothesis is true, the two samples came from the same continuous distribution, say F. Suppose that we want our test of the equality of two continuous distributions to be valid no matter what F is. In other words, suppose that we want the test to have probability α of falsely rejecting the null hypothesis of equality, for every continuous distribution F. A celebrated result in Lehmann and Romano [141, §5.8] says that a test has this property if and only if it is a permutation test. If you knew that F were, say, Normal, then there would be other valid tests; however, if the test is to be valid for every continuous F, then it must be a permutation test.

1.6.3 Tests of General Hypotheses

Initially, the hypothesis $H_{\delta_0} : \delta = \delta_0$ in (1.4) was considered for binary responses, but similar issues arise in general. In general, the hypothesis $H_{\delta_0} : \delta = \delta_0$ in (1.4) presumes that there is no interference between units so that $\delta_j = r_{Tj} - r_{Cj}$ is well defined. Presuming this, it is straightforward to test any one hypothesis $H_{\delta_0} : \delta = \delta_0$ in (1.4) when individuals are randomly assigned to treatment or control. We compute the adjusted responses, $R_j - Z_j \, \delta_{0j}$, which equal r_{Cj} if $H_{\delta_0} : \delta = \delta_0$ is true, and we apply to these adjusted responses a randomization test (1.5).

In §1.5 with binary outcomes, there were 2^N logically possible hypotheses H_{δ_0} : $\delta = \delta_0$, one of which was true. With continuous outcomes, there are infinitely many logically possible hypotheses, one of which is true.

1.7 Confidence Sets for Causal Effects

1.7.1 Confidence Sets for Treatment Effects

In principle, we could test each hypothesis $H_{\delta_0} : \delta = \delta_0$ in §1.6 using a level α randomization test, collect all the δ_0's not rejected in this way into a random set $\mathscr{C}$, and call $\mathscr{C}$ a $1 - \alpha$ confidence set for δ. In this activity, many false hypotheses would be tested, but of course we are happy to reject false hypotheses. Eventually, we would test the one true hypothesis, and because we are using a level α test, we falsely reject the one true hypothesis with probability at most α. So, with probability at least $1 - \alpha$, the random set $\mathscr{C}$ does include the true value of δ.

The set $\mathscr{C}$ would not be easy to assimilate or understand directly, as it is a subset of the set of N-dimensional real vectors. If the binary outcome in Table 1.1 were replaced by the continuous outcome of systolic blood pressure at one year, then each $\delta_0 \in \mathscr{C}$ would be a vector of dimension 20,383 causal effects, where 20,383 is the total sample size in Table 1.1. An infinite set of vectors δ_0, each of dimension 20,383, is not easy to understand.

If there is no interference between individuals, then the vector δ of causal effects exists. The confidence set $\mathscr{C}$ is conceptually important because it says that, in an experiment that randomizes assignment to treatment or control, if δ exists, then we may draw causal inferences about δ with no assumptions about the structure of δ. The confidence set $\mathscr{C}$ indicates that our technical ability to draw causal inferences in a randomized experiment far exceeds our ability to comprehend what we have done. Models or summaries are used to address our cognitive limitations; they do not address limitations of randomization inference itself. Quite often, models and summaries of treatment effects are used to say: any causal effect δ_0 with a certain specific intelligible property has been rejected; that is, any such δ_0 is not in $\mathscr{C}$.

How can we say something useful about δ given that inspection of $\mathscr{C}$ is tedious? The remainder of this section offers several answers. These answers are not mutually exclusive; rather, they are mutually supporting ways to understand $\mathscr{C}$, the set of causal effects not rejected by the data.

1.7.2 Attributable Effects with Continuous Outcomes

One approach to understanding $\mathscr{C}$ is to continue on with attributable effects, now built for continuous outcomes. These attributable effects characterize $\mathscr{C}$ in simpler terms, perhaps in terms of a one-dimensional quantity. A one-dimensional quantity A_{δ_0} is computed from the observed responses R_j and the hypothesized effects δ_{0j}; then, A_{δ_0} characterizes which hypotheses $H_{\delta_0} : \delta = \delta_0$ are rejected or not at level α, so $\mathscr{C}$ may be described in terms of A_{δ_0}. In essence, the statistic used to test the hypothesis of no effect must have a magnitude that is directly interpretable as a magnitude of the treatment effect; see, for instance, Ref. [296].

One such attributable effect is expressed in terms of quantiles of the potential outcomes, (r_{Tj}, r_{Cj}). The following argument works fairly generally [192, §3], but for a brief exposition, suppose that N is even, and the $2N$ potential responses (r_{Ti}, r_{Ci}), $i = 1, \ldots, N$, are untied, as they would be if they came from a continuous distribution. As is often the case, inferences about quantiles closely parallel inferences about binary outcomes [69, 77, 79]. The N potential responses to control have order statistics, $r_{C(1)} < r_{C(2)} < \cdots < r_{C(N)}$; however, none of these order statistics is observed. Let $r_{C\text{med}}$ be the unknown median of the N potential responses to control,

$$r_{C\text{med}} = \frac{r_{C(j)} + r_{C(j+1)}}{2} \text{ for } j = N/2,$$

so $r_{C(N/2)} < r_{C\text{med}} < r_{C((N/2)+1)}$ because there are no ties. Some individuals have $\max(r_{Tj}, r_{Cj}) \leq r_{C\text{med}}$ and will be at or below the control median under both treatment and control, while other individuals have $\min(r_{Tj}, r_{Cj}) > r_{C\text{med}}$ and will exceed the control median under both treatment and control. If Fisher's hypothesis of no effect were true, then every individual would be in one of these two groups. If Fisher's hypothesis were false, an individual with $r_{Tj} > r_{C\text{med}} \geq r_{Cj}$ would exceed the control median only if treated. Write $b_{Tj} = 1$ if $r_{Tj} > r_{C\text{med}}$ and $b_{Tj} = 0$ otherwise, noting that we cannot compute b_{Tj} because $r_{C\text{med}}$ is not observed. Write $b_{Cj} = 1$ if $r_{Cj} > r_{C\text{med}}$ and $b_{Cj} = 0$ otherwise. Write $B_j = Z_j b_{Tj} + (1 - Z_j) b_{Tj}$. With $\delta_j = b_{Tj} - b_{Cj}$, the quantity $A = \sum_{j=1}^{N} Z_j \delta_j$ is the net increase in the number of treated observations above $r_{C\text{med}}$ due to effects caused by the treatment. Under Fisher's hypothesis of no effect, $A = 0$. The task is to build a confidence set for the random variable A.

Let $\delta = (\delta_1, \ldots, \delta_N)^T$. Let $R_{(1)} < \cdots < R_{(N)}$ be the observed order statistics of the N observed responses, $R_j = Z_j r_{Tj} + (1 - Z_j) r_{Tj}$.

Consider the hypothesis $H_0 : \delta = \delta_0$ where $\delta_0 = (\delta_{01}, \ldots, \delta_{0N})^T$ is a vector whose N coordinates are -1, 0 or 1, and let $A_0 = \sum_{j=1}^{N} Z_j \delta_{0j}$. Although $r_{C\text{med}}$ is unknown, it is not difficult to show that if H_0 is true, then $R_{(N/2+1-A_0)} > r_{C\text{med}} > R_{(N/2-A_0)}$; see [192, Proposition 1].[12] So, from H_0 together with the $R_{(j)}$, we may calculate the B_j, even though $r_{C\text{med}}$ is unknown. With the B_j in hand, the problem of testing H_0 reduces to the problem addressed in §1.4 for binary responses. As in §1.4, all hypotheses $H_0 : \delta = \delta_0$ that yield the same value of $A_0 = \sum_{j=1}^{N} Z_j \delta_{0j}$ are accepted or rejected together, so a one-dimensional interval of accepted values of A_0 completely characterizes the N dimensional confidence set for δ. That confidence interval refers to the number, A, of treated responses that exceed $r_{C\text{med}}$ due to effects caused by the treatment. The corresponding interval of values of A/m refers to the proportion of treated responses that exceed $r_{C\text{med}}$ due to effects caused by the treatment.

Parallel reasoning applies for an attributable effect associated with Wilcoxon's rank sum test, considered in terms of its equivalent form, the Mann-Whitney test [140, 148]. Consider two distinct individuals, $j \neq j'$, and for a concise, uncluttered discussion, assume outcomes of distinct individuals are never tied. If Fisher's

---

[12]For other reasons in Ref. [192], it is there assumed that $r_{Tj} \geq r_{Cj}$, but this added assumption is not needed for [192, Proposition 1].

hypothesis H_0 of no effect were true, then exactly one of the following is true: $r_{Tj} = r_{Cj} > r_{Tj'} = r_{Cj'}$ or $r_{Tj} = r_{Cj} < r_{Tj'} = r_{Cj'}$, so that in exactly half of the comparisons of two distinct individuals $r_{Tj} > r_{Cj'}$. If H_0 were false, $r_{Tj} > r_{Cj'}$ might occur more than half the time. The treatment *causes* j to have a higher response under treatment than j' would exhibit under control if $r_{Tj} > r_{Cj'}$ but $r_{Cj} < r_{Cj'}$. How often does that happen? How often did a treated individual j with $Z_j = 1$ have a higher response than a control j' with $Z_{j'} = 0$ because of an effect actually caused by the treatment? There are $m \times (N - m)$ possible comparisons of an individual assigned to treatment, $Z_j = 1$, and an individual assigned to control, $Z_{j'} = 0$, so the answer, $A^\dagger$ say, is an integer between 0 and $m \times (N - m)$, and $A^\dagger / \{m \times (N - m)\}$ is the proportion of times treated subjects exhibited higher responses than controls because of effects caused by the treatment. A confidence set for $A^\dagger$ is obtained directly from the Wilcoxon test [192, §4]; indeed, this confidence set is even applicable when there is interference between individuals [203]. With some additional attention to details, ties among the outcomes do not present difficulties. In the paired case, see Ref. [197].

In brief, it is not necessary to impose structure on the N-dimensional causal effects, δ, in order to make sense of an N-dimensional confidence set $\mathscr{C}$ for δ.

Confidence intervals for quantiles of causal effects need not be formulated in terms of attributable effects, but may instead target quantiles directly [189, 191].

1.7.3 Parametric Models for δ

If δ is assumed to have a simple form expressed in terms of one or a few parameters, then it is often straightforward to build a confidence interval or set for the parameters. Fisher's hypothesis H_0 of no effect says $\delta_j = 0$ for $j = 1, \ldots, N$. This simplest alternative model is a constant effect,

$$\delta_j = \tau \text{ for } j = 1, \ldots, N; \tag{1.6}$$

then, a confidence interval is built for τ. Indeed, if the hypothesis $H_{\tau_0} : \delta_j = \tau_0$ for $j = 1, \ldots, N$ were true, then the adjusted responses, $R_j - \tau_0 Z_j$, would equal r_{Cj}, and the null hypothesis of no effect would be true for $R_j - \tau_0 Z_j$. If the test in (1.5) is applied at level α to the adjusted responses $R_j - \tau_0 Z_j$ for every τ_0, the values not rejected form a $1 - \alpha$ confidence set for τ_0, and this set may be replaced by a confidence interval defined as the shortest interval containing the confidence set. Indeed, we use the test that built $\mathscr{C}$, but apply it only to alternatives $\delta_0^T = (\tau_0, \ldots, \tau_0) = \tau_0 \mathbf{1}$. If this is done using Wilcoxon's rank sum test, it results in a familiar confidence interval for τ whose upper and lower endpoints are each the difference between the response of one treated individual and one control [139, 140]. However, any test statistic might be used; for instance, Pitman [175] used the permutation distribution of the difference in sample means.

How should the confidence interval for τ be understood? It may be understood as a conventional confidence interval under the added assumption that $\delta_j = \tau$ for $j = 1, \ldots, N$. Another interpretation is given in the next subsection of §1.7. Alternatively, the interval for τ may be understood agnostically, without added assumptions, simply as an attempt to understand and explore the N dimensional set $\mathscr{C}$ by intersecting $\mathscr{C}$ with the one-dimensional subspace $\{\tau_0 \mathbf{1} : \tau_0 \in \mathbb{R}\}$. A value τ_0 is excluded from the one-dimensional confidence interval for τ if and only if $\tau_0 \mathbf{1}$ is excluded from the N-dimensional confidence set $\mathscr{C}$ for δ. Understanding the one-dimensional confidence interval for τ is a first step in understanding the N-dimensional confidence set $\mathscr{C}$ for δ. What might be a second step?

If the outcome is always positive, as is true with systolic blood pressure, a different model for δ is multiplicative, $r_{Tj} = \beta r_{Cj}$, so that $\delta_j = r_{Tj} - r_{Cj} = (\beta - 1) r_{Cj} = (1 - 1/\beta) r_{Tj}$. If the hypothesis $\delta_j = (1 - 1/\beta_0) r_{Tj}$ were true, then the adjusted response $R_j / \beta_0^{Z_j}$ equals r_{Cj}, so we may test $H_0 : \beta = \beta_0$ by applying the same test as before in (1.5) at level α to the adjusted responses, $R_j / \beta_0^{Z_j}$, obtaining a $1 - \alpha$ confidence set for β. Indeed, we already did this test when we constructed $\mathscr{C}$. Once again, we may understand the confidence interval for β as having added the assumption of a multiplicative effect, $r_{Tj} = \beta r_{Cj}$, or we may understand it agnostically as a further exploration of the N-dimensional confidence set $\mathscr{C}$ for δ. A value of β_0 is excluded from the one-dimensional confidence interval if and only if the corresponding δ_0 with $\delta_{0j} = (\beta_0 - 1) r_{Cj}$ is excluded from the N-dimensional confidence set $\mathscr{C}$.

A two-parameter model for effect is $r_{Tj} = \tau + \beta r_{Cj}$ or $\delta_j = r_{Tj} - r_{Cj} = \tau + (\beta - 1) r_{Cj}$. If the hypothesis $H_0 : \tau = \tau_0, \beta = \beta_0$ were true, then the adjusted response $(R_j - Z_i \tau_0)/\beta_0^{Z_j}$ would equal r_{Cj}, and this H_0 could be tested in (1.5) using, for instance, LePage's [143] test. The two-dimensional set $\mathscr{L}$ of (τ_0, β_0) not rejected by a level α test forms a $1 - \alpha$ set for (τ, β). If the N-dimensional set $\mathscr{C}$ had been built using LePage's test in (1.5), then $\delta = (\delta_1, \ldots, \delta_N)^T$ with $\delta_j = r_{Tj} - r_{Cj} = \tau + (\beta - 1) r_{Cj}$ is excluded from $\mathscr{C}$ whenever (τ, β) is excluded from $\mathscr{L}$, thereby offering a two-dimensional perspective on an N-dimensional confidence set $\mathscr{C}$.

1.7.4 Stochastic Models for δ

The confidence sets described so far use randomization as the basis for inference; no additional stochastic modeling is used. Suppose, instead, that we assume the N individuals, $j = 1, \ldots, N$, were independently sampled from an infinite population in which

$$r_{Tj} = \tau + \varepsilon_j, \quad r_{Cj} = \varepsilon_j' \tag{1.7}$$

where ε_j and ε_j' have the same continuous marginal distribution, say F, but ε_j and ε_j' may be dependent for each individual j. Then, m of the N individuals were picked at random for treatment, denoted $Z_j = 1$, with remaining $N - m$ individuals receiving control, denoted $Z_j = 0$. As always, we observe (R_j, Z_j) where $R_j = Z_j r_{Tj} + (1 - Z_j) r_{Cj}$, but we do not observe (r_{Tj}, r_{Cj}) jointly. If the shared marginal distribution F of ε_j and ε_j' has finite expectation, then $\mathrm{E}(r_{Tj} - r_{Cj}) = \mathrm{E}(\delta_j) = \tau$ but generally $\tau \neq \delta_j = \tau + \varepsilon_j - \varepsilon_j'$, unlike the situation in the previous subsection.

Consider testing $H_0 : \tau = \tau_0$ in (1.7). The adjusted responses, $R_j - Z_j \tau_0$ would equal $\varepsilon_j - \varepsilon_j'$ were H_0 true, would be identically distributed, and would be independent of the Z_j. So, Wilcoxon's rank sum test could again be used, in the usual way, to test $H_0 : \tau = \tau_0$ at level α, and the τ_0 not rejected in this way would form a $1 - \alpha$ confidence set for τ; see Refs. [139, 140]. Because the same test is applied to the same data set, (R_j, Z_j), $j = 1, \ldots, N$, the confidence set from Wilcoxon's test for τ in (1.7) is exactly the same as the confidence set in the previous subsection for τ in the model of a constant effect, $\delta_j = \tau$, $j = 1, \ldots, N$. Indeed, this would be true also if Pitman's randomization test were used, where the test statistic is the difference in sample means. In fact, it is true for any permutation test (1.5). And, as noted in §1.6 and [141, §5.8], only permutation tests are valid for all continuous distributions F.

Perhaps the models $\delta_j = \tau$, $j = 1, \ldots, N$ and (1.7) are thought to differ in important ways. And yet these two different models yield exactly the same randomization-based confidence interval for τ in every dataset, and that one interval is valid if either model is true. Given any two models, we may build a third model—the disjunctive model—that asserts that either the first model or the second model is true. If the first model and the second model yield exactly the same confidence interval, then so does the disjunctive model. In this case, we might reasonably understand the confidence interval as referring to the disjunctive model, rather than to one model or the other. In this limited and specific sense, the models $\delta_j = \tau$, $j = 1, \ldots, N$ and (1.7) do not differ.

1.8   The General Situation

This chapter has emphasized experiments with two treatments and no interference between units so that each individual, j, has two potential outcomes, r_{Tj} under treatment or r_{Cj} under control, with treatment effect $\delta_j = r_{Tj} - r_{Cj}$, $j = 1, \ldots, N$. Much the same reasoning applies with more than two treatments, perhaps with interference.

In general, Fisher's hypothesis of no effect, H_0, asserts that individual j exhibits the same response under all $|G|$ treatment assignments so that all $|G|$ coordinates of r_j in (1.3) are equal to each other. Moreover, this is true for every individual, $j = 1, \ldots, N$, so the $|G|$ columns of the matrix r are all the same. We observe one column R of r, specifically column k if the randomly selected treatment assignment is g_k, but the column we observe is the same as the other columns if H_0 is true.

Consider a test statistic to test H_0, where we will reject H_0 for large values of the test statistic. That statistic is a function of the observed outcomes, R, and the randomly selected treatment assignment, g_k. As R does not change as g_k changes when H_0 is true, we might acknowledge that the test statistic depends upon R, but suppresses the dependence in the notation, writing the test statistic as $t(g_k)$. The conditional distribution of $t(g_k)$ given r, x, and u is known under H_0, because randomization means $p_{g_k} = \Pr(G = g_k \mid r, x, u) = 1/|G|$ for all $g_k \in G$. So, in principle, it is just a computational problem to determine the exact P-value testing H_0 using $t(g_k)$.

Consider testing the general hypothesis about treatment effects. Define ϕ to be the $N \times (|G| - 1)$ matrix whose $|G| - 1$ columns are the differences between column k of r and column 1 of r, $k = 2, \ldots, |G|$. Let ϕ_0 be a possible value of ϕ, and consider the hypothesis $H_{\phi_0} : \phi = \phi_0$. Every hypothesis about treatment effects is of this form. Having randomly selected g_k as the treatment assignment, and observed the kth column, $\mathbf{R}$, of $\mathbf{r}$ as the observed outcome, we may deduce all of $\mathbf{r}$ under the supposition that H_{ϕ_0} is true. Define the adjusted responses to be $\mathbf{R}$ if g_1 was the randomly selected treatment, or $\mathbf{R}$ minus column $k - 1$ of ϕ_0 if g_k was the randomly selected treatment. Were H_{ϕ_0} true, these adjusted responses would satisfy the null hypothesis of no treatment effect, so applying the above procedure for testing no effect to the adjusted responses yields a test of H_{ϕ_0}.

A $1 - \alpha$ confidence set for ϕ is formed by testing each hypothesis $H_{\phi_0} : \phi = \phi_0$ and retaining for the confidence set those value of ϕ_0 not rejected at level α.

The machinery just described is a bit abstract, but applicable in general. Commonly, to be useful in practice, the machinery needs to become less abstract by filling in some of the details. In practice, we may need computational shortcuts or approximations to calculate the P-value for testing Fisher's null hypothesis of no effect; however, many such techniques are available. Expressed in terms of ϕ, the confidence set will be a possibly infinite set of $N \times (|G| - 1)$ matrices, so it may be challenging to interpret. Commonly, computation and interpretation are aided by an assumed structure or model expressing ϕ in terms of fewer than $N \times (|G| - 1)$ parameters; for instance, the assumption of no interference imposes a great deal of structure on ϕ, and parametric models impose much more. However, an assumed structure for ϕ is not needed, providing inferences are based on attributable effects [203].

1.9 Summary: Randomization Simplifies Causal Inference

This conceptual chapter has reviewed the role that randomization plays in causal inference in randomized experiments. The chapter prepares the way for a discussion of observational studies, whose defining feature, and central problem, is that randomization was not used to assign individuals to treatments. Additionally, the chapter has introduced the notion that a treatment assignment is a permutation: it permutes N individuals into N treatment positions.

1.10 Using R

The calculations that follow were discussed in §1.5 for the ALLHAT Trial.

In R, Fisher's randomization test of no effect in the ALLHAT Trial in Table 1.2 proceeds as follows.

```
o2
                  C     L
  achieved   7434   3806
    notach   5428   3715
fisher.test(o2,alternative ="greater")
     Fisher's Exact Test for Count Data
data: o2
p-value 2.2e-16
```

To obtain the confidence interval for the attributable effect, Table 1.2 is adjusted in the sense of Table 1.5 by $A_0 = 770$ or $A_0 = 771$. We see that $A_0 = 770$ is barely rejected as too small, and $A_0 = 771$ is barely accepted as large enough, so the 95% interval is $A \geq 771$.

```
tb770
                C     L
  achieved    6664  3806
    notach    6198  3715
fisher.test(tb770,alternative = "greater")
p-value = 0.04963
```

```
tb771
                C     L
  achieved    6663  3806
    notach    6199  3715
fisher.test(tb771,alternative = "greater")
p-value = 0.05074
```

It is easier to interpret A as a fraction:

```
771/(7434+5428)
[1] 0.05994402
```

Chapter 2

Causal Inference in Observational Studies

Abstract

Selected aspects of causal inference in observational studies are reviewed. The topics discussed here are those that are relevant to evidence factors. Although adjustments for observed covariates are mentioned, the chapter emphasizes the unmeasured biases in observational studies that evidence factors seek to address. Two examples of sensitivity analyses are presented, one involving 11 pairs matched for two covariates, the other involving 2475 individuals in 104 strata defined by observed covariates, with additional robust covariance adjustment for continuous versions of the same covariates. The chapter concludes with a brief introduction to design sensitivity.

2.1 How Are Observational Studies Different from Experiments?

In 1965, William Cochran [38, p. 234] defined an observational study as an empiric investigation in which

> [t]he objective is to elucidate cause-and-effect relationships [... and ...] hypotheses about causation [... in which it ...] is not feasible to use controlled experimentation, in the sense of being able to impose the procedures or treatments whose effects it is desired to discover, or to assign subjects at random to different procedures. ... In recent years such studies have become increasingly common in medicine, public health, education, sociology and psychology. Examples are the studies of the relationship between smoking and health, studies of factors that affect the probability of injuries in motor accidents, studies of the differences in behaviour of school children under permissive and authoritarian regimes, and studies of the effects of new social programmes such as replacing slum housing by public housing.

So, the goal is the same in experiments and observational studies—inference about the effects caused by treatments—but the reasoning in Chapter 1 is not applicable, because individuals were not assigned to treatments using random numbers generated by the computer. The difficulty is evident in (1.5) where the treatment assignment probabilities play an explicit role. In (1.5), the probability of assigning treatments by treatment assignment g_ℓ is

$$p_{g_\ell} = \Pr(G = g_\ell \mid \mathbf{r}, \mathbf{x}, \mathbf{u}) = \frac{1}{|\mathsf{G}|} \text{ for all } g_\ell \in \mathsf{G}, \tag{2.1}$$

because the experimenter picked g_ℓ at random from G with equal probabilities. The key element in (1.5) and (2.1) is that treatment assignments favor no one of the N individuals over any other: despite being a conditional probability given potential outcomes, $\mathbf{r}$, observed covariates, $\mathbf{x}$, and unobserved covariates, $\mathbf{u}$, the treatment assignments g_ℓ are uniformly distributed over the set G of possible treatment assignments. The treatment an individual receives has no relationship with any attribute of that individual, whether that attribute is observed or not, simply because random numbers were used to assign treatments.

Use of (1.5) in observational studies has two aspects, one far more problematic than the other. The less problematic aspect is that $p_{g_\ell} = \Pr(G = g_\ell \mid \mathbf{r}, \mathbf{x}, \mathbf{u})$ may not be constant because it depends upon the observed covariates, $\mathbf{x}$. The deeply problematic aspect is that $p_{g_\ell} = \Pr(G = g_\ell \mid \mathbf{r}, \mathbf{x}, \mathbf{u})$ may depend also upon the $N \times |\mathsf{G}|$ array of potential outcomes, $\mathbf{r}$, and the matrix of unobserved covariates, $\mathbf{u}$. Treatment assignment is said to be ignorable [228] given observed covariates $\mathbf{x}$ if

$$\Pr(G = g_\ell \mid \mathbf{r}, \mathbf{x}, \mathbf{u}) = \Pr(G = g_\ell \mid \mathbf{x}) \tag{2.2}$$

and

$$\Pr(G = g_\ell \mid \mathbf{x}) > 0 \text{ for all } g_\ell \in \mathsf{G}. \tag{2.3}$$

Ignorable treatment assignment says treatment assignment, $\Pr(G = g_\ell \mid \mathbf{r}, \mathbf{x}, \mathbf{u})$, may depend upon the observed covariates, $\mathbf{x}$, but not upon $\mathbf{r}$ and $\mathbf{u}$. If treatment assignment were ignorable, the deeply problematic aspect of causal inference in an observational study would be absent. Notably, $\Pr(G = g_\ell \mid \mathbf{x})$ is a probability distribution for quantities, G and $\mathbf{x}$, that we observe; whereas, $\Pr(G = g_\ell \mid \mathbf{r}, \mathbf{x}, \mathbf{u})$ is a probability distribution that refers to the unobserved covariate, $\mathbf{u}$, and the potential outcomes $\mathbf{r}$ of all N individuals under all $|\mathsf{G}|$ treatment assignments, and neither of these quantities is observed. For instance, we might see in the data that women are less likely than men to smoke cigarettes, but if we recorded gender in $\mathbf{x}$, then we could compare female smokers to female nonsmokers, and male smokers to male nonsmokers. Adjusting for gender and other measured covariates in $\mathbf{x}$ requires some care and effort, but it is not deeply problematic [41]. It might be true—indeed, it is true [213]—that smokers are more likely than nonsmokers to use cocaine, heroin, and methamphetamine, so users of hard drugs are overrepresented in the smoking group, even though most smokers do not use hard drugs. If use of hard drugs is not measured, or is incompletely measured—if it is part of $\mathbf{u}$ rather than $\mathbf{x}$—then we cannot control for drug use, as we controlled for gender.

The less problematic aspect of causal inference in observational studies—i.e., adjustment for observed covariates—is important, but it has been extensively studied. In the current book, these adjustments are assumed to take simple forms, such as stratifying [39, 229] or matching [95, 97, 172, 224, 223, 265, 309] for $\mathbf{x}$, perhaps combined with model-based adjustment of outcomes for **x**; e.g., [194]. For several approaches to adjustments for **x**, see Refs. [7, 82, 102, 276, 279, 308].

If treatment assignment were ignorable, appropriate adjustment for observed co-variates **x** would suffice for causal inference [228, Theorem 4]. How can one speak to the central problem in causal inference, namely that (2.2)–(2.3) cannot be presumed true in an observational study? There are widely varied methods [195, 223], one of which is sensitivity analysis.

2.2 Sensitivity Analysis

2.2.1 Relaxing Rather than Replacing an Assumption

A sensitivity analysis in an observational study relaxes, in one way or another, the condition (2.2) that treatment assignment is ignorable. Relaxation of a condition is not replacement of that condition by an incompatible condition. Relaxing (2.2) entails assuming less than (2.2), as opposed to replacing (2.2) by a different assumption that contradicts (2.2).

When (2.2) is relaxed, the causal effect is no longer identified by the observed distributions; however, this occurs gradually, to a measured degree. Think of (2.2) as a pinnacle, reached only in a randomized experiment. Departing from (2.2) is descending a gradual slope, not falling off a cliff. Close to, but not at the pinnacle, there is no consistent estimate of the causal effect; yet, all of the possible effects are close to each other. As one moves further from the pinnacle, the set of possible effects expands. Eventually, for a large departure from (2.2), no useful inference is possible; after all, association does not logically imply causation, and statistical inference does not change that. We see this eroding identification of causal effects through a haze of sampling variability, and statistical inference does help reduce the haze.

The relaxation is quantitative: one considers an expanding neighborhood of (2.2). The question answered by a sensitivity analysis is quantitative: How far can treatment assignment depart from (2.2) without altering the qualitative causal inference that would be obtained by assuming (2.2)? What is the range of possible inferences in a quantitative neighborhood of (2.2)? What is the range of possible P-values testing the hypothesis of no treatment effect? What is the range of point estimates of the magnitude of effect? What is the range of endpoints for a 95% confidence interval for the magnitude of effect? Eventually, for a large departure from (2.2), these inferences are noninformative.[1] The question is not whether bias can explain an association as not causal—that is always possible outside randomized experiments, providing the bias is large enough. Instead, the question is: How large would the bias have to be to explain the observed association as not causal? The answer to that question varies from one observational study to the next, so we learn something by positioning the current study on a spectrum inhabited by other studies.

Are sensitivity analyses informative? They have been. In 1959, the first sensitivity analysis in an observational study concerned the effects of heavy smoking on

---

[1]This is proved in footnote 4 of Chapter 10.

lung cancer [46, 47, 81, 87]. Cornfield and colleagues [46] showed that, although association does not logically entail causation, the association between heavy smoking and lung cancer is so strong that only an enormous bias—an enormous departure from (2.2)—could explain it as anything but an effect caused by smoking. In 1959, the effect of smoking on lung cancer was still controversial. This sensitivity analysis characterized the magnitude of bias that would need to be present to explain away the observed association between smoking and lung cancer. In doing that, the sensitivity analysis made it far more difficult to propose such alternative explanations, for those alternative explanations needed to meet an empirically determined standard if they were to constitute possible explanations. In his discussion, Greenhouse [47] summarized: "No longer could one refute an observed causal association by simply asserting that some new factor (such as a genetic factor) might be the true cause. Now one had to argue that the relative prevalence of this potentially confounding factor was greater than the observed relative risk of the putative causal agent."

The inequality of Cornfield and colleagues [46] is an important conceptual advance. Association does not imply causation, and that is not going to change. However, the magnitude of bias needed to explain one association may be trivially small and entirely plausible, while the magnitude of bias needed to explain another association may be large and implausible. This is the issue examined by a sensitivity analysis: What magnitude of bias would need to be present to explain the observed association?

As a practical tool, the inequality of Cornfield and colleagues [46] is limited in several ways. It refers to binary outcomes, but not other kinds of outcomes. It ignores sampling variability, so it often mistakenly suggests that small studies with unstable estimates are insensitive to large biases. It makes no allowance for adjustments for measured covariates, though adjustments of this sort are routine in observational studies.

The method of sensitivity analysis described in this chapter is motivated by the inequality of Cornfield and colleagues [46], but it removes the limitations just described [185, 195, 221]. For discussion of various methods of sensitivity analysis in observational studies, see Refs. [70, 71, 80, 156, 227, 242, 246, 307].

2.2.2   A Small Example: DNA Damage Among Lead Workers

Fang-Yang Wu and colleagues [298] asked whether exposure to lead at work causes DNA damage. Figure 2.1 compares 11 lead workers and 11 unexposed controls matched for age and smoking. Each treatment group has three smokers and eight nonsmokers, and the age distribution is similar in Figure 2.1. Also shown in Figure 2.1 is the blood lead levels of workers and controls, and the lead workers have far more lead in their blood.[2]

In Ref. [298], potential DNA damage is measured by DNA-protein cross-links, and these are depicted in Figure 2.2. DNA-protein cross-links (DPC) occur when proteins become attached to DNA, possibly interfering with DNA replication and

---

[2]The data are available as `leadworker` in the R package `evident`.

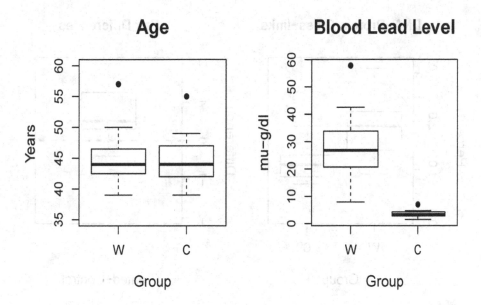

Figure 2.1 *A covariate, age, and a marker of exposure, the blood lead level in* μg/dl, *for 11 lead workers (W) and 11 unexposed controls (C), matched for age and smoking. There were 3 smokers and 8 nonsmokers in each group.*

transcription, possibly leading to mutations and cancer [273]. The left side of Figure 2.2 ignores the pairing; the right side depicts the pair differences in DPC, worker-minus-control.

In Figure 2.2, there are $N = 22$ individuals, in $S = 11$ pairs with $n_s = 2$ individuals in pair s, for $s = 1, \ldots, S$. As each pair has one worker and one control, there are $2^{11} = 2048$ possible treatment assignments in G that do not break up the pairs. In a randomized experiment, each treatment assignment in G has the same probability, namely $1/|G| = 2^{-11}$, and such a treatment assignment may be obtained by flipping a fair coin independently $S = 11$ times. Of course, Figure 2.2 is not from an experiment, and the investigator did not assign treatments using independent flips of a fair coin.

Had Figure 2.2 been the result of a trial that randomized one individual in each pair to the roles of lead worker or control, then it would constitute strong evidence that working in the lead industry causes an increase in DPC. A conventional randomization test for matched pairs is Wilcoxon's signed rank test [288], and it can be inverted to yield confidence intervals and point estimates [104, 110, 139, 140, 197]. The point estimate associated with Wilcoxon's test is called the Hodges-Lehmann estimate [104]. In Wilcoxon's signed rank test, the absolute values of the 11 pair differences are ranked from 1 to 11, with average ranks for ties, and the statistic is the sum of the ranks of the positive differences. Under Fisher's hypothesis H_0 of

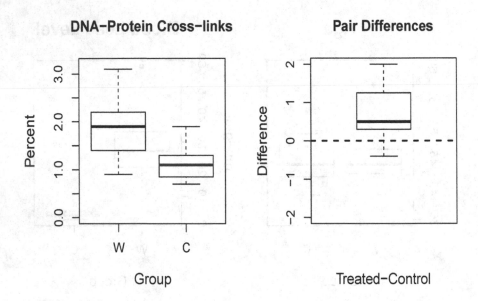

Figure 2.2 *DNA-protein cross-links in 11 lead workers (W) and 11 matched controls (C). In the boxplot of treated-minus-control pair differences, the dashed horizontal line is at zero.*

no treatment effect, randomization would create the null distribution of Wilcoxon's statistic: it is the distribution of the sum of $S = 11$ independent random variables, where random variable s is 0 with probability 1/2 and is the rank in pair s with probability 1/2. Inference for a constant or shift effect, (1.6) or (1.7), subtracts the hypothesized constant from each pair difference and applies the test for no effect to these adjusted differences, yielding by inversion the standard confidence interval and point estimate. In Figure 2.2, this yields a one-sided P-value testing no effect of 0.0049, a point estimate of a constant effect, (1.6) or (1.7), of $\hat{\tau} = 0.70$ and a one-sided 95% confidence interval of $\tau \geq 0.30$. We are not entitled to these inferences, because their validity is dependent upon random assignment of treatments, and this did not happen.

2.2.3 A Sensitivity Analysis Model for Matched Pairs

A simple model for sensitivity analysis [185, 234, Chapter 9] considers a family of departures from (2.1) formed by independently flipping $S = 11$ biased coins, where the probability π_s of assigning the first person in pair s to treatment and the second to control satisfies

$$\frac{1}{1+\Gamma} \leq \pi_s \leq \frac{\Gamma}{1+\Gamma}, \quad s = 1, \ldots, S, \tag{2.4}$$

for a real number $\Gamma \geq 1$.

If $\Gamma = 1$ in (2.4), then $\pi_s = 1/2$ as in random assignment, resulting in the usual randomization inferences that were just described. The sensitivity parameter Γ is unknown and expresses a magnitude of departure from randomization (2.1), but not a direction for the departure: it relaxes (2.1), but does not exclude (2.1) or replace it by a specific alternative. As Γ increases, (2.4) allows for larger and larger departures from randomization (2.1). The limit as $\Gamma \to \infty$ admits deterministic treatment assignment, $\pi_s = 0$ or $\pi_s = 1$, for which permutation inferences are degenerate and noninformative, in conformity with the familiar statement that association, no matter how strong, does not logically entail causation; that is, sufficiently large biases, measured by Γ, can explain any observed association between treatment received and outcome exhibited.[3] The parameter Γ is simply a yardstick for measuring departures from randomized treatment assignment, with randomization being $\Gamma = 1$ and deterministic assignment being approximated in the limit as $\Gamma \to \infty$.

Inequality (2.4) may be rewritten as

$$\frac{1}{\Gamma} \leq \frac{\pi_s}{1 - \pi_s} \leq \Gamma, \ s = 1, \ldots, S. \tag{2.5}$$

So, if you and I are in the same pair, s, then the odds are at most Γ that you receive treatment and I receive control, and those odds are at least $1/\Gamma$.

2.2.4   Inference Under the Sensitivity Analysis Model

A value of Γ in (2.4) creates a set $\mathscr{P}_\Gamma$ of possible distributions on G. As (2.4) permits $\pi_s = 1/2$ for each s, one distribution in the set $\mathscr{P}_\Gamma$ is the randomization distribution (2.1), but for $\Gamma > 1$ the set $\mathscr{P}_\Gamma$ contains other distributions as well. A probability distribution on the set of treatment assignments is a vector of dimension $|G|$

$$\mathbf{p} = \left(p_{g_1}, p_{g_2}, \ldots, p_{g_{|G|}} \right)^T \tag{2.6}$$

with

$$p_{g_\ell} \geq 0 \text{ for } s = 1, \ldots, |G| \text{ and } 1 = \sum_{\ell=1}^{|G|} p_{g_\ell}, \tag{2.7}$$

where $p_{g_\ell} = \Pr(G = g_\ell \mid \mathbf{r}, \mathbf{x}, \mathbf{u})$. In the example with eleven pairs in Figure 2.2, there are $|G| = 2^{11} = 2048$ possible treatment assignments, and each $\mathbf{p}$ in (2.6) is of dimension $|G| = 2^{11} = 2048$.

In a randomized experiment, each coordinate of $\mathbf{p}$ in (2.6) equals $1/|G|$, so this $\mathbf{p}$ satisfies both (2.4) for every $\Gamma \geq 1$ and (2.7). For $\Gamma > 1$, there are infinitely many $\mathbf{p}$ that satisfy (2.4) and (2.7), because there are infinitely many choices for each π_s in (2.4). As Γ increases, the set $\mathscr{P}_\Gamma$ grows, encompassing more and more distributions on G.

For any one $\mathbf{p} \in \mathscr{P}_\Gamma$, it is conceptually straightforward to compute the tail probability (1.5) testing the hypothesis H_0 of no effect, namely

$$\Pr\{t(G) \geq c \mid \mathbf{r}, \mathbf{x}, \mathbf{u}\} = \sum_{g_\ell \in G: t(g_\ell) \geq c} p_{g_\ell}, \tag{2.8}$$

---

[3] Again, this is proved in general in footnote 4 of Chapter 10.

albeit now without the simplification that a sum of probabilities is proportional to a count when all the probabilities are equal, as in a randomized experiment. Computing the tail probability with c set equal to the observed value of the test statistic yields a conventional P-value for the one distribution $\mathbf{p} \in \mathscr{P}_\Gamma$. Computing (2.8) for every $\mathbf{p} \in \mathscr{P}_\Gamma$, we may determine the maximum P-value, say $\overline{P}$, that a bias of Γ could produce: it is obtained from the maximum of (2.8) as $\mathbf{p}$ ranges over $\mathscr{P}_\Gamma$.[4] If there were no treatment effect, so H_0 is true, and if $\mathbf{p} \in \mathscr{P}_\Gamma$, then the probability that $\overline{P} \leq \alpha$ is at most α. As always, the test of no effect is inverted to obtain confidence intervals and point estimates. In this way, we obtain the set of possible point estimates and the set of possible confidence intervals that might be produced by a bias of Γ.

For $\Gamma = 1.25$, the interval of π_s in (2.4) is $1/(1+\Gamma) = 0.444 \leq \pi_s \leq 0.556 = \Gamma/(1+\Gamma)$. In this case, the maximum possible P-value testing no effect is 0.0116, the minimum point estimate is $\widehat{\tau}_{\min} = 0.65$, and the minimum endpoint for a one-sided 95% confidence interval is $\tau \geq 0.20$. Evidently, a bias of $\Gamma = 1.25$ would weaken the inference only slightly, leaving the qualitative impression unchanged. Table 2.1 considers other, larger biases as measured by Γ. At $\Gamma = 2.25$, there are π_s satisfying $1/(1+\Gamma) = 0.308 \leq \pi_s \leq 0.692 = \Gamma/(1+\Gamma)$ such that the hypothesis of no effect is not rejected at level $\alpha = 0.05$ as $\overline{P} = 0.0578 > 0.05$, and correspondingly the lower endpoint of the confidence interval is slightly negative, $\tau \geq -0.10$. So, Table 2.1 has compared Figure 2.2 to a yardstick measuring departures from random assignment, finding evidence of an effect on DPC for $\Gamma = 2$ but not for $\Gamma = 2.25$.

Table 2.1 *Sensitivity analysis for the effects of lead exposure on DNA-protein cross-links. For each Γ, the maximum P-value testing no effect, $\overline{P}$, is given, together with the lower endpoint of the one-sided 95% confidence interval for τ*

Γ	$\overline{P}$	95% CI
1.00	0.0049	0.30
1.25	0.0116	0.20
1.50	0.0208	0.10
1.75	0.0320	0.05
2.00	0.0445	0.00
2.25	0.0578	-0.10

2.2.5   Interpretations of Γ

We need to make quantitative sense of values of Γ besides $\Gamma = 1$ for randomization and $\Gamma \to \infty$ for infinitely large, deterministic biases. Values of Γ are tick marks on a

---

[4]Computation of $\overline{P}$ typically uses one large sample approximation or another; see Ref. [195, Chapter 4] or [204, 221]. For Wilcoxon's signed rank statistic, the approximations are straightforward and are implemented in the senWilcox and senU functions in the DOS2 package in R. For other situations and statistics, the approximations are implemented in the R packages senstrat and sensitivity2x2xk, and in the functions senm and senmCI in package sensitvitymult.

yardstick. That yardstick measures departures from random assignment (2.1); so, we need to be able to make sense of values $\Gamma = 1.25$ or $\Gamma = 2$. Here are several ways to think about Γ.

One approach uses (2.5): $\Gamma = 2$ means doubling the odds, $\pi_s / (1 - \pi_s)$, that a particular person in a pair will be the treated person, in light of the information conditioned upon by π_s, namely the observed and unobserved covariates and the potential outcomes. Just on the face of it, that does not sound like a small departure from a randomized experiment, and indeed it is not a small departure.

Another approach gains acquaintance with a new yardstick by measuring familiar things. One study of heavy smoking and lung cancer [94] became sensitive to unmeasured bias at $\Gamma = 6$ [195, Table 4.1]. A study [101] of diethylstilbestrol (DES) as a cause of vaginal cancer became sensitive to unmeasured bias at $\Gamma = 7$ [195, Table 4.9]. These are two well-established findings. A study of coffee as a cause of heart attacks [122] is sensitive to a bias of $\Gamma = 1.3$ [195, §4.4.5]; however, other studies reached different conclusions [74, 301]. Many published observational studies have small P-values from an inference that assumes there are no unmeasured confounders—i.e., from a randomization inference with $\Gamma = 1$—because of a large sample size; yet, the studies do not mention that $\overline{P} > 0.05$ for $\Gamma = 1.05$.

Imagine a logit regression of the probability of treatment on observed covariates and one unobserved binary covariate u. One might think of this as a model for the propensity score that would have been fitted if u had been observed. The coefficient γ of u in this logit regression is essentially $\gamma = \log(\Gamma)$; see Ref. [195, §4.2] for specifics.

The model (2.4) thinks in terms of biased treatment assignment conditionally given the potential outcomes. So, Γ is implicitly about the dependence of treatment assignment upon the potential outcomes. An amplification [231, 234, Table 9.1] makes this implicit dependence explicit, without altering the sensitivity analysis or the set $\mathscr{P}_\Gamma$ of distributions on G. An unobserved covariate u that increases the odds of treatment by a factor of $\Lambda \geq 1$ and increases the odds of a positive pair difference in responses to control by a factor of $\Delta \geq 1$ is equivalent to $\Gamma = (\Lambda\Delta + 1)/(\Lambda + \Delta)$. For example, $\Gamma = 2$ corresponds with an unobserved covariate that increases the odds of a positive difference in DPC by a factor of $\Delta = 3$ and increase the odds of being the lead worker rather than the control by a factor of $\Lambda = 5$ because $\Gamma = 2 = (5 \times 3 + 1)/(5 + 3) = (\Lambda\Delta + 1)/(\Lambda + \Delta)$. Actually, a single Γ corresponds with a curve of (Λ, Δ): an amplification maps a scalar into a curve. Change Γ and the curve (Λ, Δ) changes. For instance, $(\Lambda, \Delta) = (5, 3)$, $(\Lambda, \Delta) = (3, 5)$ and $(\Lambda, \Delta) = (3.73, 3.73)$ all correspond with $\Gamma = 2$. So, a one-dimensional sensitivity analysis may be compactly reported in terms of Γ, as in Table 2.1; yet, that one-dimensional analysis may be given a two-dimensional interpretation in terms of the relationships between an unobserved covariate and both treatment assignment and outcome. The value $\Gamma = 1.25$ corresponds with an unobserved covariate that doubles the odds of treatment, $\Lambda = 2$, and doubles the odds of a positive pair difference in outcomes, $\Delta = 2$, as $\Gamma = 1.25 = (2 \times 2 + 1)/(2 + 2) = (\Lambda\Delta + 1)/(\Lambda + \Delta)$; so, $\Gamma = 1.25$ is neither an enormous bias, nor a trivial one.

2.3 *Another Example of Sensitivity Analysis

2.3.1 Why a Second Example?

The example in §2.2 was exceedingly simple, eleven pairs matched for two covariates. In the current, optional section, a slightly larger, slightly less tidy example
is considered. This example involves more individuals and more covariates, and it
lacks the tidiness of matched pairs, but the sensitivity analysis takes a similar form.
This section might be skipped by a reader eager to make progress and content to
focus on the simplest case. In contrast, this section might be helpful to a reader who
would like to apply the method.

Multivariate matching may often be used, with advantage, to retain a simple form
for problems with many individuals and many covariates; see, for example [5, 257,
304, 310]. Multivariate matching is, however, a fairly large topic that is not central to
this book. For surveys of multivariate matching, see Ref. [223, Part II] and Refs. [96,
224, 265, 303]. The example that follows uses stratification and robust covariance
adjustment, not multivariate matching.

2.3.2 Cigarettes and Homocysteine

Bazzano and colleagues [14] asked whether smoking cigarettes elevates blood homocysteine levels. The example from [221] that follows updates their comparison
using data from the 2005–2006 National Health and Nutrition Examination Survey,
the most recent version that measured homocysteine.[5] For related comparisons, see
Refs. [128, 173].

Daily smokers and never smokers are compared. A daily smoker smoked every
day for the last 30 days, and smoked an average of *at least* 10 cigarettes per day.
Never smokers smoked fewer than 100 cigarettes in their lives, do not smoke now,
and had no tobacco use in the previous 5 days. Panel (a) of Figure 2.3 depicts 2475
homocysteine levels of 512 daily smokers (S) and 1963 never-smoking controls (C).
Obviously, the randomization and permutation inferences considered here need not
be applied to the homocysteine levels themselves, and could instead be applied to a
transformation of the homocysteine levels, such as the logs in panel (b) of Figure 2.3.
After all, the distributions of treatment assignments in $\Pr(G = g_\ell \mid \mathbf{r}, \mathbf{x}, \mathbf{u})$ condition
on the array of potential outcomes, $\mathbf{r}$, and this is the same as conditioning on their
logs. In Figure 2.3, base-2 logs are used, so that a difference of one unit means one
doubling, $\log_2(20) - \log_2(10) = 1$, and a difference of two means two doublings,
$\log_2(40) - \log_2(10) = 2$. Base-2 logs are a constant multiple of base-10 logs, and
a constant multiple of natural logs, but the units on a graph are easier to interpret
when base-2 logs are used. An additive effect in (1.6) of $\tau = 1$ on the base-2 log
scale is a multiplicative effect of one-doubling on the original scale. Inverting a test
of no effect for τ-adjusted responses on the log-scale yields a confidence set for a
multiplicative effect on the original scale; see §1.7. In panel (b) of Figure 2.3, the

---

[5]The data are available as hsmoke in the evident package in R. For additional detail about the data
and the analysis discussed here, see Ref. [221].

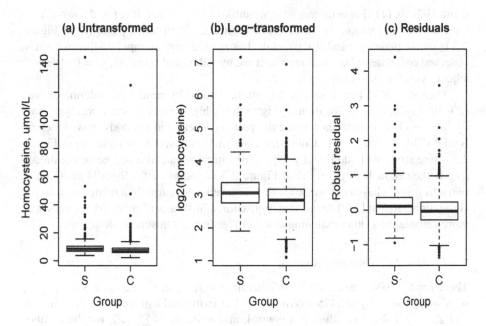

Figure 2.3 *Homocysteine levels of daily smokers (S) and never-smoking controls (C). The figure shows homocysteine levels, their base-2 logs, and the robust residuals of the base-2 logs when regressed on gender, education, and continuous covariates age, BMI, income.*

two boxplots appear to have similar shape and dispersion with different locations, consistent with a location shift on the log-scale.

Perhaps a little less obviously, the transformation of the outcome, $\mathbf{r}$, need not use $\mathbf{r}$ alone; rather, it may also involve the observed covariates $\mathbf{x}$. Another transformation of responses creates residuals adjusted for observed covariates in a model that does not include the treatment. When testing the hypothesis H_0 of no effect, we may apply a permutation or randomization test to the residual of the observed log response $\mathbf{R}$ when regressed on the observed covariate $\mathbf{x}$. We may do this because $\mathbf{R}$ equals every column of $\mathbf{r}$ when H_0 is true, and both $\mathbf{r}$ and $\mathbf{x}$ are fixed by conditioning in $\Pr(G = g_\ell \mid \mathbf{r}, \mathbf{x}, \mathbf{u})$; see [194]. Panel (c) of Figure 2.3 shows the residuals of the base-2 logs of homocysteine levels when regressed on a binary indicator of gender, a five-category integer measure of education, and three continuous covariates, namely age, family income, and the body mass index (BMI). The regression must not include the treatment—here, smoking determined by G—but the outcome may be adjusted for a hypothesized effect, τ, prior to fitting the regression, en route to building a confidence interval for τ. For instance, to test the hypothesis $H_0 : \tau = \tau_0$ that smoking increases homocysteine by 5%, we subtract $\tau_0 = \log_2(1.05) = 0.07039$ from the base-2 logs of the smoker's homocysteine levels prior to fitting the regression and obtaining the residuals, in effect, pushing down the smoker boxplot in panel (b) by 0.07039. In panel (c) of Figure 2.3, the covariance adjustment fits the regression using Huber's [115] m-estimate, so that, unlike least squares, it is not thrown off by the extreme observations in panel (b) of Figure 2.3.[6] In short, panel (c) of Figure 2.3 is unlike panels (a) and (b): panel (c) has made a first attempt to adjust for a few observed covariates when thinking about the hypothesis of no effect, $\tau_0 = 0$. We will adjust twice for these covariates.

There are 2475 individuals in 104 strata defined by gender (female/male), age (20–39, 40–60, ≥ 60), education ($\leq$ high school, high school, $\geq$ some college), family income (below or at least twice the poverty level), and the body-mass-index or BMI (< 30, 30–35, ≥ 35). Unlike the continuous adjustment in panel (c) of Figure 2.3, these strata will additionally adjust for interactions and a degree of nonlinearity. If the residuals in panel (c) of Figure 2.3 are adjusted for the 104 strata, then two adjustments have been made for the observed covariates. In a related context, in simulations, Rubin [239] found that regression adjustment of matched samples was more reliable than either matching alone or regression adjustment alone.

2.3.3 Stratified Sensitivity Analysis

There are $S = 104$ strata, with n_s individuals, $i = 1, \ldots, n_s$ in stratum s, $s = 1, \ldots, S$, so $N = n_1 + \cdots + n_S = 2475$. Write $Z_{si} = 1$ if individual i in stratum s is a smoker and $Z_{si} = 0$ if this individual is a control, and write $m_s = \sum_{i=1}^{n_s} Z_{si}$ for the number of smokers in stratum s, so $m_1 + \cdots + m_S = 512$. Write $\mathcal{Z}_s$ for the set containing the vectors of dimension n_s with m_s coordinates equal to 1 and $n_s - m_s$ coordinates equal to zero. Write $\mathcal{Z}$ for the set of vectors $\mathbf{z} = \left(z_{11}, z_{12}, \ldots, z_{S,n_S} \right)^T$ of dimension N formed by concatenating S vectors,

$$
\mathbf{z} = \begin{bmatrix} \mathbf{z}_1 \\ \mathbf{z}_2 \\ \vdots \\ \mathbf{z}_S \end{bmatrix} \quad \text{with} \quad \mathbf{z}_s \in \mathcal{Z}_s, \, s = 1, \ldots, S, \tag{2.9}
$$

so that

$$
|\mathcal{Z}_s| = \binom{n_s}{m_s} \quad \text{and} \quad |\mathcal{Z}| = \prod_{s=1}^{S} \binom{n_s}{m_s}.
$$

The connection between a treatment assignment G and the binary vector $\mathbf{Z}$ becomes explicit in (10.10) of Chapter 10; however, this level of detail can wait until it becomes useful.

In a stratified randomized experiment, $\Pr(G = g_\ell \mid \mathbf{r}, \mathbf{x}, \mathbf{u})$ picks one random treatment assignment $\mathbf{Z} \in \mathcal{Z}$ so that $\Pr(\mathbf{Z} = \mathbf{z} \mid \mathbf{r}, \mathbf{x}, \mathbf{u}) = |\mathcal{Z}|^{-1}$ for each $\mathbf{z} \in \mathcal{Z}$. Write $\mathcal{U}_s = [0, 1]^{n_s}$ for the n_s-dimensional unit cube. The sensitivity model for a stratified comparison is:

$$
\Pr(\mathbf{Z} = \mathbf{z} \mid \mathbf{r}, \mathbf{x}, \mathbf{u}) = \prod_{s=1}^{S} \frac{\exp\left(\gamma \mathbf{z}_s^T \mathbf{u}_s \right)}{\sum_{\mathbf{b}_s \in \mathcal{Z}_s} \exp\left(\gamma \mathbf{b}_s^T \mathbf{u}_s \right)} \quad \text{for} \quad \mathbf{z}_s \in \mathcal{Z}_s, \, \mathbf{u}_s \in \mathcal{U}_s, \tag{2.10}
$$

---

[6]The regression used the rlm function in the MASS package in R, with the default settings. This default for m-estimation uses Huber's $\psi(\cdot)$ function, so its influence function resembles that of a trimmed mean.

where $\gamma = \log(\Gamma) \geq 0$. When $\gamma = 0$, the model (2.10) reduces to randomization, $\Pr(\mathbf{Z} = \mathbf{z} \mid \mathbf{r}, \mathbf{x}, \mathbf{u}) = |\mathscr{Z}|^{-1}$. When $n_s = 2$ and $m_s = 1$ for $s = 1, \ldots, S$, model (2.10) becomes the sensitivity model for matched pairs in §2.2. If $S = 1$, model (2.10) describes an unstratified comparison of treated and control groups [189, 225]. When $n_s = 3$ and $m_s = 1$ for $s = 1, \ldots, S$, model (2.10) becomes a sensitivity analysis model for matched triples, one treated individual matched to two controls, and so on. The interpretation of $\Gamma = \exp(\gamma)$ in (2.10) is largely unchanged from the discussion in §2.2 for matched pairs [195, Chapter 4].

For a given Γ and $\mathbf{u}^T = (\mathbf{u}_1, \ldots, \mathbf{u}_S)^T$, a tail probability (2.8) may be calculated from (2.10). As $\mathbf{u}$ is not known, the upper bound, $\overline{P}$, on the P-value is obtained from the maximum of (2.8) over all $\mathbf{u}$ with $\mathbf{u}_s \in \mathscr{U}_s$ for $s = 1, \ldots, S$.[7] As Γ is varied, the degree of sensitivity to unmeasured bias is displayed. As noted previously, the test may be inverted to obtain a confidence set for the magnitude of effect.

2.3.4 Sensitivity Analysis for Cigarettes and Homocysteine

The most commonly used robust test statistic with strata is the Hodges-Lehmann aligned rank test [103, 140, 157]. In this test, the responses are aligned by subtracting in each stratum a stratum specific estimate of location,[8] then the responses are scored by ranking the aligned values from 1 to N, with average ranks for ties. The statistic is the sum of the ranks in the treated group. An alternative approach, perhaps more consistent with covariance adjustment by m-estimation, uses m-scores as discussed in Refs. [204, 212, 214] and Ref. [221, §5].[9]

Consider first a test of the null hypothesis H_0 of no effect of smoking on homocysteine levels using the Hodges-Lehmann aligned rank test applied to the robust residuals in Figure 2.3(c). At $\Gamma = 1$ for a randomization test, the one-sided P-value is 1.44×10^{-15}. At $\Gamma = 2$, the upper bound, $\overline{P}$, on the P-value is 0.0151. If the aligned rank test is applied, not to the residuals, but to the values in Figure 2.3(b), then $\overline{P}$ is 0.0469 at $\Gamma = 1.95$ and $\overline{P}$ is 0.0709 at $\Gamma = 2$. So, the comparison in Figure 2.3 is insensitive to moderately large unmeasured biases whether or not robust covariance adjustment is used in addition to the $S = 104$ strata. In this one example, the results are insensitive to slightly larger biases if covariance adjustment is used in addition to stratification.

The comparisons in Table 2.2 replace the aligned ranks by m-scores. More importantly, several hypotheses are tested about a multiplicative effect, β, where

---

[7]The general calculation [221] is done by the senstrat function in the senstrat package in R. For binary outcomes, the same calculation is performed more quickly by the mh and mhLS functions in the sensitivity2x2xk package [233].

[8]Hodges and Lehmann [103] subtract the stratum mean or median, but simulations by Mehrotra et al. [157] led them to align by the Hodges-Lehmann [104] location estimate, and this approach is used in the cigarettes and homocysteine example.

[9]After scaling, Huber's $\psi(\cdot)$ is applied to treated-minus-control differences in responses within the same stratum, thereby removing any stratum specific location shift. For details, see Ref. [221, §5] and the mscores function in the senstrat package in R. The default settings in the mscores function were used in the cigarettes and homocysteine example. Unlike the default settings, suitably designed and weighted m-scores can increase design sensitivity [212, 214], the limiting sensitivity to bias as $N \to \infty$. In the matched case, see also the R packages sensitivitymv, sensitivitymw, and sensitivitymult.

$H_0 : \beta = 1.05$ signifies a test of a 5% increase in homocysteine levels against the alternative that the increase is larger than 5%. Here, $\beta = 1.05$ corresponds with $\tau = \log_2(\beta) = \log_2(1.05)$ in (1.6), for an additive effect on the log scale. In Table 2.2, a 10% increase in homocysteine levels is judged too small in a randomization test, $\Gamma = 1$, a 5% increase is rejected at the 0.05 level as too small if the bias is at most $\Gamma = 1.5$, and no effect is rejected at $\Gamma = 2.25$.

Table 2.2 *Sensitivity analysis for cigarettes and homocysteine levels. Computed from m-scores of robust residuals in $S = 104$ strata. Tabulated values are upper bounds on the one-sided P-value. Hypotheses concern a multiplicative effect, so that 1 is no effect, and 1.05 is a 5 percent increase*

	$H_0 : \beta = \beta_0$		
Γ	1.00	1.05	1.1
1.00	0.000	0.000	0.023
1.25	0.000	0.000	0.392
1.50	0.000	0.027	
1.75	0.000	0.228	
2.00	0.002		
2.25	0.023		
2.50	0.115		

In brief, §2.2 and §2.3 have considered two examples, one with eleven pairs matched for two covariates, the other with $N = 2475$ individuals in 104 strata and with covariance adjustment for several observed covariates. Despite the differences between these two examples, the sensitivity analyses were similar in form and interpretation.

2.4 Design Sensitivity

2.4.1 *Anticipating the Results of a Sensitivity Analysis*

Can we anticipate the results of a sensitivity analysis? Can we know in advance that data from one study design will tend to be less sensitive to unmeasured bias than data from a different design? Can we know in advance that one statistical method will tend to exaggerate the degree of sensitivity to unmeasured bias, so that another method is preferable?

A sensitivity analysis is computed from the observed data, so its behavior is determined by distributions of observable data. In a crude way, we could simulate data in various circumstances, from various study designs when analyzed by various methods, and study how the sensitivity analysis turns out in many simulated data sets. There is no difficulty in doing this in principle. Unfortunately, simulation without guidance from theory can resemble throwing darts in the dark: it is difficult to know whether one has checked enough cases, the important cases, the aspects that are critical. In a less crude way, we could develop a theoretical scaffolding that would anticipate how all such simulations would turn out.

We should consider clear cases. If there is a treatment effect and no unmeasured bias, then we cannot be sure of this from observed data, but we hope to report that the evidence in favor of an effect is insensitive to small and moderate unmeasured biases. So that is one clear case, worth understanding. Call this case the "favorable situation." It is favorable in that the treatment did work, and straightforward analyses are not misleading, because there is no unmeasured bias. It is favorable in that things are the way they appear: the higher response of treated individuals is effects caused by a treatment that did work. Alas, if we were in the favorable situation, we would not know it. The same observable distributions could reflect a bias in treatment assignment with no treatment effect. The design sensitivity, $\tilde{\Gamma}$, is a theoretical quantity that refers to this clear case.

In another clear case, there is no treatment effect, and the association between treatment received and outcome exhibited is entirely due to bias in treatment assignment. In this alternative clear case, we have no desire to report that results are insensitive to small or moderate biases. In this case, we hope that the sensitivity analysis will caution us against making incorrect claims about the effectiveness of the treatment. The design sensitivity, $\tilde{\Gamma}$, concerns our ability to distinguish these two clear cases.[10] In these two clear cases, we know what we want the sensitivity analysis to do, and the only question is whether it succeeds or fails.

2.4.2 What Is Design Sensitivity?

The design sensitivity, $\tilde{\Gamma}$, is a theoretical quantity that describes how a sensitivity analysis will turn out in the favorable situation [198, 223, Part III]. The design sensitivity could be determined numerically by simulation in particular situations, but there is often a formula that covers all situations. Described informally, the design sensitivity is the limiting sensitivity to unmeasured bias as the sample size increases, computed in some favorable situation. The numerical value of the design sensitivity, $\tilde{\Gamma}$, depends upon the study design and the methods of analysis, so we could learn to prefer designs and methods that yield larger values of $\tilde{\Gamma}$.

Described more formally, consider a sequence of favorable situations with increasing sample sizes, N. Perhaps there are $S = N/2$ matched pairs sampled at random from an infinite population of matched pairs, and let $N \to \infty$. Consider the upper bound on the P-value, $\bar{P}_{\Gamma,N}$, computed from N observations with the sensitivity parameter set to Γ. Then there is often a number $\tilde{\Gamma}$ such that $\bar{P}_{\Gamma,N}$ converges in probability to zero for $\Gamma < \tilde{\Gamma}$, and $\bar{P}_{\Gamma,N}$ converges in probability to one for $\Gamma > \tilde{\Gamma}$. When this occurs, the number $\tilde{\Gamma}$ is called the design sensitivity. If the sample size is large enough, we are all but certain to report insensitivity to biases smaller than $\tilde{\Gamma}$, and all but certain to report sensitivity to biases larger than $\tilde{\Gamma}$.

Consider the simplest favorable situation. There are $S = N/2$ matched pairs, yielding S treated-minus-control pair differences Y_s in outcomes, $s = 1, \ldots, S$, with

---

[10]This section is a very brief introduction to design sensitivity, with a view to its use in later chapters. Detailed discussion is available in Ref. [223, Part III]. See the discussion in the Preface of sections with an asterisk (*) for more about the role of §2.4.

random assignment of treatments within pairs, and a constant (1.6) or shift (1.7) effect, τ. Suppose further that the pairs, the Y_s, are independently sampled from an infinite population with a continuous distribution. Then, the Y_s are symmetric about τ, independent, and identically distributed, free of ties. Take two different observations, Y_s and $Y_{s'}$, with $s \neq s'$, and define η to be the probability that their sum is positive. In this situation, the design sensitivity of Wilcoxon's signed rank test is [99, Expression (4)]:

$$\widetilde{\Gamma} = \frac{\eta}{1-\eta} \quad \text{where} \quad \eta = \Pr(Y_s + Y_{s'} > 0). \tag{2.11}$$

Indeed, (2.11) is true whether or not there is a shift effect, τ. For instance, if Y_s is Normal with expectation τ and variance 1, $Y_s \sim N(\tau, 1)$, then Wilcoxon's test has $\widetilde{\Gamma} = 3.171$ for $\tau = 1/2$. We could see this by simulation. Taking a sample of $S = 100000$ pair differences, $Y_s \sim N(0.5, 1)$, and performing the sensitivity analysis using Wilcoxon's test, at $\Gamma = 3, 3.1, 3.2$ and 3.3, upper bounds $\overline{P}_{\Gamma,N}$ on the P-value are 3.8×10^{-11}, 0.00379, 0.851, and 1.000, so the P-value takes a step up from near zero to near one in the vicinity of $\widetilde{\Gamma} = 3.17$. What can we learn from design sensitivity?

2.4.3   Heterogeneity and Causality

In an observational study, are you better off with fewer but more stable Y_s? Or with more but less stable Y_s? Which situation is better if the goal is to report insensitivity to small and moderate biases whenever the favorable situation arises? Is money better spent on more observations? Or on better observations?

Laboratory scientists are fanatical about driving out heterogeneity, for instance, using genetically engineered, nearly identical mice. In his "method of difference," John Stuart Mill argued that causal inference depended upon eliminating heterogeneity, but in his *Design of Experiments*, Fisher ridiculed Mill's method [200, 223, §16.1]. Fisher believed that our ability to reduce heterogeneity is limited, and that randomization in experiments makes heterogeneity unrelated to treatment assignment. Of course, Fisher was thinking about randomized experiments, not observational studies.

Let us level the playing field by taking $Y_s \sim N(\tau, 1)$ for $s = 1, \ldots, 4S$ and $Y_s' \sim N(\tau, 1/4)$ for $s = 1, \ldots, S$, so that the standard deviation of Y_s' is half the standard deviation of Y_s, but there are four times as many Y_s. In this case, the means,

$$\overline{Y} = \frac{1}{4S}\sum_{s=1}^{4S} Y_s \quad \text{and} \quad \overline{Y}' = \frac{1}{S}\sum_{s=1}^{S} Y_s' \quad \text{both have distribution } N\left(\tau, \frac{1}{4S}\right). \tag{2.12}$$

Because of (2.12), if the variances were known, the standard confidence intervals for τ based on inverting the z-test would have the same expected length and the same distribution for $\overline{Y}$ and $\overline{Y}'$; moreover, unknown variances would produce negligible differences in the confidence intervals formed by inverting the t-test when S is large.

Despite (2.12), the boxplots of Y_s and Y_s' would look very different, with their boxes centered at τ, but with the length of the box for Y_s' being half the length of the box for Y_s. Does that matter?

Applying (2.11) with $\tau = 1/2$, we again find $\widetilde{\Gamma} = 3.171$ for the Y_i, but now $\widetilde{\Gamma} = 11.715$ for Y_s'. As $S \to \infty$, between $\Gamma = 3.171$ and $\Gamma = 11.715$, the power of Wilcoxon's test applied to Y_s is tending to zero, but if applied instead to Y_s' then the power is tending to one. Expressed differently, at $\Gamma = 2$ as $S \to \infty$, the point estimate and confidence limits for $\tau = 1/2$ formed by inverting Wilcoxon's test are tending to the real interval $[0.195, 0.805]$ if computed from Y_s, but are tending to $[0.348, 0.652]$ if computed from Y_s', so unmeasured bias creates less ambiguity in large samples if there is less heterogeneity [200, 223, §16.3]

Are there genetically engineered, nearly identical mice available for observational studies in economics and business? Indeed, there are. A common business strategy called replication rapidly reproduces highly similar retail outlets that operate in widely varied economic environments [291]. Think of Starbucks, Carrefour, Zara, or Lidl. For example, Card and Krueger [34] studied the employment effects of changes in the minimum wage by comparing Burger King restaurants in US states with different minimum wage laws. They also made comparisons within three other restaurant chains: KFC, Roy Rogers, and Wendy's. Their study is examined further in §4.4 and §6.2.

Devices that reduce heterogeneity can increase insensitivity to unmeasured bias. For instance, if matching balances many covariates, but pairs closely for a few covariates highly predictive of the outcome, then there can be a visible increase in insensitivity to unmeasured bias, when compared to matching for the same covariates without distinguishing their distinct roles. In Ref. [312], the same treated and control individuals, matched once by cardinality matching, are paired in two different ways—so the covariate balance is the same—but one pairing emphasizes highly predictive covariates, and that pairing reports greater insensitivity to unmeasured biases.

2.4.4 Doses, Transformations, and Design Sensitivity

A treatment may be applied at different doses in different matched pairs; see the examples in §4.1 and §4.3. The manner in which doses are used in the analysis affects the design sensitivity [198, 223, §18.4]. If the treatment effect is larger at higher doses—a big if—then emphasizing pairs with high doses can increase insensitivity to unmeasured biases. Conversely, if doses are irrelevant, then de-emphasizing low doses can be detrimental; see the example in §4.5. Greater emphasis may mean either a test statistic that gives a larger weight to pairs with higher doses [190, 196, 277], or it may mean simply ignoring low-dose pairs. For calculations of $\widetilde{\Gamma}$ for various statistics in various situations with doses, see Ref. [223, §18.4].

In Figure 2.3, the treated and control groups appear shifted once logarithms are taken. Transformations can also affect the design sensitivity.

Because the impact of doses or transformations on $\widetilde{\Gamma}$ depends upon the process that generated the data, an investigator may find it difficult to guess, prior to examining data, which analysis will report the greatest insensitivity to unmeasured bias. If more than one analysis is performed, corrections are needed to reflect multiple testing. In this context, the corrections for multiple testing are often quite small, much smaller than the common corrections using the Bonferroni inequality, because several analyses asking the same question of the same data are often highly correlated. In Ref. [211], an adaptive method performs twelve analyses—with and without doses, with and without a log transformation, with three test statistics—locating the most insensitive comparison, while paying only a small price for multiple testing. The adaptive method has the largest design sensitivity of its component tests. Adaptive methods perform well in large samples, because $\tilde{\Gamma}$ is affected by doses, transformations and the choice of test statistic, but $\tilde{\Gamma}$ is not affected by the necessary corrections for multiple testing. Corrections for multiple testing do affect power, but with diminished consequences as the sample size increases, whereas $\tilde{\Gamma}$ continues to affect the power of a sensitivity analysis even as the sample size increases without bound. See also Refs. [113, 210, 222]. This issue arises with evidence factors in §6.3, where an example is discussed.

2.4.5 *Design Sensitivity and the Choice of Test Statistic

Is Wilcoxon's signed rank statistic a good statistic? Does it achieve high design sensitivity in the favorable situation? Is its sensitivity analysis efficient when compared to other test statistics?

Using (2.11), we saw that $\tilde{\Gamma} = 3.171$ for Wilcoxon's statistic if $Y_s \sim N(\tau, 1)$ with $\tau = 1/2$. In the same sampling situation, how does that compare with the design sensitivity for other test statistics? The sign test statistic is much worse with $\tilde{\Gamma} = 2.24$, but a statistic due to Brown [29] is better with $\tilde{\Gamma} = 3.60$; see Ref. [210, Table 2]. Noether [166] proposed a simple generalization of the sign test statistic: it counts the number of positive Y_s among the $100\zeta\%$ of the Y_s with the largest $|Y_s|$. With $\zeta = 1/3$, Noether's statistic uses $1/3$ of the Y_s with the largest $|Y_s|$, and it has much higher design sensitivity than Wilcoxon's statistic with $\tilde{\Gamma} = 4.97$. Although $\tilde{\Gamma}$ varies with τ, the comparative performance of these statistics is similar for $\tau = 1/4$, $\tau = 1/2$ and $\tau = 3/4$; see Ref. [210, Table 2]. Similar patterns for $\tilde{\Gamma}$ occur if the errors have longer tailed distributions, the logistic distribution or the t-distribution with 3 degrees of freedom [210, Table 2]. For methods closely related to those of Noether [166] and Brown [29], see Gastwirth [78], Groeneveld [89], and Markowski and Hettmansperger [154].

For $Y_s \sim N(\tau, 1)$, Noether's statistic with $\zeta = 1/3$ has poor Pitman efficiency relative to Wilcoxon's statistic in a randomization test, $\Gamma = 1$, but, with $\tau = 1/2$, for $3.171 < \Gamma < 4.97$ the power of the sensitivity analysis for Wilcoxon's test is declining to zero with increasing sample size, while the power of Noether's test is increasing to one. For $\Gamma < 3.171$, the P-value bounds $\overline{P}$ from both tests tend to zero with increasing sample size. Which $\overline{P}$ tends to be smaller for $\Gamma < 3.171$? This is the question addressed by the Bahadur efficiency [9] of a sensitivity analysis, which is derived from the rate at which $\overline{P} \to 0$ when $\Gamma < \tilde{\Gamma}$. For $\tau = 0.5$, at $\Gamma = 2$, the bound $\overline{P}$ for Noether's statistic is declining to zero at a faster rate, and Wilcoxon's statistic is only 68% as efficient as Noether's statistic [215, Table 2]. Pitman efficiency is determined by letting $\tau \to 0$ as the sample size increases, but this is not applicable to a sensitivity analysis, because small effects τ are always sensitive to small biases Γ. In contrast, Bahadur efficiency keeps τ fixed as the sample size increases.

Can statistics be built to have high design sensitivity? Wilcoxon's signed rank statistic is nearly identical to a certain U-statistic [139, Appendix §5, Example 21]. Consider all pairs of two distinct pair differences, Y_s and $Y_{s'}$, with $s \neq s'$. Record a 1 if $Y_s + Y_{s'} > 0$ and a 0 otherwise. Equivalently, record a 1 if $|Y_s| > |Y_{s'}|$ and $Y_s > 0$, record a 1 if $|Y_{s'}| > |Y_s|$ and $Y_{s'} > 0$; otherwise, record 0. Let U be the total count over all $\binom{S}{2}$ choices of distinct Y_s and $Y_{s'}$. Then inferences based on U are virtually identical to inferences based on Wilcoxon's signed rank statistic. Here, U is one member of Hoeffding's [105] class of U-statistics.

This representation of Wilcoxon's statistic as a U-statistic may be generalized to produce a class of related statistics, some of which have higher design sensitivities than Wilcoxon's statistic [208]. Consider m distinct pair differences, $Y_{s_1}, \dots Y_{s_m}$, and sort these into increasing order by $|Y_{s_j}|$. In this revised order, count the number of positive Y_{s_j} among those in positions $\underline{m}, \underline{m} + 1, \dots, \overline{m}$ where $1 \leq \underline{m} \leq \overline{m} \leq m$. Define U to be the total count over all choices of distinct $Y_{s_1}, \dots Y_{s_m}$; so, U is another member of Hoeffding's [105] class of U-statistics. The U-statistic for Wilcoxon's test has $(m, \underline{m}, \overline{m}) = (2, 2, 2)$; see the preceding paragraph. The statistic $(m, \underline{m}, \overline{m}) = (1, 1, 1)$ is the sign-test statistic. The statistic $(m, \underline{m}, \overline{m}) = (m, m, m)$ for general m was proposed by Stephenson [262].

If $Y_s \sim N(\tau, 1)$ in a randomized experiment, then the statistic $(m, \underline{m}, \overline{m}) = (5, 4, 5)$ has the same Pitman efficiency as Wilcoxon's statistic; however, for $\tau = 1/2$, the statistic $(5, 4, 5)$ has higher design sensitivity of $\widetilde{\Gamma} = 3.9 > 3.171$; see [208, Tables 1 and 3].[11] Better still is the statistic $(m, \underline{m}, \overline{m}) = (8, 7, 8)$ with $\widetilde{\Gamma} = 5.08$, so its design sensitivity exceeds that of Noether's statistic, 4.97, and its Bahadur efficiency at $\Gamma = 2$ is 19% higher than Noether's statistic and 75% higher than Wilcoxon's statistic [215, Table 2]. For an adaptive choice of the test statistic $(m, \underline{m}, \overline{m})$, see [211]. A suitable choice of $(m, \underline{m}, \overline{m})$ can strengthen some weak instruments [100].

In brief, Wilcoxon's statistic tends to exaggerate sensitivity to unmeasured biases; so, other statistics are preferable. It is not difficult to understand why this happens [206].

2.5 Summary: Biased Treatment Assignment

This chapter is intended to make the book self-contained. The chapter has discussed a few aspects of causal inference in observational studies that are relevant to later parts of the book. Two examples of sensitivity analyses were considered. The first concerned matched pairs. The second example combined strata and covariance adjustment. The design sensitivity and the Bahadur efficiency of a sensitivity analysis were briefly described.

---

[11]In R, the $(m, \underline{m}, \overline{m})$ statistic is implemented with examples in the senU function of the DOS2 package. The function provides the upper bound $\overline{P}$ on the P-value, together with a confidence interval and a point estimate. For Wilcoxon's statistic, use the senWilcox function in the same package.

2.6   Using R

2.6.1   The leadworker Example

Consider again the leadworker example in §2.2. The data are in the evident package, and the analysis uses functions from the DOS2 package associated with Ref. [206]. Under its default setting, the senWilcox function in the DOS2 package produces results for Wilcoxon's signed rank test similar to results produced by wilcox.test in the standard stats package.[12] However, senWilcox will also do a sensitivity analysis [185, 188, 195, 206] by setting the gamma parameter to be a number greater than 1.

```
library(evident)
library(DOS2)
data(leadworker)
attach(leadworker)
y<-dpc[group==1]-dpc[group==0]
senWilcox(y,conf.int=TRUE)
pval
[1] 0.0049
estimate
 low high
0.70 Inf
ci
 low high
0.30 Inf
```

These results are similar to results from wilcox.test:
```
wilcox.test(y,alternative = ''greater'' ,conf.int=T,
correct=FALSE).
```

```
Wilcoxon signed rank test with continuity correction
data: y
V = 62, p-value = 0.00489
alternative hypothesis: true location is greater than 0
95 percent confidence interval:
 0.2999315 Inf
sample estimates:
(pseudo)median
 0.7000666
```

The following calculations set the sensitivity parameter to $\Gamma = 2$. The maximum

---

[12]The functions senWilcox and wilcox.test handle zeros differently: wilcox.test removes zeros before ranks are computed, while senWilcox removes zeros after ranks are computed. In this example, no pair difference equals zero.

P-value testing the hypothesis of no effect is 0.0445 if the bias in treatment assignment is at most $\Gamma = 2$, the minimum point estimate of an additive effect is 0.50, and
the one-sided 95% confidence interval barely excludes zero.

```
senWilcox(y,gamma=2,conf.int=TRUE)
pval
[1] 0.0445
estimate
 low high
0.50 Inf
ci
 low high
0.00 Inf
```

2.6.2   The Homocysteine Example

The homocysteine and smoking data in §2.3 are in the evident package as hsmoke.
The analysis uses the senstrat package for stratified sensitivity analyses [221].
The analysis is done taking as the outcome residuals from a robust regression of
the base 2 logs of homocysteine levels when regressed on covariates, *without* the
treatment indicator [194]. So, the adjustment for covariates is done twice, once using
covariance adjustment, and a second time using strata. The covariance adjustment
is fit using Huber's m-estimation as implemented in the rlm function in the MASS
package. The calculations that follow reproduce two of the upper bounds on P-values
in Table 2.2, namely the 0.023 bound testing no effect in column $H_0 : \beta = 1$ for $\Gamma = 2.25$ and the 0.027 bound for $H_0 : \beta = 1.05$ for $\Gamma = 1.50$. In the case of $H_0 : \beta = 1.05$,
the hypothesized effect must be removed before covariance adjustment.

```
library(evident)
library(senstrat)
data(hsmoke)
attach(hsmoke)
l2h=log2(homocysteine)
```

Consider testing no effect or $H_0 : \beta = 1$ for $\Gamma = 2.25$ in Table 2.2.

```
mod=MASS::rlm(l2h~female+age+povertyr+bmi+education)
l2hr=mod$residual
madjr=senstrat::mscores(l2hr,z,st=st)
senstrat(madjr,z,st,gamma=2.25)$Result
P-value
   0.023
```

Now, consider testing $H_0 : \beta = 1.05$ for $\Gamma = 1.5$ in Table 2.2. Because l2h is the base 2 log of the homocysteine level, $\log_2(1.05)$ must be subtracted from these values for smokers, that is, individuals with $z_j = 1$.

```
adj=l2h-(log2(1.05)*z)
mod=MASS::rlm(adj~female+age+povertyr+bmi+education)
adjr=mod$esiduals
madjr=senstrat::mscores(adjr,z,st=st)
senstrat(madjr,z,st,gamma=1.5)$Result
P-value
   0.027
```

2.7   Exercises

Exercise 2.1. *Do a sensitivity analysis using the shinyapp at*

$$https://rosenbap.shinyapps.io/learnsenShiny/$$

that runs R in the background, requiring no knowledge of R.

Exercise 2.2. *Use Wilcoxon's signed rank statistic to perform a sensitivity analysis for the matched observational study in the* help *file for the* senWilcox *function in the R package DOS2.*

Exercise 2.3. *Repeat Exercise 2.1 in R using the* help *files for the* senm *and* senmCI *functions in the* sensitivitymult *package.*

Exercise 2.4. *Use the* mh *function in the* sensitivity2x2xk *package to perform sensitivity analyses for a 2×2 table and for a $2 \times 2 \times 2$ table. This* help *file for* mh *concerns the BRCA1 mutation and breast cancer risk. It is a simple example, but it illustrates several issues, including effect modification.*

Exercise 2.5. *If matched pair differences, Y_s, $s = 1, \ldots, S$, are independently drawn from a Normal distribution with expectation $\tau = 1/2$ and standard deviation 1, then the design sensitivity of Wilcoxon's signed rank test is $\widetilde{\Gamma} = 3.17$. Satisfy yourself that this is true by (i) using* rnorm *in R to sample a million observations from this distribution, and (ii) apply the* senWilcox *function in the DOS2 package to this sample, using* gamma=3.0 *and* gamma=3.3*. That is, perform two sensitivity analysis with Γ slightly below and slightly above the design sensitivity $\widetilde{\Gamma} = 3.17$. Using the same sample and the same values of Γ, replace Wilcoxon's test by the U-statistic [208] defined by $(8,7,8)$ in the* senU *function in the DOS2 package. (In that function, you must set* m=8, m1=7, m2=8.*)*

Exercise 2.6. *Continuing Exercise 2.5, check the claims about heterogeneity and causality in §2.4 and [200] as follows. Use* rnorm *in R to sample a quarter of a million observations from the Normal distribution with expectation $\tau = 1/2$ and standard deviation 1/2. Apply the* senWilcox *function in the DOS2 package to this sample, using* gamma=3.0, gamma=3.3, gamma=5 *and* gamma=10*. Repeat both exercises, but now with a sample size of 1000 for Exercise 2.5 and sample size 250 for the* *current exercise. Produce parallel boxplots of the two simulated samples. Finally, compare the conventional confidence intervals for τ based on the t-test for these two samples.*

Exercise 2.7. *Use the* `adaptmh` *function in the* `sensitivity2x2xk` *package [233] to perform adaptive sensitivity analyses for $2 \times 2 \times k$ tables, in which the data choose the test statistic. The* `help` *file for* `adaptmh` *illustrates adaptive inference in three simple observational studies.*

Exercise 2.8. *Use the* `tt` *function in the* `testtwice` *package [211] to perform adaptive sensitivity analyses for matched pairs, in which the data choose the test statistic. The* `help` *file for* `tt` *illustrates adaptive inference using the example from Ref. [211].*

Chapter 3

Replication and Its Limits

Abstract

Replication is an attempt to resolve the principal sources of uncertainty that linger from previous studies. There is little or no point in repeating a study if doing so reproduces the same uncertainty. Rather, a replication should eliminate or reduce or disrupt or at least vary a principal source of uncertainty. An example is given of a sequence of large observational studies that reproduced the same ambiguity, thereby failing to strengthen the evidence provided by the initial study in the sequence. Concerning the importance of variety in evidence, a brief review is given of the perspectives of a statistician, an epidemiologist, a mathematician and two philosophers. Several examples are given of replications of observational studies that successfully vary the evidence.

3.1 Biases Can Replicate

3.1.1 How Effective Is Treatment for Addiction?

Between 1969 and 2000, several large studies examined the effectiveness of treatments for addiction, primarily addiction to heroin, but also with some attention to cocaine. Between 1969 and 1972, the Drug Abuse Reporting Program (DARP) collected data about 44,000 people in 139 separate treatment programs funded by the US Federal Government. Between 1979 and 1981, the Treatment Outcomes Prospective Study (TOPS) collected data concerning 12,000 people in 41 treatment programs. In the 1990's, the Drug Abuse Treatment Outcome Studies (DATOS) collected data concerning 10,000 people in 96 treatment programs.[1] These data were analyzed by several investigators in the hope of shedding light on the effectiveness of programs to reduce addiction. For example, Hubbard and colleagues [114, p. 268] wrote:

> The general finding from DARP and TOPS that treatment duration of at least three months is associated statistically and clinically with more positive outcomes supports the inference of treatment effectiveness. The following analysis retests this hypothesis...

using DATOS, and reaching essentially the same conclusion. So, this is a claim of "treatment effectiveness" based on an observational comparison involving treatment

---

[1]http://www.datos.org/background.html#DARP

for at least three months. Moreover, the claim is that finding this same association in DARP, TOPS, and DATOS materially strengthens the conclusion that might have been reached from one study, say from the earliest using DARP.

How should we assess this claim?

3.1.2   An Assessment by the US National Academy of Sciences (NAS)

In 1999, Manski and colleagues [149] produced a report for the NAS assessing various studies based, in part, on DARP, DATOS, and TOPS. In particular, they wrote [149, pp. 17–18]:

> The RAND study compares the post-treatment average drug use of members of the TOPS sample who completed their treatment programs with ... drug use of TOPS subjects who began treatment but dropped out within 3 months .... Suppose, however, that treatment dropouts are more predisposed to drug use than are those who complete treatment. If dropouts are more severely addicted or less motivated or have fewer social supports than those who complete treatment, the observed differences in post-treatment drug use of dropouts and completers may reflect differences in characteristics of these two groups, not the effect of treatment programs. ... The people who complete their treatment program may be those who are more likely to reduce their drug use, whether or not they receive treatment. The true post-treatment effect may be smaller than estimated by RAND, or even zero.

Several aspects of this assessment deserve attention:

- The comment above is not about whether treatment is or is not effective; rather, it is about the strength of the evidence of effectiveness that is provided by comparing people who stay in treatment for at least three months and people who dropped out before three months. How strong is this evidence?

- The comment above raises an alternative explanation, besides a treatment effect, for the observed association between staying in treatment and having better outcomes. This alternative explanation does not involve sampling variability or a limited sample size: a small P-value, a large point estimate, a small standard error, and a short confidence interval are all beside the point. The alternative explanation accepts that the observed association is fairly strong and not attributable to chance. Rather, the alternative explanation speculates that a person intending to resume use of heroin might be inclined to drop out of a treatment program that monitors use of heroin. In contrast, a person determined to end an addiction might be more inclined to remain in treatment. The observed association between treatment effectiveness and duration of treatment could reflect an effect caused by treatment. However, it could alternatively reflect the decision by one person to exit treatment and resume use of heroin, and the decision by another person to tough it out and quit using heroin. The same pattern of observed associations is compatible with both explanations. The observed association is compatible with a treatment effect and no bias in treatment assignment, but it is also compatible with biased treatment assignment and no treatment effect.

- The rival explanations of an observed association between treatment and outcome are not addressed by seeing the same association in three studies of similar design. The same rival explanation is plausible each time, in DARP, TOPS, and DATOS.

If biases can replicate, is replication beside the point? Is there more to replication than repetition?

3.2 Some Perspectives

3.2.1 Addressing Uncertainty that Does Not Arise from Sampling Variability

In §3.1, the NAS report [149] emphasized uncertainty that did not arise from sampling variability, from a limited sample size.

How does one address uncertainty that does not arise from a limited sample size? Presumably, increasing the sample size will not help. Certain other things will not help either. The Pitman efficiency of one statistical procedure in comparison to another measures relative performance in terms of the ratio of the sample sizes needed to achieve the same standard error or power [140, §A.6]. Useful as that is in other contexts, if an increase in efficiency equates with an increase in sample size, presumably an increase in Pitman efficiency will not help either. A sensitivity analysis quantifies the magnitude of uncertainty from certain sources other than sampling variability; see Chapters 2 and 10, but it does not, by itself, reduce that uncertainty.[2]

What might we seek in a replication if the main worry is not sampling uncertainty? This section collects perspectives of a statistician, an epidemiologist, a mathematician and two philosophers.

3.2.2 A Statistician: William G. Cochran

In his survey of observational studies, Cochran [38, pp. 252–253] wrote:

> The combined evidence on a question that has to be decided mainly from observational studies will usually consist of a heterogeneous collection of results of varying quality, each bearing on some consequence of the causal hypothesis . . . [The investigator] cannot avoid an attempt to weigh the evidence for and against, since some results are so vulnerable to bias that they should be given low weight even if supported by routine tests of significance.

Note, in particular, the emphasis on a variety of consequences of the causal hypothesis, and the reluctance to take something seriously simply because a possibly biased P-value is small. Cochran continues [38, pp. 252–253]:

> [W]hen constructing a causal hypothesis one should envisage as many different consequences of its truth as possible, and plan observational studies to discover whether each of these consequences is found to hold. Of course, the number and variety of consequences depends on the nature of the causal hypothesis,

---

[2]In contrast, increasing the design sensitivity, $\tilde{\Gamma}$, and the Bahadur efficiency of a sensitivity analysis may reduce uncertainty from unmeasured biases; see §2.4 and Ref. [223, Part III].

but imaginative thinking will sometimes reveal consequences that were not at first realized, and this multi-phasic attack is one of the most potent weapons in observational studies. In particular, the task of deciding between alternative hypotheses is made easier since they may agree in predicting some consequences but will differ in others.

See also Ref. [216].

3.2.3   An Epidemiologist: Mervyn Susser

A similar emphasis on variety was expressed by Mervyn Susser:

> The epidemiologist [. . . seeks . . .] consistency of results in a variety of repeated tests. . . Consistency is present if the result is not dislodged in the face of diversity in times, places, circumstances, and people, as well as of research design [267, p. 148]. The strength of the argument rests on the fact that diverse approaches produce similar results [268, p. 88].

3.2.4   The Henle-Koch Postulates

Working in the late 1800's, Jacob Henle and Robert Koch were among the pioneers in the discovery that bacteria are the cause of many diseases [282, Chapter 12]. The famous Henle-Koch postulates constituted a list of varied evidence to be collected and checked in an effort to establish that a specific bacterium caused a specific disease [64, 65]. The list included the presence of the bacterium in naturally occurring cases of the disease, and the ability to isolate the bacterium and use it to induce disease in a healthy animal. New versions of the Henle-Koch postulates were proposed as new causes of disease were discovered [65], including viruses [182] and prions [281], as new technologies were developed [31], and with growing concern for chronic diseases [144, 302].

The Henle-Koch postulates are best viewed as endorsing consideration of varied evidence in general, rather than as an immutable set of rules. Rivers [182] wrote: "Thus, in regard to certain diseases, particularly those caused by viruses, the blind adherence to Koch's postulates may act as a hindrance instead of an aid." What is of enduring value in the Henle-Koch postulates is the thought that investigators benefit from a list of suggestions for varied evidence, suitable to a particular scientific context, at a particular state of scientific development. Yet, any such list is transient: open to criticism, amendment, evolution, obsolescence.

3.2.5   A Mathematician: George Polya

A mathematical proof is unaffected by sampling uncertainty. And yet, before a proof is known, there can be uncertainty about the truth or falsity of a conjecture. For example, in 1782, Euler conjectured that there is no Graeco-Latin square of order $4t + 2$ for $t = 0, 1, 2, 3, \ldots$, that is, no Graeco-Latin square of order 2, 6, 10, 14,.... Euler was a bit off: there is no Graeco-Latin square of order $4t + 2$ for $t = 0, 1$, but for $t \geq 2$, or for $4t + 2 \geq 10$, such a square exists, as was demonstrated in 1959 by Bose and Shrikhande [25] and Parker [169]; see also Ref. [76].

Mathematical heuristics refer to the kinds of reasoning that precede the existence of a proof. Between 1782 and 1959, anyone interested in Euler's conjecture was engaged in heuristics.

George Polya wrote several books and articles about heuristics; see, in particular Refs. [176, 177]. Polya uses Bayes' theorem and likelihood ratios qualitatively. He claims one situation provides stronger evidence than another because, if you filled in the numbers in Bayes' theorem that Polya left out, then Bayes' theorem would confirm the ordering that Polya asserts [176]. For example, Polya [176, p. 464] wrote:

> Our confidence in a theorem can only increase as a new consequence of the theorem is established. The increase in our confidence brought about by a new confirmation, or, if we wish, the inductive evidence furnished by this new confirmation, will vary inversely as the plausibility of the new consequence appraised in light of the previously verified consequences ... That consequence which, on the basis of the preceding verifications, stands the best chance of refuting the given theorem will disclose the strongest inductive evidence if it is confirmed in spite of forebodings ... this will be the case when this consequence has no immediate relation with the old ones, when it is removed from the preceding, when this new consequence is not only new, but of a new kind.

Polya, too, is emphasizing variety; however, he is sharpening the claim. The variety we seek is a new consequence that would be implausible were the theorem false, a consequence that is not rendered plausible by the previously verified consequences. In Ref. [177, p. 6], he writes:

> A circumstance which has a great influence on the strength of inductive evidence [is] the variety of the consequences tested. The verification of a new consequence counts more if the new consequence differs more from the formerly verified consequences.

When we do not yet have a proof, we nonetheless have reasons or grounds for suspecting that the conjecture is true. Polya [177, p. 20] writes: "Our confidence in a conjecture can only diminish when a possible ground for the conjecture is exploded." We may also have reasons or grounds for doubting that the conjecture is true, in which case [177, p. 20]: "Our confidence in a conjecture can only increase when an incompatible rival conjecture is exploded." So, Polya is saying that heuristic evidence, unlike proof, engages our reasons for suspecting the conjecture is true or false.

Dretske [58, pp. 20–22] makes a similar point about strengthening or weakening evidence for a conjecture indirectly by strengthening or weakening evidence for the reasons that support the conjecture:

> If Q is a reason for believing P true, then although P need not be true, Q must be. We can, and often do, give reasons — sometimes very good reasons — for believing something that is not true. ... Any challenge to the truth of Q is simultaneously a challenge to the acceptability of Q as a reason.

Staley [261] also discusses indirect strengthening of one conclusion by direct strengthening of claims that support that conclusion.

See Ref. [201] for an empirical evaluation of reasons for a treatment effect, in the context of the possible effects of gun buy-back programs on gun violence.

3.2.6   Two Philosophers: Wittgenstein and Haack

The Preface and §3.1 recalled the familiar fact that association does not, by itself, imply causation. Outside of a randomized experiment, an observed association between treatment received and outcome exhibited may reflect an effect caused by the treatment, or it may reflect bias in the assignment of treatments to unaffected individuals. Given this, ask: How can an observational study demonstrate that a treatment has an effect? How do we establish that we see an effect, not a bias, if an effect and a bias look the same in observable data?

Wittgenstein [292, #115] remarked: "A picture held us captive. And we could not get outside it, for it lay in our language and language seemed to repeat it to us inexorably."

What is this picture? It is the picture of proof, of demonstration, of settling the matter once and for all at the end of an empirical article. It is the picture of a headline in the newspaper: "New research demonstrates this or that." It is the picture in which scientific conclusions are settled on the day of publication. It is the picture that asks: "If the article isn't conclusive, why publish it? Surely, competent peer review should sort reports of observational studies into two piles, those that got it right, and those that got it wrong, and should reject those that got it wrong." Or, at least, that is the picture embedded in our language of demonstration and proof.

Philosophers loosen the grip of a picture by offering alternative pictures. The new pictures do not substitute for the old. Rather, the limitations of the first picture are revealed by the existence of alternative pictures that have alternative limitations.

Susan Haack [91, pp. 81–82] offers this picture:

> The model is not ... how one determines the soundness or otherwise of a mathematical proof; it is, rather, how one determines the reasonableness or otherwise of entries in a crossword puzzle ... [T]he crossword model permits pervasive mutual support, rather than, like the model of a mathematical proof, encouraging an essentially one-directional conception ... The clues are the analogues of the subject's experiential evidence; already filled in entries, the analogues of his reasons. The clues don't depend upon the entries, but the entries are, in variable degrees, interdependent ... How reasonable one's confidence is that a certain entry in a crossword is correct depends on: how much support is given to this entry by the clue and any intersecting entries that have already been filled in; how reasonable, independently of the entry in question, one's confidence is that those other already filled-in entries are correct; and how many of the intersecting entries have been filled in.

Haack is making several points best understood by considering a puzzle, say the one in Figure 3.1. There, 1-across is "1970s rubber burning transport" in eight

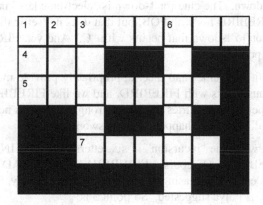

Across

1. 1970s rubber burning transport

4. Dug up

5. Bonkers

7. Of warships

Down

1. Electronic key

2. Anger

3. Seen before

6. Incursion

Figure 3.1 *A crossword puzzle.*

letters. It isn't a MUSTANG, with seven letters, but it might be a CORVETTE or a FIREBIRD or perhaps something else. So point 1 is:

1. The individual clues—the data—do not identify the individual entries. The clue for 1-across is compatible with at least two very different entries for 1-across. Repeated reexamination of the clue for 1-across will not settle the matter.

So, we look at 1-down. The clue for 1-down is "electronic key" in three letters, perhaps a "FOB." FIREBIRD fits with FOB, but that does not settle the matter: perhaps there is a solution to 1-down that begins with "C." And yet, FIREBIRD-FOB looks promising. So point 2 is:

2. Two entries that fit their clues and meet appropriately provide mutual support. We like FOB because it fits with FIREBIRD, and we like FIREBIRD because it fits with FOB, although both entries might be wrong. That does not happen in a mathematical proof, but it does happen in a crossword puzzle.

Consider 6-down with clue "incursion" in six letters. Perhaps, INROAD. That again fits with FIREBIRD. Of course, FIREBIRD-FOB-INROAD could all be wrong, yet our confidence is increasing as more and more unlikely, unrelated predictions turn out true, as Polya suggested. So point 3 is:

3. The clues do not identify the entries, and that is not going to change, but in an odd way, the lack of identification is getting smaller as more entries fit together.

Let's try 5-across, with clue "bonkers," in seven letters. BERSERK fits the space and meets FOB and INROAD appropriately. This leads to point 4:

4: Coherence and mutual support lack sharp boundaries. BERSERK and FIRE-BIRD do not intersect, yet provide mutual support, because they each intersect FOB and INROAD appropriately.

We could have made a mistake. Why not? People do crossword puzzles in pencil for a reason. So let us review the evidence. It feels uncomfortable that we trust FOB because it meets FIREBIRD appropriately, and we trust FIREBIRD because it meets FOB appropriately. If the only evidence we had for FOB is that it meets FIREBIRD appropriately, and the only evidence we had for FIREBIRD is that it meets FOB appropriately, then we would not have much evidence. So, let us demarcate the evidence. Let us ask: What evidence do we have for FIREBIRD that does not involve FOB? The clue for 1-across fits FIREBIRD, and FIREBIRD intersects INROAD appropriately, and INROAD intersects BERSERK appropriately, and the clues for 6-down and 5-across do fit with INROAD and BERSERK. So, the evidence for FIREBIRD is extensive, if still inconclusive, without relying on FOB. And similarly, the evidence for FOB is extensive, without relying on FIREBIRD. This leads to point 5:

5. We can, perhaps should, set aside—demarcate—parts of the evidence provided by mutual support, setting aside one or more entries to examine the strength of the evidence that remains.

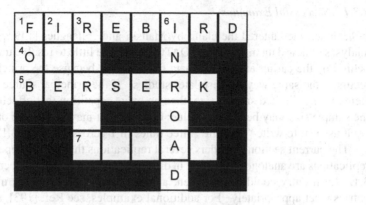

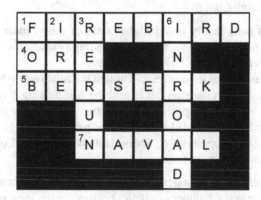

Figure 3.2 *A crossword puzzle.*

Figure 3.2 completes the puzzle. Perhaps someone more clever than I could construct one substantial crossword that could be completed in two incompatible ways that fit the same clues. It is not inconceivable that Figure 3.2 could be filled in differently, yet appropriately, but the possibility seems remote. At what moment in filling in the puzzle did we become all but certain of FIREBIRD? Was there such a moment? Wittgenstein [293, #141]: "Light dawns gradually over the whole."

3.3 Replications that Disrupt Some Potential Biases

3.3.1 Successful Examples

In §3.1, we encountered the claim by Manski and colleagues [149, pp. 17–18] that analyses of new data in TOPS and DATOS had done little to resolve uncertainties left behind by the earlier analyses of data from DARP, because the principal ambiguity recurs in the same way in these later studies. If the principal source of uncertainty stems from a limited sample size, then an exact repetition that effectively increases the sample size may be of great value; otherwise, it may be of little or no value. Of what use is it to write "Corvette" three times in 1-across in Figure 3.1?

The current section considers several replications that are not repetitions. These replications are analogous to filling in different, perhaps intersecting entries in Figure 3.1. Each entry could be mistaken, and yet conviction grows as more and more entries meet appropriately. For additional examples, see Ref. [193], and for related discussion, see Refs. [24, 98, 119, 135, 161, 168].

3.3.2 Smoking and Lung Cancer

Observational studies consistently found higher rates of lung cancer among heavy smokers than among nonsmokers [57, 94]. This finding is insensitive to quite large biases in who chooses to smoke [46, 47].

Most smokers do not die of lung cancer. Though the relationship between heavy smoking and lung cancer is quite strong, it is nothing like flicking a switch and seeing a light come on. Are there aspects of the relationship that resemble flicking a switch? Auerbach and colleagues [8] examined for pathology the lung tissue from 402 autopsies, including autopsies of 63 individuals who had died of lung cancer. They summarized their findings as follows:

> From the standpoint of carcinogenesis, what impressed us most was the tremendous increase in the number of atypical cells with the increased amount of smoking. The number of sections of atypical cells in the bronchial epithelium of heavy smokers who died of diseases other than lung cancer approximated the number of sections of atypical cells in the remaining bronchial epithelium of men who died of lung cancer. ... In our opinion the histologic evidence from this study greatly strengthens the already overwhelming body of epidemiologic evidence that cigarette smoking is a major factor in the causation of bronchogenic carcinoma. [8, p. 267]

Though many heavy smokers die of cardiovascular diseases, other cancers, accidents, and so on, the vast majority have lungs that exhibit cellular pathology of the kinds that pathologists believe to be precursors to cancer. An older heavy smoker who dies in a car accident is quite unlikely to have healthy lungs.

Traditionally, women were much less likely than men to smoke cigarettes, but in the 1960s, the tobacco industry sought to change that with products and marketing campaigns aimed at women. For instance, beginning in 1967, the Virginia Slims brand was marketed under the slogan "You've come a long way baby," with ads that showed independently minded, slender, glamorous women smoking cigarettes in defiance of tradition. Thirty years later, in 1997, Bailar and Gornik [10, p. 1571] wrote: "For lung cancer, death rates for women 55 or older have increased to almost four times the 1970 rate," but rates for males over 55, and rates for other cancer sites, show no such dramatic change. An induced change in smoking behavior among women was followed, after an appropriate interval of time, by higher rates of lung cancer among women.

The three patterns just noted are all compatible with one explanation, namely that smoking causes lung cancer. The three patterns are also compatible with selection bias, but it would take three very different selection biases acting in concert to misleadingly produce what appears to be an effect caused by smoking.

3.3.3 Minimum Wages and Employment

Card and Krueger [34] asked about the possible effect of increasing the minimum wage on the employment of individuals who receive that wage. They looked at four fast-food restaurant chains, such as Burger King, before and after the US state of New Jersey increased its minimum wage by almost 20%, from \$4.25 to \$5.05 per hour, on 1 April 1992. They compared the change in employment in New Jersey to the change in employment in adjacent Pennsylvania, where the minimum wage remained at the US Federal minimum wage. Amid much controversy, they found no indication that an increase in the minimum wage depressed employment. Their data will be examined in greater detail in §4.4 and §6.2.

A basic concern is that New Jersey opted to increase its minimum wage, while Pennsylvania declined to do so. Perhaps there were good reasons these states, and other states, handle the minimum wage in the way they do. Perhaps New Jersey was more worried about wages than about full employment, perhaps because unemployment was under control, and perhaps the situation in Pennsylvania was different despite its proximity to New Jersey. Perhaps states exceed the Federal minimum wage only when they anticipate little harm as a result. New Jersey and Pennsylvania chose their treatments, and perhaps latitude to choose a treatment always creates a biased comparison. Perhaps we should worry that every nonrandomized treatment misleadingly appears to be more effective than it is, because rational agents always select for themselves the course of action that will be of greatest benefit to them.[3]

A few years later, on 1 October 1996, the US Federal minimum wage was increased from \$4.25 to \$4.75. This forced a reluctant Pennsylvania to increase minimum wages, but made no demands on New Jersey as its state minimum of \$5.05 was higher than the new Federal minimum wage. The issue of treatment choice is now reversed. So, Card and Krueger [35, II.A] replicated their own study, again finding no indication of depressed employment following the wage increase. Card and Krueger found similar results, whether a state chose to increase its minimum wage or was forced to do so.

For various perspectives and studies, see Refs. [32, §3] and [1, 163].

---

[3]This worry is sometimes expressed in economics. However, recall from §3.1, the alternative worry that individuals most in need of assistance in ending their addictions were those least likely to accept assistance. For yet another possibility, see Ref. [33].

3.3.4   The Effect of Advertising on Prices

Does advertising create price competition that reduces prices? This is a difficult question to answer, because it entails observing similar situations with and without advertising.

On 13 May 1996, the US Supreme Court struck down Rhode Island's ban on the advertising of liquor prices. Milyo and Waldfogel [158] compared liquor prices in Rhode Island before and after the Supreme Court decision. They also compared Rhode Island to adjacent parts of Massachusetts, where it was legal to advertise prices before and after the court action.

Between 10 August 1978 and 5 October 1978, a strike closed three of New York City's major newspapers, eliminating that era's main source of advertising of food prices. The main newspaper, Newsday, in the adjacent suburb of Nassau county was unaffected by the strike. Glazer [83] compared changes in food prices in New York City and Nassau County to assess the effect of advertising on prices.

These two comparisons each face the problems observational studies commonly face. And yet, the biases that might attend a Supreme Court decision have no obvious reason to align with the biases that might attend a newspaper strike.

3.4   Instruments and Replication

3.4.1   What Is an Instrument?

An instrument is a haphazard push to receive one treatment or another, in which the push affects the outcome only if it alters the treatment received [4].

The most basic example of an instrument is a placebo-controlled randomized trial with imperfect compliance. In this case, the instrument, randomization, is not merely haphazard: it is truly random, statistically independent of every pretreatment attribute of the individuals under study. Because compliance is imperfect, randomization pushes individuals towards treatment or control, but does not completely determine the dose of the treatment received. Because there is a placebo, individuals do not know whether they received treatment or control, so the hidden random assignment can only affect outcomes indirectly by altering the consumed dose of the active treatment.

For instance, the "ACE-Inhibitor After Anthracycline" (AAA) study tried to preserve cardiac function of children who had received anthracyclines as a treatment for cancer [256]. The children were randomized to either an active drug, enalapril, or to placebo. Perhaps because enalapril was taken for several years to prevent future symptoms, there was some noncompliance: some children took less than the prescribed dose of enalapril or placebo. A comparison of the groups randomly assigned to enalapril or placebo is straightforward—this is the so-called intent-to-treat analysis—but it estimates the effects of being encouraged to take a medication, rather than the effects of actually taking the prescribed dose. There is, however, a randomization inference for the effect at full dose [88], formed by attributing the intent-to-treat effect to compliers [4].

Angrist, Imbens, and Rubin [4] used the Vietnam era draft lottery as an instrument for military service in a study of the effects of military service on mortality. The draft lottery was essentially randomized, but it did not determine military service, because some people volunteered without being drafted, and others found ways to evade the draft. So, their study resembles a randomized trial with imperfect compliance.

Most instruments are less compelling than a lottery or randomization with noncompliance. The typical instrument may itself be biased.

3.4.2 Different Instruments May Be Biased in Different Ways

For some treatments, the bias is almost inevitably in the same direction. Disrupting the bias in a replication may be impossible.

For instance, it is of interest to know the effects of, say, a college education on income, but the biases in a straightforward comparison are almost inevitably in the same direction. A college education may affect income, but it is also true that young adults who go to college typically have parents with more income, more education, and a greater concern with education; moreover, these young adults typically have done well in high school and have personal qualities that allow them to succeed in school, possibly ambition, self-discipline, and intelligence. It is difficult to imagine a study that adequately measures and controls for all of these attributes. Observing higher incomes among those with a college education leaves us in doubt about the effect caused by education, as distinct from the many attributes that get a young person into and through college.

In this context, Imbens and I wrote [118, §1.1]:

> Compare two sequences of studies of the same self-inflicted treatment: one sequence without instruments comparing treated with untreated; the other sequence using a variety of different instruments to manipulate the treatment. Throughout the first sequence, the comparison is likely to be biased in the same way. A repeated finding that people with more education earn more than people with less education does little to isolate the effects that are caused by education from the consequences of unmeasured ambition, perseverance and talent that led to extended education—the same bias appears repeatedly. However, if different instruments are used to manipulate education—a lottery, a temporal discontinuity in educational policy or a regional discontinuity in educational policy—and if each instrument is plausible but not certain, there may be no reason why these different instruments should be biased in the same direction. In replicating observational studies, the goal is to replicate whatever treatment effects may exist without replicating whatever biases may coexist [193], and this goal is sometimes achievable by using a variety of instruments ... subject to different biases.

Use of evidence factors with instruments is discussed in Ref. [127]. There, two instruments and a direct comparison of treated and control groups yields three evidence factors.

3.5   Summary: Replication Is Not Repetition

This chapter has separated replication from repetition, making the following specific points.

1. Replication, if it is to be of service, should eliminate, or address, or attempt to disrupt one of the principal sources of uncertainty that linger from previous studies.

2. If the sole source of uncertainty is a limited sample size, then an exact replication that increases the effective sample size will be what is needed. This is an uncommon situation in an observational study because, more or less by definition, an observational study faces uncertainty about biases that arise when treatments are not assigned at random to individuals.

3. If the competence, honesty, and objectivity of the original investigators is the principal source of uncertainty, then a replication that is exact but for replacing the investigators may be useful. Alas, this situation is not as uncommon as one might wish.

4. In the typical situation in an observational study, the principal source of uncertainty stems from the absence of random assignment; that is, from the nearly inevitable possibility that adjustments for measured covariates may have failed to render comparable the treatment groups being compared. This is a substantial source of uncertainty even if the sample size is large and the investigators are competent, honest and objective. In this case, it is of little or no value to repeat a study so that the principal sources of uncertainty recur in their original forms; see §3.1.

5. In replicating an observational study, one seeks to remove or disrupt or at least vary some source of potential bias, to determine whether the ostensible effects of the treatment reappear or vanish.

6. Despite lack of identification, conviction grows that a treatment did cause its ostensible effects if widely varied sources of evidence are readily explained by a causal effect, but difficult to explain in any other way; see §3.2–§3.3 and Ref. [193].

A question arises if replication is not repetition. Can a single observational study replicate itself? Can it provide varied and essentially independent evidence, evidence that becomes more difficult to attribute to bias because of its variety? Can a single study carry out two very different analyses that can be combined as if they came from two unrelated studies? Can we measure and quantify the resulting strengthening of the evidence for an effect and against a bias? These are the questions addressed in the remainder of this book.

Part II

Evidence Factors in Practice

Chapter 4

Examples of Studies with Evidence Factors

Abstract

This chapter takes a first look at several examples of observational studies with two or more evidence factors. The studies vary in structure, yet share certain elements. In each example, treatment assignment has two or more aspects. One might conduct an analysis based on the first aspect, ignoring the second aspect. Alternatively, one might fix the first aspect and ask what is added by the second aspect. Later chapters will return to these examples. There are three goals: (i) to make the subject tangible with reference to particular empirical studies, (ii) to sketch in informal terms certain technical results developed in later chapters, and (iii) to provide some informal intuition in support of the technical results in later chapters.

4.1 Smoking and Periodontal Disease

4.1.1 Treatment/Control Pairs, with Doses Varying Among Pairs

Cigarette smoking is believed to cause periodontal disease [271]. Figure 4.1 depicts 441 pairs of a daily cigarette smoker and a never-smoker from the 2011–2012 National Health and Nutrition Examination Survey (NHANES) [219, 220]. A daily smoker is a person who has smoked every day for the past 30 days. On average, daily smokers have smoked for 30 years, and 90% began smoking more than 14.9 years ago. To be a never-smoker, a person cannot have smoked 100 cigarettes in his or her life, must not smoke now, and must have no tobacco exposure in the previous five days. Smokers and nonsmoking controls were matched for age, income, education, sex, and black race, and Figure 4.1 depicts the three continuous covariates.

As in Ref. [271], periodontal disease is assessed at six locations on each of 28 teeth, if present, and a location is diseased if there is evidence of a separation of tooth and gums at that location, specifically either a loss of attachment of ≥ 4 mm or a pocket depth of ≥ 4 mm. The outcome is the percent of locations judged diseased, 0% to 100%.

Figure 4.2 depicts the 441 smoker-minus-control pair differences in periodontal disease, -100% to 100%. In panel (a) of Figure 4.2, there is a boxplot of the 441 pair differences, and these tend to be positive, indicating typically more extensive

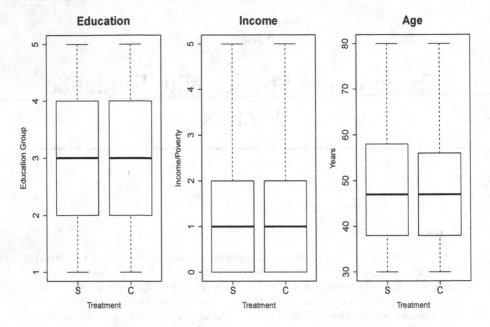

Figure 4.1 *Daily smokers (S) and never-smoking controls (C) in 441 pairs matched for age, income, education, sex, and black race. Education is scored 1 for less than 9th grade, 2 for no high school degree, 3 for high school or equivalent, 4 for some college, 5 for at least a BA degree. Income is the ratio of family income to the poverty level, capped at 5 times the poverty level.*

periodontal disease for the smoker in the pair. In panel (b) of Figure 4.2, the same 441 pair differences are plotted against the number of cigarettes smoked by the smoker in each pair. For brevity, refer to the number of cigarettes smoked by the smoker in a pair as the "dose." Figure 4.2(b) includes a lowess smooth indicative of the general trend [37]. In pairs in which the smoker smoked more cigarettes, the smoker-minus-control difference in periodontal disease is larger.

In brief, there are two patterns consistent with an effect of smoking on periodontal disease: (a) more extensive disease among smokers than nonsmokers, (b) a larger difference between smokers and nonsmokers when the smoker smokes more.[1]

Recall that Wilcoxon's signed rank statistic takes the 441 pair differences in Figure 4.2(a), ranks their absolute values from 1 to 441, with average ranks for ties, and sums the ranks of the positive differences [110, 140, 288]. The statistic tends to be large, suggesting a positive effect, when positive differences outnumber negative differences, and when large positive differences occur more often than large negative differences. In randomized experiments, Wilcoxon's test is a close second to the optimal t-test when the pair differences are sampled from a Normal distribution, but Wilcoxon's test is much better—has higher power—than the t-test when the pair

---

[1]The data are available in the evident package in R as periodontal.

differences come from a distribution with longer tails than the Normal. Computing Wilcoxon's signed rank statistic from Figure 4.2(a) and comparing it to its randomization distribution in a paired randomized experiment, we obtain a one-sided P-value of $\leq 2.2 \times 10^{-16}$ testing no effect, and a one-sided 95% confidence interval for an additive effect of $\geq 10.7\%$.

Kendall's rank correlation statistic [110, 140] looks at the $441 \times 440/2$ pairs of two points in Figure 4.2(b): the test statistic is the number of positive slopes between two points minus the number of negative slopes between two points. Computing Kendall's rank correlation in Figure 4.2(b) and comparing it to its randomization distribution in an experiment that randomly assigned doses of cigarette smoking to pairs, we obtain a one-sided P-value of 0.0064 testing no effect. The patterns in Figure 4.2 are not easily dismissed as due to chance. Neither Wilcoxon's statistic nor Kendall's statistic is the best test to use in an observational study, and other tests will be considered later.

Had doses of cigarettes been randomly assigned to pairs, and one individual in each pair picked at random to be the smoker, then Wilcoxon's signed rank statistic and Kendall's statistic would be independent in the absence of a treatment effect [207]. It is as if the two P-values came from two separate studies, of different data, by different investigative teams, even though the two P-values were produced by analyzing the same data twice. As a consequence, the two P-values, from Wilcoxon's test and Kendall's test, may be combined using meta-analytic techniques originally intended to combine results from unrelated studies. The exact independence of the Wilcoxon and Kendall tests is a somewhat specialized property of certain rank tests, but the property needed for meta-analytic combination is weaker than independence and is applicable with a wide variety of tests; see Chapter 7 and in particular Definition 2.

Of course, we are not entitled to the two P-values just quoted. Those P-values would be appropriate if randomization had been used to pick the smoker in each pair in Figure 4.2(a) and had been used to assign doses to pairs in Figure 4.2(b), and neither randomization took place. It seems quite possible that smokers, by virtue of smoking, express less concern for their health than do nonsmokers, and that might manifest itself in a wide variety of health-related behaviors, perhaps reduced brushing or flossing of teeth, or fewer visits to the dentist. Perhaps smokers do have more periodontal disease than nonsmokers, but perhaps that is not an effect caused by smoking.

Because we are not entitled to the two P-values just quoted, we conduct two sensitivity analyses, one for Figure 4.2(a), the other for Figure 4.2(b). With some attention to detail, these two sensitivity analyses for the two factors, Figure 4.2(a) and Figure 4.2(b), may be combined by meta-analytic techniques, as if they came from unrelated studies; see Chapter 11 and in particular Theorem 9. The combined sensitivity analysis employs precisely the assumptions already present in the separate sensitivity analyses, but no additional assumptions are made when combining them. If the separate sensitivity analyses are valid, so is the joint analysis. As we will see, a joint sensitivity analysis for Figure 4.2(a) and Figure 4.2(b) reports greater insensitivity to unmeasured bias than does either of its components: the joint analysis

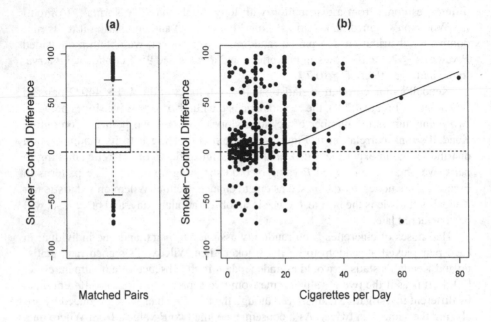

Figure 4.2 *Smoker-minus-control matched-pair differences in periodontal disease. (a) Boxplot of the 441 pair differences. (b) Pair differences plotted against the amount smoked by the smoker. The solid line is a lowess smooth.*

provides measurably stronger evidence that Figure 4.2(a) and Figure 4.2(b) reflect an effect caused by smoking, not a bias in treatment assignment. Equally important, the combination will entertain the possibility that either factor faces infinite bias, that either Figure 4.2(a) or Figure 4.2(b) is infinitely biased in its treatment assignments, asking what evidence remains from the other factor.

4.1.2   Building Intuition: Two Factors, Not Two Tests with the Same Factor

Two analyses of Figure 4.2(a) would not produce two evidence factors. If we did two tests of no effect versus harm from smoking in the boxplot in Figure 4.2(a), then those two tests would be strongly dependent, highly correlated, and they could not be combined as if they came from independent studies. By and large, those two tests would repeat the same information twice, wasting space in a journal article. For example, in Figure 4.2(a), the Wilcoxon test and the paired t-test repeat much of the same information, and so they could not be combined using meta-analytic techniques, as if they came from different studies. Both the Wilcoxon test and the paired t-test take note of the pattern in Figure 4.2(a) that smoker-minus-control differences in periodontal disease tend to be positive, and both yield small P-values because of that pattern. However, this is the same evidence repeated twice, not new evidence.

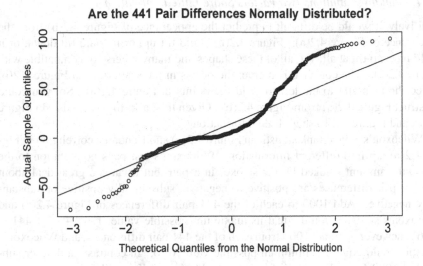

Figure 4.3 *Normal quantile plot of the 441 pair differences in periodontal disease. For data from a Normal distribution, the points should fall approximately along a straight line, but this is not true here. Based on the departure from a straight line, the Shapiro-Wilk test [255] rejects the null hypothesis that the data are from a Normal distribution with a P-value of* 3.1×10^{-16}.

4.1.3   Building intuition: One Good Statistic for Each Factor

Is there any reason to do both the Wilcoxon signed rank test and the paired t-test? Arguably, there is good reason to do neither test. Wilcoxon's signed rank test is not a good test to use in a sensitivity analysis in an observational study: compared to some other tests, including rank tests, Wilcoxon's test has inferior design sensitivity and Bahadur efficiency; see §2.4 and Refs. [206, 208, 215]. That is, Wilcoxon's test tends to suggest an observational study is sensitive to smaller unmeasured biases than is actually the case. In Figure 4.2(a), the t-test would not be a good choice of test statistic even in a randomized experiment, because the assumptions that would make the t-test an efficient test in a randomized experiment are obviously false in Figure 4.2(a). This is evident in the Normal quantile plot in Figure 4.3: it clearly indicates that the 441 pair differences are not from a Normal distribution. This is further confirmed by the Shapiro-Wilk [255] test of Normality: it rejects the null hypothesis that 441 pair differences were sampled from a Normal distribution with a P-value of 3.1×10^{-16}. This chapter serves to introduce evidence factors, and it makes reference to conventional test statistics—Wilcoxon's test, Kendall's test, and the t-test—which might be used with evidence factors. Later chapters select more appropriate test statistics, whether familiar or not. We should apply to each evidence factor one appropriate test; we should not express our confusion about what makes a test appropriate by reporting the same information again and again with varied test statistics.

4.1.4   Building Intuition: Two Factors Share Little Information

Intuitively, it would be difficult to predict the appearance of Figure 4.2(b) from the appearance of Figure 4.2(a). Figure 4.2(b) could tilt up, or it could tilt down, or it could have no tilt at all; yet, all of these shapes and many others are compatible with Figure 4.2(a). The converse is untrue: the points in the scatterplot in Figure 4.2(b) project horizontally to the left to yield the points in Figure 4.2(a). So, you could construct Figure 4.2(a) from Figure 4.2(b). Given this, ask: In what sense do Figure 4.2(a) and Figure 4.2(b) share little information?

Wilcoxon's signed rank statistic in Figure 4.2(a) and Kendall's correlation in Figure 4.2(b) tap into different information. Wilcoxon's test pays no attention to the doses, the amount smoked by the smoker in a pair, but it cares a great deal about whether pair differences are positive or negative, substantially positive or substantially negative. Add 1000 to each of the 441 pair differences in Figure 4.2(a) and Wilcoxon's statistic would equal its maximum possible value, $1 + 2 + \cdots + 441 = 97461$; however, subtract 1000 from each of the 441 pair differences, and Wilcoxon's statistic would equal its minimum possible value of 0. In contrast, adding or subtracting 1000 from the pair differences would change Kendall's correlation not at all. Kendall's correlation cares whether the pair differences are ordered in the same way as the doses, not whether the pair differences are positive. Indeed, if Fisher's hypothesis of no effect were true in an experiment that randomized both doses and smoker/control, then Wilcoxon's statistic and Kendall's statistic would be independent.[2] In that rather specific sense, Wilcoxon's statistic and Kendall's statistic share no information.

Suppose that we replaced Wilcoxon's signed rank statistic and Kendall's correlation by the mean of the pair differences and the Pearson's correlation of pair differences with doses. Again, suppose Fisher's hypothesis of no effect is true, that 441 doses are randomly assigned to pairs, and independently smoker/control is randomly assigned to individuals within each of the 441 pairs. Given the 441 pair differences, Pearson's correlation has expectation zero, because doses are permuted at random; so Pearson's correlation has expectation zero given any function of the 441 pair differences, and hence is uncorrelated with any function of the pair differences, including their mean. However, sign changes among the 441 pair differences affect the shape of the distribution of differences—the shape of the boxplot in Figure 4.2(a)—and thereby can affect the distribution of Pearson's correlation: uncorrelated statistics may be dependent; see Refs. [106, 109, 179, 295] for various arguments of this general form. If a bivariate central limit theorem applied to the joint distribution of the mean and Pearson's correlation, then zero correlation in the finite sample bivariate distributions would entail independence of the asymptotic joint distribution. This is a different sense in which the mean in Figure 4.2(a) and Pearson's correlation in Figure 4.2(b) share little information.

A better approach to saying that Figures 4.2(a) and 4.2(b) share little information is through Theorem 9 in Chapter 11: it requires *none* of the following: (i) random assignment of doses to pairs, (ii) random assignment of smoker/control within pairs,

---

[2]Strictly speaking, this claim requires the additional assumption that the data are free of ties.

(iii) large samples, (iv) a central limit theorem for the joint distribution of two statistics.

4.2 Antineoplastic Drugs and DNA Damage

4.2.1 Background

There is concern that antineoplastic drugs—cancer chemotherapies—may cause genetic damage to health professionals who prepare or administer them to patients. Kopjar and Garaj-Vrhovac [131] compared hospital workers who handle antineoplastic drugs to unexposed controls using a measure of DNA damage, the comet assay [43, 259]. The comet assay is so-called because the assay produces an image resembling the tail of a comet, the magnitude of the tail being taken as a measure of the extent of DNA damage. In the comet assay, DNA from cells in a blood sample is placed in an electrically charged field that does little to move large intact strands of DNA, but pulls broken strands into an elongated pattern, the comet's tail. The outcome used here is the tail moment of the comet assay, where larger values signify greater damage.

In Ref. [131], there were three groups with at least 19 individuals, and a few much smaller groups; so, the analysis here focuses on the three groups that were not small. These three larger groups are: 20 unexposed controls comprised of students and office workers, 20 exposed individuals who were protected only by latex gloves, and 19 exposed individuals who were protected by both latex gloves and a safety cabinet with vertical air-flow. A worker stands or sits with gloved hands inside the cabinet but head outside the cabinet, as a vertical flow of air draws fumes into the hood, away from the face. Most of the health professionals were nurses, but a few were physicians.

Figure 4.4 depicts the level of DNA damage, with the $59 = 20 + 20 + 19$ individuals grouped in various ways.[3] Factor 1 compares exposed and control groups, ignoring the issue of a ventilated hood. Factor 2 focuses on exposed workers, distinguishing workers with both gloves and a ventilated hood from workers with gloves alone.

This might be a good moment to review the subsection of §1.1 that discussed how a randomized trial with three groups contains two trials with two groups. That situation has parallels in factors 1 and 2 in Figure 4.4.

4.2.2 Two Factors

Health professionals are potentially exposed to a variety of biochemically active substances besides antineoplastic drugs, such as other drugs, anesthetic agents, antiseptics, and diagnostic radiation, so the comparison labeled factor 1 in Figure 4.4 may not isolate the effects of antineoplastic drugs. Factor 2 in Figure 4.4 compares two groups of health professionals handling antineoplastic drugs, but it depends upon the

---

[3]The data are available in the `evident` package in R as `antineoplastic`.

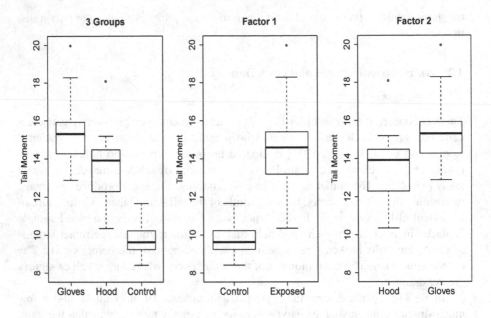

Figure 4.4 *DNA damage in workers exposed to antineoplastic drugs and unexposed controls. Workers are subdivided into those who were protected by latex gloves and those protected by both latex gloves and a safety cabinet with a laminar hood.*

premise that the laminar hood substantially decreases exposure to the drugs. Additionally, hospitals that provide their staff with better safety equipment for handling antineoplastic drugs may protect their staff in other ways as well, say providing better protection from diagnostic radiation. So the two comparisons, factors 1 and 2 in Figure 4.4 may each be biased, though the biases appear to have different origins. It is, therefore, informative that both comparisons find reduced levels of DNA damage associated with reduced exposure to antineoplastic drugs.

For factor 1 in Figure 4.4, if Wilcoxon's rank sum statistic is computed and compared to its randomization distribution, then the one-sided P-value testing no effect is 7.85×10^{-10}, and the one-sided 95% confidence interval for a shift is $\tau \geq 4.0$. For factor 2 in Figure 4.4, if Wilcoxon's rank sum statistic is computed and compared to its randomization distribution, then the one-sided P-value testing no effect is 0.0007132 with 95% confidence interval for a shift of $\tau' \geq 0.88$. Of course, we are not entitled to these inferences, because randomization was used in neither factor.

4.2.3   Building Intuition: The Two Factors Share Little Information

Two analyses by different methods of the typical level of DNA damage in factor 1 in Figure 4.4 would largely repeat the same information twice, and would therefore waste space in a scientific journal. This is not true of two analyses, one of factor 1, the other of factor 2. In parallel with §4.1 whose structure is quite different, factors 1 and 2 in Figure 4.4 share little information. Can this be understood with greater precision?

Consider, first, the simplest possible case, three treatment groups, A, B, and C, each containing one individual. The three individuals, 1, 2, and 3, are randomly assigned to groups. There are $3! = 3 \times 2 \times 1 = 6$ ways to permute the three individuals to assign them to the treatment groups, and each permutation has probability $1/6$ in this randomized experiment. Suppose the three individuals have outcomes $y_1 = 15.34$, $y_2 = 18.28$ and $y_3 = 13.18$, which are actual values from Ref. [131, Table 1]. Fisher's hypothesis of no effect is true, so randomization moves individuals from one treatment group to another, but their outcomes do not change. (If the outcomes changed, then Fisher's hypothesis would be false, and the treatment would have some effect.)

The Wilcoxon rank sum statistic, W_A, for group A compared to the combination of groups B and C is the rank of y_j for the individual j assigned to treatment A. That is equally likely to be the rank of y_1 or y_2 or y_3, so it is equally likely to be 2, 3, or 1. So, $\Pr(W_A = k) = 1/3$ for $k = 1, 2, 3$. In the same way, the Wilcoxon statistic, W_B, comparing group B to group C takes the value 1 or 2, depending upon whether the individual assigned to group B has a lower or a higher response than the individual assigned to group C, so $\Pr(W_B = k) = 1/2$ for $k = 1, 2$. Much more important than these two marginal distributions of W_A and W_B is the observation that W_A and W_B are independent in a randomized experiment in which Fisher's hypothesis is true. It is easy to see this. No matter who is picked for group A, the conditional distribution of W_B is the same, namely $\Pr(W_B = k) = 1/2$ for $k = 1, 2$, so the conditional distribution of W_B does not depend upon who is picked for A, and so does not depend upon W_A. This is the simplest instance of a very old result due to Alfred Renyi about partial ranks, nicely described by Alam [3] and Resnick [181, §4.3.1].

A little more thought yields the same conclusion when the three treatment groups, A, B, and C, are larger, with sample sizes $m_A \geq 1$, $m_B \geq 1$ and $m_C \geq 1$. Suppose that Fisher's hypothesis of no effect is true, and that $N = m_A + m_B + m_C$ individuals are randomly divided into groups A, B, and C of sizes m_A, m_B and m_C. Then, Wilcoxon's rank sum statistic W_A for group A compared to the combination of groups B and C is independent of Wilcoxon's rank sum statistic W_B comparing group B to group C.[4] Intuitively, no matter which m_A individuals are picked for treatment group A, the distribution of W_B is the same: it is the distribution of the total of m_B numbers picked at random without replacement from $1, 2, \ldots, m_B + m_C$. An analogous result holds with more than three treatment groups. For proof in the general case, see Dwass [60] or Marden [152]. Related ideas are discussed by Hogg [107, 108] and Savage [244].

---

[4]As before, strictly speaking this requires the outcomes to be untied, as was true of $y_1 = 15.34$, $y_2 = 18.28$ and $y_3 = 13.18$. This slightly tedious requirement will soon disappear by way of Definition 2 and Theorem 9 in later chapters.

4.2.4 Building Intuition: Either Factor Could Be Biased When the Other Is Not

The previous subsection divided $N = m_A + m_B + m_C$ individuals at random to form groups A, B, and C with fixed sizes m_A, m_B, and m_C. Suppose, instead, that we picked m_A individuals from N individuals for group A, then subdivided the remaining $N - m_A$ individuals into m_B individuals for group B and m_C individuals for group C. If each of the two splits were done by simple random sampling without replacement, then we would again have randomly assigned individuals to A, B, and C with all $N! / (m_A! \times m_B! \times m_C!)$ possible assignments having the same probability.

Suppose, however, that we selected m_A individuals from N individuals for group A at random, but then subdivided the remainder into B and C in a very biased manner. If Fisher's hypothesis of no effect were true, then Wilcoxon's statistic W_A comparing group A to the combination of groups B and C has its usual randomization distribution, and provides a valid test of no effect. However, W_B may be severely biased by the biased subdivision that formed groups B and C. Importantly, one factor may be biased when the other is not.

Conversely, suppose the selection of m_A individuals from N individuals for group A was extremely biased, but the subdivision of the remaining $N - m_A = m_B + m_C$ individuals to form groups B and C was done at random, with all $(m_B + m_C)! / (m_B! \times m_C!)$ assignments having the same probability. If Fisher's hypothesis of no effect were true, then Wilcoxon's statistic W_B comparing group B to group C has its usual randomization distribution, and provides a valid test of no effect. So, W_A may be biased when W_B is not.

The sense in which the two factors provide separate information is stronger than statistical independence: it is about bias too. Biased treatment assignment, no matter how strong, affecting one factor does nothing to invalidate the other factor. True, both factors may be biased, but it takes two biases, a bias when selecting for group A, and another bias when subdividing what is left, to bias both factors.[5] Moreover, to provide misleading confirmation, the two biases must align so they mistakenly suggest compatible treatment effects.

4.2.5 Building Intuition: Are Rank Tests Essential?

Rank tests are not essential. Here and in §4.1, two rank tests were exactly independent under Fisher's hypothesis of no effect in a randomized experiment, providing there were no ties. Rank tests are essential for exact independence, but exact independence is of no importance at all. What is needed to combine two factors as if they were independent are Definition 2 in Chapter 7 and Theorem 9 in Chapter 11; however, rank tests play no role in this definition and theorem.

To build some intuition, return to the example of three individuals, 1, 2, and 3, randomly assigned to treatment groups A, B, and C by a random permutation, with outcomes $y_1 = 15.34$, $y_2 = 18.28$ and $y_3 = 13.18$, under Fisher's hypothesis of no effect. Suppose that we look at two contrasts, C_A and C_B, among group means, where C_A is the mean in group A minus the mean in the combination of

---

[5]This section illustrates the use of the pick matrices and the subpick matrices in Chapter 8.

groups B and C, and C_B is the mean in group B minus the mean in group C. If I told you that individual 1 was assigned to group A, then you would know that $C_A = y_1 - (y_2 + y_3) = 15.34 - (18.28 + 13.18)/2 = -0.39$ and C_B is equally likely to be $y_2 - y_3 = 18.28 - 13.18 = 5.1$ and $y_3 - y_2 = -5.1$. If I told you that individual 2 was assigned to group A, then you would know that $C_A = y_2 - (y_1 + y_3) = 18.28 - (15.34 + 13.18)/2 = 4.02$ and C_B is equally likely to be $y_1 - y_3 = 2.16$ and $y_3 - y_1 = -2.16$. If I told you that individual 3 was assigned to group A, then you would know that $C_A = y_3 - (y_1 + y_2) = 13.18 - (15.34 + 18.28)/2 = -3.63$ and C_B is equally likely to be $y_1 - y_2 = -2.94$ and $y_2 - y_1 = 2.94$. Moreover, these six possibilities each have probability 1/6. There are several consequences. One less important consequence is that $E(C_A) = 0 = E(C_B)$. Another less important consequence is that C_A and C_B are strongly dependent. Indeed, if $|C_B| = 5.1$, then $C_A = -0.39$; if $|C_B| = 2.16$, then $C_A = -4.02$; if $|C_B| = 2.94$, then $C_A = -3.63$. Permute data, and the permuted data exhibit strong forms of dependence, unlike partial ranks. There is one important consequence: the conditional distribution of C_B given C_A is symmetric about zero, favoring neither treatment group B nor treatment group C; see [295].

More generally, suppose that $N = m_A + m_B + m_C$ individuals are divided at random to form groups A, B, and C with fixed sizes m_A, m_B, and m_C, under Fisher's hypothesis of no effect. Define the contrasts of means, C_A and C_B, as above. The marginal distribution of C_A has the randomization distribution of the difference of two means, one based on m_A observations, the other based on $m_B + m_C$ observations, so there is a valid randomization test based on C_A. Conditionally given the identities of the individuals selected for group A, the second contrast C_B has the randomization distribution of the difference of two means, one based on m_B observations, the other based on m_C observations. So, conditionally given the identities of the individuals selected for group A, there is a valid randomization test based on C_B. These two tests are not independent: they both depend on the identities of the individuals selected for group A; however, Proposition 2 in Chapter 7 shows that their P-values may be combined as if they came from unrelated studies. Moreover, this fact is general: contrasts of means play no special role, nor does randomization, as seen in Theorem 9 in Chapter 11.

4.2.6 Age Strata

In Ref. [131], DNA damage appears to be greater for older individuals, as seen in Figure 4.5. Does this invalidate the comparison in Figure 4.4? Figure 4.4 paid no attention to age.

Figures 4.6 and 4.7 divide the two factors in Figure 4.4 by three age groups. Generally, the patterns seen in Figure 4.4 persist within each age group, although the data becomes thin as 59 people are divided into smaller groups. For instance, in Figure 4.6, at age 40–55, the control boxplot describes just three individuals. To be useful, the information in the three age groups needs to be combined into a single analysis.

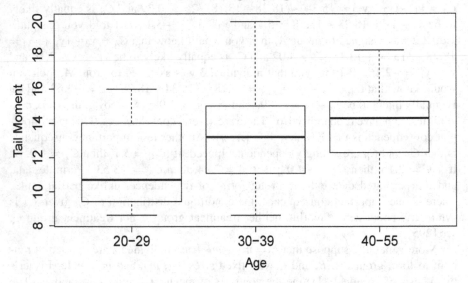

Figure 4.5 *DNA damage in three age groups.*

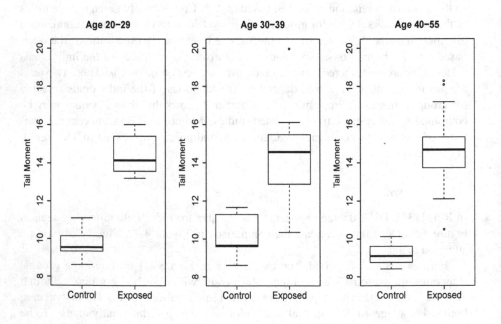

Figure 4.6 *DNA damage in workers exposed to antineoplastic drugs and unexposed controls in three age groups.*

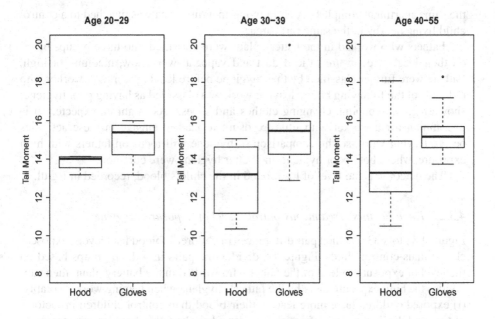

Figure 4.7 *DNA damage by age group in exposed workers using gloves alone or gloves plus a laminar hood.*

Later, Figure 4.4 will illustrate an analysis with two evidence factors for three groups. Figures 4.6 and 4.7 will illustrate a stratified analysis with two evidence factors.

4.3 Lead Absorption in Children

4.3.1 Parent's Occupational Exposure to Lead and Child's Blood Lead Level

Does a parent's exposure to lead at work affect the level of lead in the employee's children? If it does, then regulations governing occupational exposure to lead need to consider children who may never visit the worksite. It is possible that a parent exposed to lead at work brings lead home in clothing and hair, thereby exposing children.

Morton et al. [159] asked this question of a battery plant in Oklahoma. The study examined 33 matched pairs of a child whose father worked in the battery plant and a control child of the same age living in a different, nearby household in the same neighborhood. In addition to lead from the battery plant, lead may be present also at home: in the air or in the physical structure of the home. Particular attention was given to matching for neighborhood characteristics that might involve exposure to lead at home. For instance, if "the residence of the lead worker was located along a major traffic street, the control child was selected from the same side of that street [159, p. 550]." A child in an apartment complex was matched to a control child from the same apartment complex. A child living in a rural area was matched to a control child living nearby in the same rural area.

Fathers who worked in the battery plant were classified into three groups based on their level of exposure to lead dust and vapor at work: low, medium, or high. Fathers were further classified by their hygiene before leaving work. A worker who did none of the following before leaving work was classified as having poor hygiene: showering, shampooing, changing clothes and shoes. As might be expected, it is uncommon for a worker with little exposure to lead to engage in these activities before leaving work, so the comparison of hygiene will focus on fathers with high exposure, where both poor hygiene and better hygiene were common.

The outcome is the level of lead found in the child's blood, recorded in μg/dl.

4.3.2   Three Factors: Treatment/Control, Level of Exposure, Hygiene

Figure 4.8 plots 33 matched pair differences in children's blood lead levels, exposed-child-minus-control-child. Figure 4.8 divides the pairs into three groups based on the level of exposure to lead of the father who worked in the battery plant, then subdivides the high exposure pairs by the father's hygiene when leaving work. Notably: (i) exposed children have more lead in their blood than control children in factor 1 of Figure 4.8, (ii) the pair difference is larger when the father has higher exposure to lead in factor 2 of Figure 4.8, and (iii) the pair difference is larger when the father has poor hygiene in factor 3 of Figure 4.8. [6]

Unlike the examples in §4.1 and §4.2, Figure 4.8 has not two but three factors. Specifically, Figure 4.8 has pair differences and a classification of pair differences by dose, like Figure 4.1, but it also has repeated refinements of the treatment group, like Figure 4.4.

In both Figures 4.4 and 4.8, a potentially harmful exposure appears to be mitigated by an activity intended to reduce harm, the laminar hood in Figure 4.4 or good hygiene in Figure 4.8. The comparison of jobs with high and low exposure to lead may be biased—perhaps, higher paying jobs have lower lead exposure. There could also be bias in the comparison of high exposure fathers who wash up before going home and those who practice poor hygiene. However, there is no immediately obvious reason that the same biases should recur in these two comparisons.

Is there more? The children were paired for age and similar nearby housing. The meaning and impact on lead levels of matching for neighborhood is not evident in Figure 4.8. Figure 4.9 looks at lead levels for exposed and control children separately, rather than matched-pair differences, though the children in Figure 4.9 are still paired for age and neighborhood. Each boxplot in the first row of Figure 4.9 contains children of the same age and neighborhood as the boxplot immediately below in the second row. It is evident from Figure 4.9 that the pattern in Figure 4.8 is produced by characteristics of exposed fathers, because that pattern is not evident in control children of the same age, living in the same neighborhood.

---

[6]The data are available in the evident package in R as lead.

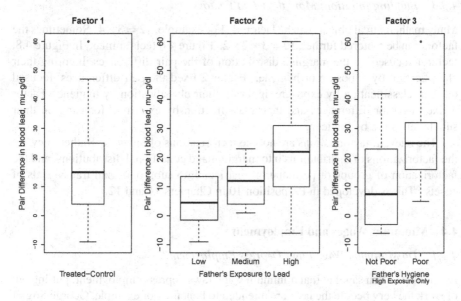

Figure 4.8 *Exposed-minus-control matched pair differences in levels of lead in 33 pairs of two children. The 33 pairs are divided by the father's exposure to lead at work, low (n=8), medium (n=6), and high (n=19), 33 = 8 + 6 + 19. The 19 high exposure pairs are further divided by the father's hygiene upon leaving work, poor (n=13) and not poor (n=6), 19 = 13 + 6.*

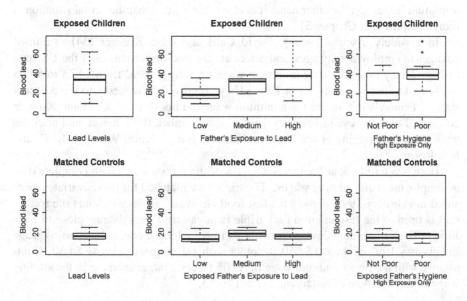

Figure 4.9 *Separate plots for children whose fathers were exposed to lead and their matched controls. Lead levels are depicted, not pair differences in lead levels.*

4.3.3   Building Intuition: More than Two Factors

Many mathematical objects can be factored. For example, $12 = 3 \times 4$. Sometimes the factors can be factored further, $12 = 3 \times 2 \times 2$. Figure 4.8 feels similar. In Figure 4.8, factor 1 focused on the marginal distribution of the pair differences, ignoring their classification by exposure or hygiene. Factor 2 fixed the pair differences, focused on their classification by exposure, ignoring their classification by hygiene. Factor 3 fixed the pair differences and their classification by exposure, focusing on their subclassification by hygiene.

The relevant factorizations are not the factorizations of integers. Rather, they are the factorizations of distributions into marginal and conditional distributions, and the factorization of groups of permutation matrices into subgroups and transversals of cosets. This is developed in Proposition 10 in Chapters 11 and 12.

4.4   Minimum Wages and Employment

4.4.1   Do Minimum Wage Laws Depress Employment?

Economists often say that that minimum wage laws depress employment, putting out of work the very people the laws are intended to benefit. For example, George Stigler [263] wrote: "Each worker receives the value of his marginal product under competition . . . it must therefore have one of two effects: first, workers whose services are worth less than the minimum wage are discharged [or] second the productivity of low-efficiency workers is increased." Stigler then argued that the second alternative, an increase in productivity, is not a plausible consequence of an increase in the minimum wage. On the other hand, it is also often argued that the actual situation is more complex [32, Chapter 3].

In a widely discussed study, David Card and Alan Krueger [34] examined changes in employment, wages, and prices at fast food restaurants after the US state of New Jersey raised its state minimum wage on 1 April 1992 from $4.25 to $5.05 per hour, an increase of $0.80 or 19%. They compared New Jersey to the adjacent state of Pennsylvania where the minimum wage did not change. Card and Krueger conducted two surveys in February 1992 and November 1992, before and after the wage increase, looking at four fast food chains, Burger King, Wendy's, KFC, and Roy Rogers.

Here, we will look at 66 matched triples of three restaurants with complete data on employment and starting wages. The triples are matched for two covariates measured in February 1992, namely the fast food chain and number of hours the restaurant is open. One restaurant in each triple is in eastern Pennsylvania, close to New Jersey. Each triple contains two restaurants in New Jersey, one with a starting wage in February 1992 of at most $4.50, the other with a starting wage above $4.50. Compliance with the new minimum wage of $5.05 forces a larger increase in the starting wage in the first type of restaurant, at least $0.55.

Starting Wages in February 1992, Before the Wage Increase in NJ

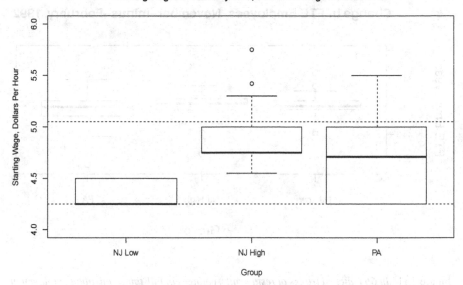

Figure 4.10 *Starting wages in 66 matched triples of three fast food restaurants, in February 1992, before New Jersey (NJ) raised its minimum wage from $4.25 to $5.05 (horizontal dashed lines), while Pennsylvania's (PA) minimum wage remained unchanged. Each triple contains two restaurants from New Jersey, one with a starting wage of at most $4.50, the other with a starting wage above $4.50.*

The match used an approximation algorithm developed by Bikram Karmaker and colleagues in [126].[7] This algorithm is intended for use in constructing evidence factors. The new match improves upon a related match described in Ref. [207, §2.2] in producing greater separation in starting wages of the two groups from New Jersey; see Figure 4.10. In Figure 4.10, the 66 NJ-Low restaurants needed a substantial increase in their starting wage to comply with the new law, the 66 NJ-High restaurants needed either a smaller or no increase, and no increase was required of the 66 PA restaurants.[8]

4.4.2 What Do We Expect to See?

People often cross the Delaware River that separates New Jersey and Pennsylvania, and some people do so to work or dine. It seems somewhat less likely, though not impossible, that someone would cross the Delaware River to work or dine at a Burger King in an adjacent state. Burger Kings are similar in the two states, as are other fast food chains; moreover, the cost and inconvenience of commuting between states would limit the value of a higher minimum wage for someone who must travel out-

---

[7]In R, this is Karmakar's approxmatch package.

[8]The data are available in the evident package in R as ck.

Change in FTE Employees, November–minus–February, 1992

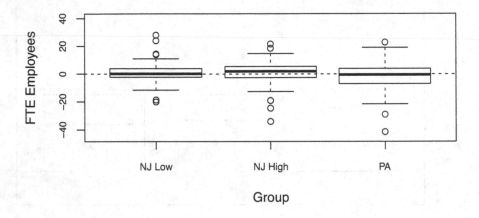

Figure 4.11 *In 66 matched triples of restaurants, changes in full-time equivalent employment, after the minimum wage increase minus before the increase. The horizontal dashed line is at zero.*

of-state to receive it. For these reasons, one expects to see in Pennsylvania Burger Kings little effect of an increase in the minimum wage in New Jersey.

A simple interpretation of Stigler's [263] argument says that one expects to see some decline in employment at fast food restaurants in New Jersey following the increase in the minimum wage. If it really were true that wages in February 1992 more closely reflected the marginal value of labor, then an increase in the minimum wage should more severely distort wages in restaurants whose starting wage was quite low in February 1992, so one expects to see a larger decline in employment in such restaurants. This yields a prediction about the change in employment in the three groups of restaurants in Figure 4.10.

Conversely, if one doubted Stigler's [263] argument, then one might expect little change in employment in the three groups of restaurants.

A large change in employment in Pennsylvania restaurants, whether up or down, would suggest that forces were at work between February 1992 and November 1992 besides the change in the minimum wage in New Jersey.

4.4.3   Change in Employment

Figure 4.11 depicts the changes in employment in the $198 = 3 \times 66$ fast food restaurants in Figure 4.10. In terms of the centers of the distributions, there is little indication of a decline in employment in any of the three groups. A few of the changes seem

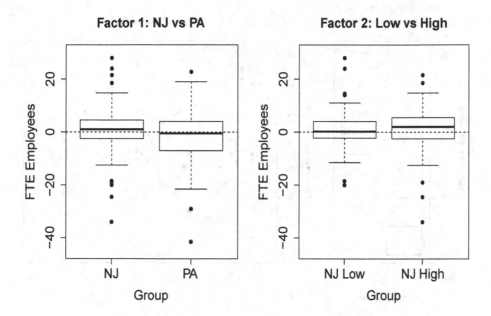

Figure 4.12 *Reorganization of Figure 4.11 into two factors, 132 New Jersey restaurants versus 66 Pennsylvania restaurants in Factor 1, and 66 low wage New Jersey restaurants versus 66 high wage New Jersey restaurants in Factor 2.*

implausibly large, perhaps indicating that a few survey respondents misunderstood a question.

Figure 4.12 reorganizes Figure 4.11 into two factors. If raising the minimum wage reduces employment, then we expect to see larger declines in employment in New Jersey than in Pennsylvania in factor 1, and larger declines inside New Jersey among restaurants with a lower starting wage prior to the wage increase in factor 2. In fact, the median changes are close to zero throughout Figure 4.12, and the direction is the opposite of the prediction in factor 1.

4.4.4 Building Intuition: Do Confidence Intervals Concur?

As is familiar [141, Chapter 3], and as discussed in §1.5 and §1.7, a confidence interval is formed by testing hypothesized treatment effects and retaining those effects that are not rejected by the test. Figure 4.12 provides two essentially independent tests of each hypothesized effect, one from factor 1, the other from factor 2. Factors 1 and 2 may or may not concur in their assessment of the hypothesis of no effect, and in the same way, factors 1 and 2 may or may not concur about whether particular magnitudes of effect are plausible. This issue is examined in §6.2.

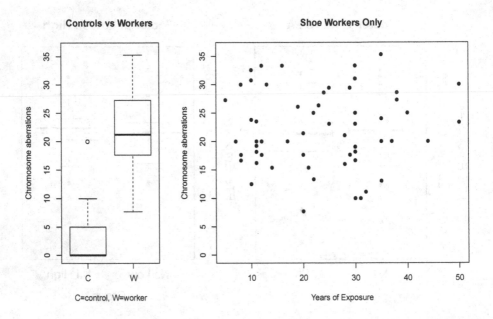

Figure 4.13 *Total chromosome aberrations, including gaps, in 58 shoe workers exposed to benzene and 20 unexposed controls.*

4.5 Benzene and Chromosome Aberrations

4.5.1 *Shoe Workers Exposed to Benzene in Turkey*

Workers who manufacture shoes are often exposed to benzene, a carcinogen. Tunca and Egeli [275] compared 58 shoe workers in Bursa, Turkey to 20 unexposed residents of Bursa in terms of chromosome aberrations in blood lymphocytes. Figure 4.13 makes two comparisons of total chromosome aberrations: (i) on the left, shoe workers are compared to unexposed controls; (ii) on the right, shoe workers are distinguished based on years of exposure to benzene. The 58 points on the right for shoe workers project horizontally to the boxplot for the 58 shoe workers.

Although there are two sources of evidence in Figure 4.13, they are not, in this case, mutually supporting. The 58 shoe workers have much higher levels of chromosome aberrations than the 20 unexposed controls. If Wilcoxon's rank sum statistic is used to compare shoe workers and controls, the one-sided P-value is 1.2×10^{-10}, and the one-sided 95% confidence interval for a shift is $\tau \geq 16.7$. On the other hand, Kendall's correlation between chromosome aberrations and duration of exposure for shoe workers is 0.03 with one-sided P-value 0.39 when testing no association.[9] These tests would be appropriate in an infeasible experiment that randomly assigned individuals to worker and control groups, and randomly assigned workers to dura-

---

[9]The data are available in the evident package in R as benzene.

tions of exposure. Many lymphocytes are short-lived, so it is possible that only recent exposure to benzene affects the level of chromosome aberrations in lymphocytes.

The comparison in the scatter plot in Figure 4.13 does not strengthen the comparison in the boxplots. Does the evidence in the scatter plot detract from the evidence in the boxplots? To what extent, if at all, does "failure to strengthen" constitute "weakening"? Or is "failure to strengthen" merely "failure to strengthen"? To what extent can this be clarified by statistical analysis? Does the choice of analytic methods affect the answer?

The benzene example is discussed further in §5.4.

4.5.2 Building Intuition: Exposure Duration and Age in Paired and Unpaired Factors

Figures 4.2 and 4.13 both make two comparisons, one involving exposed and unexposed groups, the other involving duration of exposure, but there is an important difference. In Figure 4.2, smokers and nonsmokers were matched for several covariates, including age. If smoking had no effect on periodontal disease, and if the two comparisons in Figure 4.2 were free of unmeasured biases, then there is no reason that pair differences in periodontal disease should increase as the duration of smoking increases for the smoker. True, smokers who have smoked for 40 years cannot be 25 years old, but in Figure 4.2, 25-year-old smokers are compared to 25-year-old nonsmokers. Perhaps we should adjust twice for age in Figure 4.2, as will be done in §5.3, but we have adjusted once by matching for age.

The situation in Figure 4.13 is different. Someone who has been a shoe worker for 50 years is certainly not 30 years old. There is no adjustment for age in Figure 4.13, so duration of exposure could be misleadingly associated with chromosome aberrations if age is associated with chromosome aberrations. So, an adjustment for age is needed here.

4.6 Summary: Mutually Supporting, Unrelated Comparisons

This chapter has discussed several observational studies that each have more than one comparison with the potential to provide mutually supporting evidence. These comparisons may each be biased by the absence of random assignment, but the biases affecting different comparisons lack an obvious reason for aligning to produce misleading evidence of an effect. In the example of children of fathers exposed at work to lead in §4.3, ask: Why should exposed/control, level of exposure at work, and hygiene leaving work align to one another in such a way as to suggest an effect on children if there is truly no effect? In the example of occupational exposure to antineoplastic drugs in §4.2, ask: Why should exposed/control and the presence or absence of ventilating hood align to one another to suggest DNA damage from exposure? Perhaps there are reasons for misleading alignment that are not obvious, but it is worth a moment's thought about what such reasons might be.

The examples feel both ordinary and clever at the same time. The examples are ordinary in the sense that nothing astonishing is being done: everyday matters are being considered. The investigators whose examples these are seem clever because they have materially strengthened causal conclusions from observational data by bringing into focus ordinary considerations that most investigators miss. That the examples feel ordinary suggests that evidence factors are often available, but pass unnoticed through inattention.

Later chapters will return to these examples in an effort to quantify whether the evidence has actually been strengthened. To what extent, if any, does alignment strengthen causal claims?

It is not a forgone conclusion that two factors will align, as seen in the example in §4.5, where all of the evidence of harm from benzene comes from the comparison of exposed workers and unexposed controls. Does the absence of alignment weaken a causal claim? If so, to what quantitative degree? Or is the absence of alignment the absence of strengthened evidence, not weakened evidence? See §5.4 for discussion.

With appropriate statistical tools used in appropriate contexts, there are clear answers to these questions.

4.7 Using R

4.7.1 Periodontal Disease and Smoking

The data [220] for the example in §4.1 is available as periodontal in the R package evident. As is customary in sensitivity analyses, one-sided inferences are calculated by default; however, two-sided tests and confidence intervals are an option. A one-sided P-value can be doubled for a two-sided test [49]. The randomization inferences using Wilcoxon's signed rank statistic and Kendall's correlation appear below.

```
library(evident)
library(DOS2)
data(periodontal)
attach(periodontal)
y=pcteither[z == 1] - pcteither[z == 0]
senWilcox(y,gamma=1,conf.int=TRUE,alternative="greater")
$pval
[1] 0
$estimate
low   high
11.05 Inf
$ci
low high
8.60 Inf

x=cigsperday[z==1]
cor.test(y,x,method="kendall",alternative="greater")
z = 2.4914, p-value = 0.006361
```

In Chapter 5, Kendall's test of independence will be replaced by the crosscut test [218], which has excellent design sensitivity:

```
crosscut(x,y,ct=.2)
$output$pval
[1] 0.002199
```

4.7.2 Antineoplastic Drugs and DNA Damage

The data [131] in §4.2 is available in the R package evident as antineoplastic. The two factors in Figure 4.4 were analyzed using Wilcoxon's rank sum statistic:

```
library(evident)
data(antineoplastic)
attach(antineoplastic)
z=1-z1
wilcox.test(tailmoment~z,conf.int=T,alternative="greater",
correct=FALSE)
W = 767, p-value = 7.85e-10
alternative hypothesis: true location shift is greater than 0
95 percent confidence interval:
 4.009979 Inf

z=1-z2
wilcox.test(tailmoment[f2]~z[f2],conf.int=T,
alternative="greater",correct=FALSE)
W = 303.5, p-value = 0.0007132
alternative hypothesis: true location shift is greater than 0
95 percent confidence interval:
 0.8799933 Inf
```

For Wilcoxon's rank sum statistic, the function sen2sample in the senstrat package performs a sensitivity analysis that will appear in Chapter 5. Here, it is illustrated with $\Gamma = 1$ for a randomization test. Notice that sen2sample requires you to replace tailmoment by its ranks to obtain the rank sum statistic; otherwise, it will permute the observations, not the ranks, yielding Pitman's permutational t-test.

```
library(senstrat)
sen2sample(rank(tailmoment[f2]),z2[f2],gamma=1)
$pval
[1] 0.0007132
```

4.8 Exercises

Exercise 4.1. *Trivalent chromium is often used in the tanning of leather, but chromium may also damage the DNA of workers who are exposed to it. Zhang, Chen, Chen, Zou, Lou, and He [306] used the comet assay to compare 90 individuals in 30 matched sets of three individuals. In each matched set, one individual worked in the tannery department of a tannery, where exposure to chromium was high. A second individual worked in the finishing department of the tannery, where chromium exposures were lower. A third individual was an unexposed control who did not work in the tannery. The data are in* tannery *in the* evident *package in R. Suggest two evidence factors. Become familiar with the data by plotting it in various ways. Later chapters have exercises that continue the examination of the* tannery *data. For two evidence factor analyses of the* tannery *data, see Ref. [209] and Refs. [223, §20.2].*

Exercise 4.2. *Is the risk of suicide higher following the purchase of a handgun? Grassel, Wintemute, Wright and Romero [86] compared cases of suicide in California in 1998 to deaths from causes other than suicide, firearms and unintentional injuries. So, this is a so-called case-control study – really, a case-noncase comparison – comparing handgun purchases among cases and noncases of suicide. Their thought is that allowing the purchase of a handgun is unlikely to cause a death from a myocardial infarction, but it might cause a suicide that would not otherwise have occurred. Because it is not always clear whether a death is a suicide – a drug overdose or a car crash might possibly be a veiled suicide – there are subtleties when counting suicides and comparing them to other deaths [199]; however, omit these considerations for the purpose of this exercise. There are three treatment groups: (i) purchase of a handgun within the year before death, (ii) purchase of a handgun within the three years before death but not in the most recent year, (iii) no purchase of a handgun within the three years before death. Table 4.1 contains summary data.*

How are Tables 4.2 and 4.3 obtained from Table 4.1? Can Table 4.1 be recovered from Tables 4.2 and 4.3? Do Tables 4.2 and 4.3 together have more, less or the same information as Table 4.1? Show that Tables 4.2 and 4.3 are not independent. (Hint: Compare column 1 of Table 4.2 to the column of totals in Table 4.3.) Would the information in Table 4.2 provide much information about the odds ratio in Table 4.3? Is there any sense in which the people in Table 4.3 have something in common that many people in Table 4.2 lack?

Exercise 4.3. *Use Fisher's test for a 2×2 table to perform a one-sided randomization test of no effect in Table 4.2. Do the same in Table 4.3. In R, the test is implemented as* fisher.test.

Table 4.1 *Data from Ref. [86] for exercise 4.2. Deaths from suicide and other causes in California in 1998, classified by whether the most recent handgun purchase occurred in the year before death, 2 to 3 years before death, and all other situations including purchases in the distant past and no purchases ever*

	Handgun Purchase			Total
	Within 1 Year	2 or 3 Years Ago	Other	
Suicide	179	58	2798	3035
Other death	369	518	207851	208738
Total	548	576	210649	211773

Table 4.2 *Factor 1 from Table 4.1: Any purchase within 3 years*

	Handgun Purchase		Total
	Within 3 Years	Other	
Suicide	237	2798	3035
Other death	887	207851	208738
Sum	1124	210649	211773

Table 4.3 *Factor 2 from Table 4.1: Timing of the handgun purchase*

	Handgun Purchase		Total
	Within 1 Year	2 or 3 Years Ago	
Suicide	179	58	237
Other death	369	518	887
Sum	548	576	1124

Chapter 5

Simple Analyses with Evidence Factors

Abstract

The simplest analysis with two evidence factors is considered. This analysis begins with one analysis for the two factors jointly, and it may continue via closed testing to separately examine the two component hypotheses. In both examples, the joint analysis is insensitive to larger unmeasured biases than are the two components of the joint analysis. In both analyses, infinite bias invalidating either factor would leave behind fairly strong, fairly insensitive evidence from the complementary factor. Analyses strongly control the family-wise error rate at level α despite performing several tests, each at level α.

The situation in which two factors do not concur is discussed. In this case, there are two possibilities that should be distinguished: (i) the factors actively disagree; (ii) one factor fails to provide much information.

5.1 Structure of the Simple Analyses

5.1.1 Two Factors Viewed in Combination and Separately

In Chapter 4, in connection with smoking and periodontal disease, it was suggested that the two comparisons in panels (a) and (b) of Figure 4.2 share little information, so the information they provide could be combined as if they came from two unrelated studies. Similarly, it was suggested that, in connection with antineoplastic drugs and DNA damage, factors 1 and 2 in Figure 4.4 share little information, so the information they provide could be combined as if they also came from unrelated studies. These informal suggestions become precise in Theorem 9 of Chapter 11.

The current chapter presents the simplest analyses with two evidence factors. These simplest analyses are sometimes too simple, a topic discussed in Chapter 6.

5.1.2 One P-value Residing on the Unit Interval

Let P be a P-value testing some null hypothesis, H_0. The definition of a valid P-value requires that, if the null hypothesis is true, then $\Pr(P \leq \alpha) \leq \alpha$ for all $0 \leq \alpha \leq 1$; that is, the P-value must be stochastically larger than the uniform distribution on the unit interval, $[0, 1]$. At the conventional $\alpha = 0.05$ level, a valid P-value satisfies $\Pr(P \leq 0.05) \leq 0.05$ if H_0 is true, so if H_0 is rejected when $P \leq 0.05$, then the probability of falsely rejecting H_0 is at most 5%. The P-value is more informative than a binary report, "rejected at 0.05," in the limited sense that the P-value indicates the smallest level α that would lead to rejection [49]. For instance, a P-value of 0.001 indicates that H_0 would be rejected at level $\alpha = 0.05$, also at levels $\alpha = 0.01$ and $\alpha = 0.001$, but not at $\alpha = 0.0005$.

5.1.3 Two P-values Residing on the Unit Cube

Let P and P' be two valid P-values from unrelated studies testing null hypotheses H_0 and H_0', respectively; so, $\Pr(P \leq \alpha) \leq \alpha$ for all $0 \leq \alpha \leq 1$ if H_0 is true, and $\Pr(P' \leq \alpha) \leq \alpha$ for all $0 \leq \alpha \leq 1$ if H_0' is true. Two valid statistically independent P-values, P and P', from unrelated studies satisfy a strong consequence of their independence: if H_0 and H_0' are both true, then (P, P') are jointly stochastically larger than the uniform distribution on the unit square, $[0, 1] \times [0, 1] = [0, 1]^2$. What does this mean? Let me mention a consequence of being larger than uniform, then state the precise definition. Consider the probability, $\Pr(P \leq \alpha, P' \leq \alpha')$, that $P \leq \alpha$ and $P' \leq \alpha'$. If (P, P') are larger than uniform on $[0, 1]^2$, then one consequence is that $\Pr(P \leq \alpha, P' \leq \alpha') \leq \alpha\alpha'$ for all $0 \leq \alpha \leq 1$ and $0 \leq \alpha' \leq 1$.

5.1.4 Larger than Uniform on the Unit Cube

Although stochastic ordering implies $\Pr(P \leq \alpha, P' \leq \alpha') \leq \alpha\alpha'$, the definition of stochastic ordering is somewhat stronger. Let (Q, Q') be two random variables that actually *are* uniformly distributed on the unit square, so $\Pr(Q \leq \alpha, Q' \leq \alpha') = \alpha\alpha'$ for all $0 \leq \alpha \leq 1$ and $0 \leq \alpha' \leq 1$. Here, (Q, Q') may be quite unlike (P, P'). For instance, if P is a P-value taken from a table of the binomial cumulative distribution, then P is discrete: there is a set containing finitely many real numbers such that P is certainly in that set; however, Q is continuous, in fact uniform on $[0, 1]$.

A function $f(p, p')$ on $[0, 1]^2$ is monotone increasing if $f(p, p') \leq f(q, q')$ whenever $p \leq q$ and $p' \leq q'$. Let $\mathcal{M}$ be the set of monotone increasing functions defined on the unit square, $[0, 1]^2$.

By definition, $(P, P') \in [0, 1]^2$ is stochastically larger than the uniform distribution on $[0, 1]^2$ if and only if

$$\mathrm{E}\{f(P, P')\} \geq \mathrm{E}\{f(Q, Q')\} \text{ for every } f \in \mathcal{M}. \tag{5.1}$$

Condition (5.1) is understood to mean: whenever the expectations exist, the stated inequality holds. There are many equivalent forms of condition (5.1)—see Refs. [155, 254]—but (5.1) is one convenient form.

Larger than Uniform Two, possibly *dependent*, P-values, (P, P'), are jointly larger than two *independent* uniform random variables, (Q, Q'), if condition (5.1) holds.

To clarify (5.1), consider a specific monotone increasing function f defined on the unit square, $[0, 1]^2$. Let $f(p, p') = 1$ if either $p > \alpha$ or $p' > \alpha'$, and

$f(p, p') = 0$ otherwise; then, f is monotone increasing. If (5.1) is true, then $\mathrm{E}\{f(P, P')\} \geq \mathrm{E}\{f(Q, Q')\}$, where $1 - \mathrm{E}\{f(Q, Q')\} = \mathrm{Pr}(Q \leq \alpha, Q' \leq \alpha') = \alpha \alpha'$ and $1 - \mathrm{E}\{f(P, P')\} = \mathrm{Pr}(P \leq \alpha, P' \leq \alpha')$, with the consequence noted above, namely $\mathrm{Pr}(P \leq \alpha, P' \leq \alpha') \leq \alpha \alpha'$.

5.1.5   Fisher's Method of Combining Independent P-values

Fisher proposed combining independent uniform P-values by producing a new statistic, their product $P \times P'$, working out the distribution of $P \times P'$, and obtaining a single combined P-value from the observed value of $P \times P'$, rejecting for small values of $P \times P'$. For instance, if $P = 0.05$ and $P' = 0.05$, then $P \times P' = 0.05 \times 0.05 = 0.0025$, and the chance that two independent, uniform random variables have a product less than or equal to 0.0025 turns out to be 0.017, much smaller than each of the two component P-values. Of course, $P \times P'$ is a monotone increasing function of (P, P') on the unit square, so condition (5.1) is relevant to its behavior.

We are less interested in the expectation of $P \times P'$ than in the probability that $P \times P'$ is small. So, let $f(p, p') = 1$ if $p \times p' > k$, and $f(p, p') = 0$ otherwise; so, f is monotone increasing on $[0, 1]^2$. If (5.1) is true, then $\mathrm{Pr}(P \times P' > k) = \mathrm{E}\{f(P, P')\} \geq \mathrm{E}\{f(Q, Q')\} = \mathrm{Pr}(Q \times Q' > k)$, so that $\mathrm{Pr}(P \times P' \leq k) \leq \mathrm{Pr}(Q \times Q' \leq k)$.

In words, suppose (5.1) were true, and suppose we applied Fisher's method for combining independent uniform P-values to (P, P') despite the fact that (P, P') are not uniform on $[0, 1]^2$; then, the resulting test would be, at worst, conservative, with $P \times P' \leq k$ occurring with probability at most $\mathrm{Pr}(Q \times Q' \leq k)$. Indeed, the same logic and conclusion applies to any method of combining independent uniform P-values that rejects when a monotone increasing function $f(\cdot, \cdot)$ is small.

Fisher's method acts as if P-values were uniformly distributed, but the upper bounds on P-values that occur in sensitivity analysis can be quite large. As discussed in greater detail later in §5.1, other methods, such as the truncated product of P-values [305] often exhibit better performance when applied to upper bounds on P-values [112, Tables 2–3].

5.1.6   Dependent P-values; Sensitivity Analysis

Condition (5.1) is what we need to combine two P-values, (P, P'), as if they came from two independent studies. Importantly, (5.1) can be true of two P-values, (P, P'), even if P is not independent of P', and the two P-values do not come from different studies. This is fortunate. Panels (a) and (b) of Figure 4.2 are not independent: the points in panel (b) project horizontally to the left to the corresponding points in panel (a), so panel (b) determines panel (a). Nonetheless, Proposition 2 of Chapter 7 shows that many tests applied to panels (a) and (b) produce dependent P-values that satisfy condition (5.1). We may act as if such P-values came from two independent studies.

In an observational study, there are true P-values, (P, P'), but they depend upon the true but unknown distribution of treatment assignments, so these true P-values, (P, P'), are unknown. So, we conduct a sensitivity analysis, with two sensitivity parameters, Γ for P in the first factor, Γ' for P' in the second factor. The sensitivity parameters, Γ and Γ', are also unknown, but the sensitivity analysis varies their values, thereby indicating the degree to which unknown biases of various magnitudes might alter the conclusions. If the bias in the first factor is at most Γ, then we determine an observed sharp upper bound, $\overline{P}_\Gamma \geq P$, where equality holds for some bias of magnitude Γ. If the bias in the second factor is at most Γ', then we determine an observed sharp upper bound, $\overline{P}'_{\Gamma'} \geq P'$, where equality holds for some bias of magnitude Γ'.

Clearly, if $\overline{P}_\Gamma \geq P$ and $\overline{P}'_{\Gamma'} \geq P'$, and if (P, P') is stochastically larger than uniform, then $\left(\overline{P}_\Gamma, \overline{P}'_{\Gamma'}\right)$ is stochastically larger than uniform. From this, we can say: if the bias in the first factor is at most Γ, if the bias in the second factor is at most Γ', if Fisher's hypothesis of no effect is true, then there is at most an α chance that an upper bound on the single combined P-value from $\left(\overline{P}_\Gamma, \overline{P}'_{\Gamma'}\right)$ is less than or equal to α. There are some technical details in this claim that are clarified in Part III, but for now let us proceed without the details.

Write H_Γ for the hypothesis that there is no treatment effect and the bias in treatment assignment in the first factor is at most Γ. Write $H'_{\Gamma'}$ for the hypothesis that there is no treatment effect and the bias in treatment assignment in the second factor is at most Γ'. Write $H_\Gamma \wedge H'_{\Gamma'}$ for the conjunction hypothesis that asserts H_Γ and $H'_{\Gamma'}$ are both true.[1] With this notation, the above discussion may be stated concisely: Suppose $H_\Gamma \wedge H'_{\Gamma'}$ is true; then, the chance that the combined P-value is $\leq \alpha$ when computed from $\left(\overline{P}_\Gamma, \overline{P}'_{\Gamma'}\right)$ is at most α.

5.1.7 Truncated Product Method of Combining P-values

We could combine $\left(\overline{P}_\Gamma, \overline{P}'_{\Gamma'}\right)$ using Fisher's method, as discussed in the previous subsection, but there is a better approach. In conventional problems, without sensitivity analysis, Fisher's method has some optimal properties in terms of Bahadur efficiency, but these optimal properties are shared with a large class of related methods [19], so these properties do not determine the best method of combination. In sensitivity analyses, $\overline{P}_\Gamma$ or $\overline{P}'_{\Gamma'}$ may be much larger than uniform; indeed, $\overline{P}_\Gamma \to 1$ as $\Gamma \to \infty$ and $\overline{P}'_{\Gamma'} \to 1$ as $\Gamma' \to \infty$, and for even sufficiently large but fixed Γ or Γ' this happens as the sample size increases to infinity. At times, we will let $\Gamma' \to \infty$ to ask: What information is provided by the first factor if the second factor is presumed to be utterly biased? Fisher's method pays for uniform P-values, so it often overpays with sensitivity bounds $\left(\overline{P}_\Gamma, \overline{P}'_{\Gamma'}\right)$ that are larger than the uniform.

The truncated product of P-values was proposed by Zaykin, Zhivotovsky, Westfall and Weir [305]. Where Fisher's method is the product of all P-values, $f(P, P') = P \times P'$, the truncated product statistic is the product of those P-values less than or

---

[1] In logic, for propositions A and B, the proposition $A \wedge B$ is read "A and B"; it denotes the new proposition asserting that A and B are both true. In parallel, the disjunction, $A \vee B$, is read "A or B" and denotes the new proposition asserting that either A or B or both are true.

Table 5.1 *Combining two or three P-values, (P_1, P_2) or (P_1, P_2, P_3), using the truncated product, with three truncation points, including Fisher's method that does not truncate with $\kappa = 1$. The three columns on the right give the three pooled P-values at different truncation points. The smallest P-value in each situation is in* **bold**

Situation	P_1	P_2		$\kappa = 1$	$\kappa = 0.2$	$\kappa = 0.1$
1	0.020	0.900		0.090	0.066	**0.046**
2	0.020	0.500		0.056	0.066	**0.046**
3	0.020	0.200		0.026	**0.020**	0.046
4	0.050	0.100		0.031	0.023	**0.017**
5	0.050	0.050		0.017	0.013	**0.010**
	P_1	P_2	P_3	$\kappa = 1$	$\kappa = 0.2$	$\kappa = 0.1$
6	0.003	0.900	0.900	0.061	0.039	**0.026**
7	0.003	0.500	0.900	0.040	0.039	**0.026**
8	0.030	0.100	0.900	0.066	0.039	**0.026**
9	0.050	0.100	0.900	0.095	0.054	**0.036**
10	0.050	0.050	0.900	0.058	0.035	**0.023**
11	0.040	0.210	0.210	**0.048**	0.181	0.125

equal to a threshold, κ, perhaps $\kappa = 0.1$ or $\kappa = 0.2$. For $\kappa = 1$, the truncated product equals Fisher's product. The truncated product is defined to be 1 if both P-values exceed κ. The truncated product statistic equals the product if both P-values are less than or equal to κ; otherwise, the truncated product statistic is larger than Fisher's product statistic. Because of this, the truncated product statistic is compared to a different null distribution; see Refs. [305] and [112, Expression (6)].[2] So, the resulting combined P-values from the truncated product can be larger or smaller than the combined P-values obtained by Fisher's method.

> **Truncated Product of P-values** Unlike Fisher's method, the truncated product focuses on smaller P-values, ignoring the large P-value bounds that may arise in a sensitivity analysis.

Generally, Fisher's method produces larger combined P-values when one P-value is large and the other is small, but Fisher's method produces smaller combined P-values when one P-value barely exceeds κ. With $\kappa = 0.1$, $P = 0.02$, and $P' = 0.9$, Fisher's method produces a combined P-value of 0.090, while the truncated product produces a P-value of 0.046. In contrast, with $\kappa = 0.1$, $P = 0.02$, and $P' = 0.11$, Fisher's method produces a combined P-value of 0.016, while the truncated product produces the same combined P-value of 0.046. With two or three P-values, Table 5.1 compares the combined P-values produced by Fisher's method and the truncated product. Other methods of combination are discussed in §7.4.

---

[2]In R, this is implemented in the `truncatedP` or `truncatedPbg` functions in the `sensitivitymv` package.

Large P-value bounds are common in sensitivity analyses. Simulation suggests that the truncated product has higher power in sensitivity analyses than does Fisher's method [112, Tables 2–3].

It is useful to compare the truncated product method with $\kappa = 0.1$ to the Simes [258] procedure for two independent P-values testing a global null hypothesis[3] at overall level $\alpha = 0.05$. The Simes procedure rejects if

$$\min \left(\overline{P}_\Gamma, \overline{P}'_{\Gamma'} \right) \leq \alpha/2 = 0.025 = 1/40 \qquad (5.2)$$

or if

$$\max \left(\overline{P}_\Gamma, \overline{P}'_{\Gamma'} \right) \leq \alpha = 0.05 = 1/20. \qquad (5.3)$$

The truncated product with $\kappa = 0.1$ rejects[4] if

$$\min \left(\overline{P}_\Gamma, \overline{P}'_{\Gamma'} \right) \leq 0.0222 = 1/45 \qquad (5.4)$$

or if

$$\max \left(\overline{P}_\Gamma, \overline{P}'_{\Gamma'} \right) \leq 0.1 = 1/10. \qquad (5.5)$$

So, the truncated product demands a tiny bit more in (5.4) than in (5.2) from the minimum P-value—that it be less than or equal to $1/45 = 0.0222$ rather than $1/40 = 0.025$—but it is much more lenient in (5.2) than in (5.3) about the maximum P-value—that it be less than or equal to $1/10$ rather than $1/20$. Under the global null hypothesis, two independent P-values are both less than or equal to $1/10$ with probability at most $1/100 = 1/10 \times 1/10$, and the truncated product suggests that this is evidence against the global null hypothesis.

5.1.8   What if $\overline{P}_\Gamma$ and $\overline{P}'_{\Gamma'}$ Are Both Small?

If $\left(\overline{P}_\Gamma, \overline{P}'_{\Gamma'} \right) = (0.05, 0.05)$, then the truncated product of P-values with $\kappa = 0.1$ produces a combined P-value bound of 0.011, so $H_\Gamma \wedge H'_{\Gamma'}$ is rejected at the conventional $\alpha = 0.05$ level. Can more be said? Indeed, it can. If we reject $H_\Gamma \wedge H'_{\Gamma'}$ at level α, ask: Can we test H_Γ and $H'_{\Gamma'}$, each at level α? Or, does conducting three tests increase the chance of at least one mistake to a level well above α? What follows is the simplest case of "closed testing" due to Marcus, Peritz, and Gabriel [151], in which component hypotheses are tested only if their conjunction is rejected. Closed testing will be described in greater detail in §6.1.

---

[3]When there are several component null hypotheses, the global null hypothesis is the null hypothesis that asserts that all of the component hypotheses are true.

[4]In R,

```
library(sensitivitymv)
truncatedP(c(1/45,1),trunc=.1)
0.05
truncatedP(c(.1,.1),trunc=.1)
0.028
```

> **Closed Testing Enhances a Joint Analysis by Also Examining its Components**
> The general method [151] called "closed testing" coordinates the testing of several
> hypotheses, each at level α, so the chance of falsely rejecting at least one true
> hypothesis is at most α. With two evidence factors, closed testing may examine
> both the joint P-value and its two components.

If $\left(\overline{P}_\Gamma, \overline{P}'_{\Gamma'}\right) = (0.05, 0.05)$, then $H_\Gamma \wedge H'_{\Gamma'}$, H_Γ and $H'_{\Gamma'}$ can all be rejected at the
conventional $\alpha = 0.05$ level, and the chance of at least one false rejection in three
tests is at most $\alpha = 0.05$, even though three tests have been done, each at the 0.05
level. That is, $\left(\overline{P}_\Gamma, \overline{P}'_{\Gamma'}\right) = (0.05, 0.05)$ leads to rejection at level $\alpha = 0.05$ of the
disjunction hypothesis $H_\Gamma \vee H'_{\Gamma'}$ that either H_Γ or $H'_{\Gamma'}$ is true. In other words, rejecting
$H_\Gamma \vee H'_{\Gamma'}$ says: (i) if the bias in the first factor is at most Γ, then no treatment effect
has been rejected by the first factor and we do not need the second factor; (ii) if the
bias in the second factor is at most Γ', then no treatment effect has been rejected by
the second factor and we do not need the first factor. That is a considerably stronger
statement than: "H_Γ has been rejected at level α."

5.1.9   Intersection-Union Tests

The disjunction hypothesis $H_\Gamma \vee H'_{\Gamma'}$ is also called a union hypothesis—it is true if
either subhypothesis is true—and an intersection-union test of $H_\Gamma \vee H'_{\Gamma'}$ rejects the
union hypothesis at level α if both P-values are at most α. If $H_\Gamma \vee H'_{\Gamma'}$ is true, the
chance that $H_\Gamma \vee H'_{\Gamma'}$ is falsely rejected in this way is at most α despite doing two
tests [16, 17, 138].

5.1.10   What If $\overline{P}'_{\Gamma'}$ Is Small, but $\overline{P}_\Gamma$ is Not?

The simple procedure with two factors will now be defined. It is a simple version of
closed testing [151]. The steps are as follows. Step 4 is the intersection-union test.

1. If the combined P-value from $\left(\overline{P}_\Gamma, \overline{P}'_{\Gamma'}\right)$ is at most α, then reject $H_\Gamma \wedge H'_{\Gamma'}$ and
   continue to step 2. Otherwise, stop, rejecting no hypothesis at level α.
2. If $\overline{P}_\Gamma \le \alpha$, then reject H_Γ.
3. If $\overline{P}'_{\Gamma'} \le \alpha$, then reject $H'_{\Gamma'}$.
4. If $\overline{P}_\Gamma \le \alpha$ and $\overline{P}'_{\Gamma'} \le \alpha$, then reject $H_\Gamma \vee H'_{\Gamma'}$.

For instance, if $\left(\overline{P}_\Gamma, \overline{P}'_{\Gamma'}\right) = (0.90, 0.02)$, then the truncated product with truncation $\kappa = 0.1$ produces a combined P-value bound of 0.046, so $H_\Gamma \wedge H'_{\Gamma'}$ is rejected
at level $\alpha = 0.05$ in step 1, and testing continues in step 2. As $\overline{P}_\Gamma = .90 > 0.05$,
the first factor does not reject in step 2: H_Γ is not rejected at level $\alpha = 0.05$. As
$\overline{P}'_{\Gamma'} = 0.02 < 0.05$, the second factor does reject in step 3: $H'_{\Gamma'}$ is rejected at level

$\alpha = 0.05$. As $\overline{P}_\Gamma = .90 > 0.05$, the union hypothesis $H_\Gamma \vee H'_{\Gamma'}$ is not rejected at $\alpha = 0.05$ in step 4.

What would have happened if Fisher's method had been used in place of the truncated product? If $\left(\overline{P}_\Gamma, \overline{P}'_{\Gamma'}\right) = (0.90, 0.02)$, then Fisher's method produces a combined P-value bound of 0.090, so $H_\Gamma \wedge H'_{\Gamma'}$ is not rejected at level $\alpha = 0.05$ in step 1, and no hypothesis is rejected by steps 1–4. See again situations 1–5 in Table 5.1 for the situations in which various methods reject $H_\Gamma \wedge H'_{\Gamma'}$ in step 1.

It is easy to see [151] that the probability that steps 1–4 reject at least one true hypothesis is at most α.[5] This is true despite testing several hypotheses, each at level α.

If both factors are insensitive, closed testing never alters this. More precisely, if $\left(\overline{P}_\Gamma, \overline{P}'_{\Gamma'}\right) \leq (0.05, 0.05)$, then the truncated product with truncation $\kappa \geq 0.05$ leads to rejection of $H_\Gamma \wedge H'_{\Gamma'}$ at level 0.05; so, step 2 of closed testing rejects H_Γ at level 0.05, step 3 rejects $H'_{\Gamma'}$ at level 0.05, and step 4 rejects $H_\Gamma \vee H'_{\Gamma'}$ at level 0.05.

Evidence factors and closed testing If both factors are insensitive to bias, closed testing never alters this conclusion. It may add that the two factors are jointly insensitive to larger biases that would invalidate either factor on its own.

When H_Γ and $H'_{\Gamma'}$ are both substantially false, the power in step 1 will often exceed the power in step 2 or step 3 alone.[6] Steps 2 and 3 apply the usual standard to test H_Γ and $H'_{\Gamma'}$. Rejection of $H_\Gamma \vee H'_{\Gamma'}$ in step 4 is a stronger statement than rejecting either hypothesis alone. There is some loss of power in step 1 if one hypothesis, H_Γ or $H'_{\Gamma'}$, is true and the other is false, but the loss is often tolerable when the combined test uses the truncated product with a fairly small κ.

5.2   Antineoplastic Drugs and DNA Damage

5.2.1   Two Factors: Worker-Control; Workers With or Without Ventilation

Recall the study in §4.2 by Kopjar and Garaj-Vrhovac [131] of possible DNA damage from handling drugs used to treat cancer. Figure 4.4 depicted the tail moment of the comet assay in health care workers exposed to antineoplastic drugs. There were two factors: (i) a comparison of workers and unexposed controls, and (ii) a comparison of

---

[5]Consider the possible cases, one at a time. If H_Γ and $H'_{\Gamma'}$ are both false—that is, if $H_\Gamma \vee H'_{\Gamma'}$ is false— then there is nothing to prove: there is no true hypothesis to reject. If $H_\Gamma \wedge H'_{\Gamma'}$ is true, then the probability of rejecting it in step 1 is at most α, and unless $H_\Gamma \wedge H'_{\Gamma'}$ is rejected in step 1 no hypothesis is rejected. So, suppose $H_\Gamma \wedge H'_{\Gamma'}$ is false. Then step 1 cannot reject a true hypothesis. Two cases remain. If $H_\Gamma \wedge H'_{\Gamma'}$ is false but $H_\Gamma \vee H'_{\Gamma'}$ is true, then exactly one of H_Γ or $H'_{\Gamma'}$ is true; suppose H_Γ is true. Then false rejection of a true hypothesis occurs in steps 2 and 4 if and only if $\overline{P}_\Gamma \leq \alpha$, which happens with probability at most α if H_Γ is true. The remaining case, with H_Γ false and $H'_{\Gamma'}$ true is analogous.

[6]More precisely, when H_Γ and $H'_{\Gamma'}$ are both false, the Bahadur efficiency of the joint test will exceed the Bahadur efficiency of each component test [19].

workers with and without ventilation from a laminar hood. In both factors, greater exposure predicted greater indications of DNA damage in the tail moment of the comet assay. How sensitive are the two comparisons to bias from nonrandomized treatment assignment?

The answer is in Table 5.2. The table gives the sensitivity bounds $\left(\overline{P}_{\Gamma}, \overline{P}'_{\Gamma'}\right)$ for the two factors separately; then, in the interior of the table, combines the bounds using the truncated product with truncation at $\kappa = 0.1$. For both factors in Table 5.2, the test statistic is Wilcoxon's rank sum with its associated sensitivity analysis [225].

Table 5.2 *Evidence factors for antineoplastic drugs and DNA damage. The interior of the table is the combined P-value from the truncated product with Truncation at $\kappa = 0.1$. The largest P-value ≤ 0.05 in a row and column is in* ***bold***

Factor 2 With/Without Ventilation		Factor 1: Worker-versus-Control Γ						
		1	10	25	50	125	150	∞
					$\overline{P}_{\Gamma}$			
Γ'	$\overline{P}'_{\Gamma'}$	0.000	0.001	0.008	**0.029**	0.094	0.112	1.000
∞	1.000	0.000	0.004	**0.024**	0.062	0.179	1.000	1.000
5	0.117	0.000	0.004	0.024	0.062	0.179	1.000	1.000
4	0.074	0.000	0.000	0.003	0.009	**0.022**	0.143	0.143
3	**0.037**	0.000	0.000	0.002	0.005	0.013	0.076	0.076
2	0.011	0.000	0.000	0.001	0.002	0.005	0.030	**0.030**
1	0.001	0.000	0.000	0.000	0.000	0.001	0.004	0.004

Consider factor 1 alone. The first factor is insensitive to enormous unmeasured biases. At $\Gamma = 50$, the bound on the *P*-value is $\overline{P}_{\Gamma} = 0.029$. If instead of randomization, $\Gamma = 1$, people could differ by a factor of $\Gamma = 50$ in their odds of becoming a worker rather than a control, then the maximum possible *P*-value for testing no effect is $\overline{P}_{\Gamma} = 0.029$. For comparison, the association between heavy smoking and lung cancer in one well-known study [94] is sensitive to a bias of $\Gamma = 6$; see Ref. [195, Table 4.1].

Consider factor 2 alone. The second factor is insensitive to large unmeasured biases. At $\Gamma = 3$, the bound on the *P*-value is $\overline{P}'_{\Gamma'} = 0.037$.

The two factors provide separate information, as if they came from unrelated studies. The combined analysis is insensitive to larger biases than either component. The combined *P*-value from $\left(\overline{P}_{\Gamma}, \overline{P}'_{\Gamma'}\right)$ is 0.022 at $(\Gamma, \Gamma') = (125, 4)$.

Infinite bias affecting either factor leaves its counterpart providing strong evidence against the hypothesis of no effect. At $(\Gamma, \Gamma') = (\infty, 2)$, the joint *P*-value is 0.030, and at $(\Gamma, \Gamma') = (25, \infty)$, the joint *P*-value is 0.024.

If we adjust by closed testing for testing several hypotheses, the component hypotheses are not diminished. Closed testing rejects both component hypotheses, H_{Γ} and $H'_{\Gamma'}$, and their union $H_{\Gamma} \vee H'_{\Gamma'}$, at the $\alpha = 0.05$ level for $(\Gamma, \Gamma') = (50, 3)$.

5.2.2   Two Factors, with Adjustments for Age

In Figure 4.5, the comet assay found higher levels of DNA damage at older ages. Could this explain away the pattern in Figure 4.4? The stratified analysis that follows makes the comparisons in Figure 4.4 within each of three age strata, as depicted in Figures 4.6 and 4.7.

The sample sizes become small inside individual strata; so, it is important to combine evidence over strata. Here, this will be done with a traditional test due to Hodges and Lehmann [103, 140, §3.3] called the aligned rank test. The aligned rank test subtracts the median value of the outcome, the tail moment, within each of the three age strata, then ranks these aligned responses for $N = 59 = 20 + 20 + 19$ individuals from 1 to $N = 59$, with average ranks for ties. The resulting ranks are called aligned ranks. When comparing two groups, the aligned rank statistic is the sum of the aligned ranks belonging to the first group. The statistic is compared to a permutation distribution that permutes individuals within the same stratum. When applied to matched pairs, the aligned rank test is almost the same as Wilcoxon's signed rank test [103]. See Ref. [157] for a comparison of the aligned rank test and various competing tests. Sensitivity bounds for the aligned rank test and other stratified tests are discussed in Ref. [221].[7]

Table 5.3 *Evidence factor analysis for antineoplastic drugs and DNA damage, adjusting for age strata. The analysis uses the aligned rank test of Hodges and Lehmann [103]*

Factor 2 With/Without Ventilation		Factor 1: Worker-versus-Control				Γ
		1	20	35	60	∞
Γ'	$\bar{P}_{\Gamma'}$			$\bar{P}_\Gamma$		
		0.000	0.018	**0.049**	0.100	1.000
∞	0.148	0.000	**0.042**	0.098	0.189	1.000
4	0.100	0.000	0.008	0.017	**0.028**	0.190
2.75	**0.045**	0.000	0.004	0.010	0.016	0.092
2	0.020	0.000	0.002	0.005	0.009	**0.046**
1	0.002	0.000	0.000	0.001	0.001	0.009

Table 5.3 shows the resulting analysis. The qualitative sense here is similar to Table 5.2, but somewhat smaller unmeasured biases could produce the patterns in Table 5.3. Nonetheless, (i) the joint test is insensitive to a larger bias, $(\Gamma, \Gamma') = (60, 4)$, than its separate components, $\Gamma = 35$ and $\Gamma' = 2.75$; (ii) even infinite biases affecting either factor alone leave rejection of H_0 insensitive to fairly large biases in the remaining factor; (iii) as always, closed testing leaves insensitive findings undiminished, rejecting H_Γ, $H'_{\Gamma'}$ and the union hypothesis, $H_\Gamma \vee H'_{\Gamma'}$ at the $\alpha = 0.05$ level for $(\Gamma, \Gamma') = (35, 2.75)$.

In this example, an adjustment for age did not greatly alter the conclusions obtained without an adjustment for age, but rejection of the hypothesis of no effect became sensitive to somewhat smaller unmeasured biases. Does this always

---

[7]The sensitivity analysis is implemented in the R package senstrat.

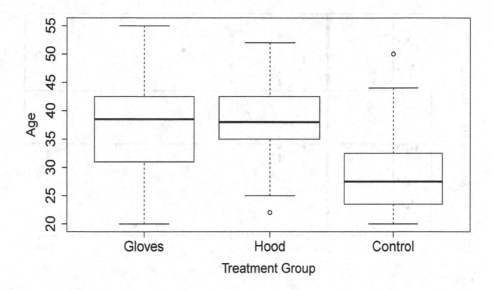

Figure 5.1 *Age distribution in three treatment groups for antineoplastic drugs and DNA damage.*

happen? It does not. Figure 4.5 showed that age predicts the level of DNA damage. Figure 5.1 shows that the controls are distinctly younger than the workers, although the two groups of workers had similar ages. No surprise then: adjustment for age had a larger impact on factor 1, worker-versus-control, than on factor 2, with-or-without ventilation.

We can look at Figures 4.5 and 5.1 because age was measured. Had age not been measured, there would be no way to see from Figure 5.1 that factor 1 is biased by age, but factor 2 is not.

5.3   Smoking and Periodontal Disease

5.3.1   *Two Factors: Smoker/Control and the Dose of Cigarettes*

Recall the example in §4.1 linking cigarette smoking and periodontal disease, and in particular the two factors in Figure 4.2. Panel (a) of Figure 4.2 depicted 441 smoker-minus-control pair differences in a measure of periodontal disease, with positive differences being more common than negative differences. Panel (b) of Figure 4.2 plotted these same 441 pair differences against the number of cigarettes smoked per day by the smoker in each pair. In panel (b), the smoker-minus-control difference tended to be larger in pairs in which the smoker smoked more. Here, the simple evidence factor analysis is performed for Figure 4.2.

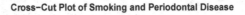

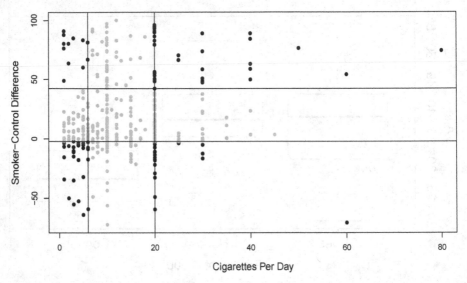

Figure 5.2 *Pair differences in periodontal disease plotted against cigarettes-per-day for the smoker in each pair. The plot is cut at the outer 20%.*

The analysis of Figure 4.2(a) uses the U-statistic discussed in §2.4 that generalizes Wilcoxon's signed rank statistic [208, 262]. Wilcoxon's statistic judges Figure 4.2(a) to become sensitive to unmeasured bias at about $\Gamma = 2.75$, where the one-sided P-value is 0.047 and the one-sided 95% confidence interval for an additive effect is $\tau \geq 0.00$. As predicted by its superior design sensitivity [208, Table 3], at the same $\Gamma = 2.75$, the U-statistic $(8,7,8)$ has a one-sided P-value of 0.000083 and confidence interval $\tau \geq 5.4$. The U-statistic $(8,7,8)$ judges Figure 4.2(a) to become sensitive to a much larger unobserved bias of $\Gamma = 4.35$, where the P-value is 0.049 and the confidence interval is $\tau \geq 0.04$.

Figure 5.2 cuts Figure 4.2(b) at the outer 20% or outer quintiles, and Table 5.4 counts the points in the outer corners of Figure 5.2. The analysis is comparing smokers who smoke at least a pack-a-day (≥ 20 cigarettes) to smokers who smoke less than a third of that (≤ 6). The odds ratio in Table 5.4 is $3.65 = (28 \times 36) / (23 \times 12)$. In a randomized experiment, the crosscut test [218] compares Table 5.4 to the hypergeometric distribution, yielding a one-sided P-value of 0.0022. The crosscut test is a generalization of the corner test of Olmstead and Tukey [167]. The crosscut test is so-named because it cuts a cross from a scatterplot. The sensitivity analysis for the crosscut test [218] compares Table 5.4 to the extended hypergeometric distribution with parameter Γ'. In large samples, the crosscut test will often exhibit insensitivity to unmeasured bias even with a modest correlation between dose and response, because it focuses on the outer corners where both the dose difference and the response difference are extreme.[8]

The crosscut analysis of Figure 5.2 becomes sensitive to unmeasured bias at about $\Gamma' = 1.6$ with a one-sided P-value of 0.044. Had we cut at the outer 33.3% rather than the outer 20%, we would have compared ≥ 15 cigarettes to ≤ 10 cigarettes, so more people would have entered into the test, but even in a randomized trial ($\Gamma' = 1$) the one-sided P-value is 0.058.

Table 5.4 *Crosscut counts for smoking and periodontal disease. Cutting at the outer 20%, the counts relate the pair difference, smoker-minus-control, in periodontal disease to the number of cigarettes smoked per day by the smoker in a matched pair*

	Periodontal Disease		Total
Cigarettes	≤ -2.2	≥ 42.3	
≤ 6	28	12	40
≥ 20	23	36	59
Total	51	48	99

Table 5.5 combines the two sensitivity analyses into one. The two separate analyses each barely reject at $\alpha = 0.05$ the hypothesis H_0 of no effect at $(\Gamma, \Gamma') = (4.35, 1.6)$, but the pooled analysis rejects H_0 at $(\Gamma, \Gamma') = (4.7, 1.9)$. Rejection of H_0 is insensitive to $(\Gamma, \Gamma') = (\infty, 1.4)$ and to $(\Gamma, \Gamma') = (4, \infty)$; that is, rejection of H_0 would occur even if either factor were invalidated by infinitely large biases. The separate analyses are undiminished by correction for multiple testing: at $(\Gamma, \Gamma') = (4.35, 1.6)$, closed testing rejects H_Γ, $H'_{\Gamma'}$ and the union hypothesis, $H_\Gamma \vee H'_{\Gamma'}$ while controlling the family-wise error rate at $\alpha = 0.05$.

5.3.2   Two Factors, with Repeated Adjustments for Age and Gender

The analysis in Table 5.5 controls for age, gender and other covariates by matching smokers to similar controls. So, the analysis in Table 5.5 has adjusted for age and gender once. Should one adjust twice? If yes, how?

Younger male smokers tend to smoke somewhat more cigarettes (median 13 cigarettes) than older male smokers (10), younger female smokers (10), or older female smokers (10), a difference judged too large to be due to chance by the Kruskal-Wallis test [110, 140], with P-value 0.023.

Table 5.5 permuted doses—cigarettes per day—among 441 smoker/control pairs in all 441! ways, but perhaps that was not reasonable. Perhaps the doses should have been permuted within strata defined by age and gender, but not across such strata. Table 5.6 stratifies the pairs by the average age in the pair and by gender,[9] thereby permuting doses within but not across strata.

---

[8]More precisely, the crosscut test often has a large design sensitivity $\tilde{\Gamma}'$. For instance, with bivariate Normal dose and response, cutting at the outer 20%, a correlation of 0.2 yields a design sensitivity of $\tilde{\Gamma}' = 5.0$, while a correlation of 0.4 yields a design sensitivity of $\tilde{\Gamma}' = 32.1$; see Ref. [218, Table 3]. To understand this, it helps to imagine cutting the elliptical shape of the bivariate Normal at the outer quintiles.

[9]Eight of 441 pairs are not exactly matched for gender, and are grouped with the female-female pairs.

Table 5.5 *Evidence factor analysis for smoking and periodontal disease. Factor 1 uses the U-statistic applied to smoker-minus-control pair differences. Factor 2 uses the crosscut statistic. The interior of the table reports P-values combined using the truncated product, with truncation 0.1. The largest P-value ≤ 0.05 in a row and column is in* **bold**

Factor 2		Factor 1: Smoker-versus-Control Γ				
Dose of		1	4	4.35	4.7	∞
Cigarettes				$\overline{P}_\Gamma$		
Γ'	$\overline{P}_{\Gamma'}$	0.000	0.021	**0.049**	0.094	1.000
∞	1.000	0.000	**0.048**	0.097	0.180	1.000
2	0.122	0.000	0.048	0.097	0.180	1.000
1.9	0.099	0.000	0.009	0.017	**0.027**	0.188
1.6	**0.044**	0.000	0.005	0.009	0.015	0.090
1.4	0.021	0.000	0.003	0.005	0.009	**0.048**
1	0.002	0.000	0.000	0.001	0.001	0.009

A stratified crosscut test performs a sensitivity analysis [233] for the exact version [23] of the Mantel-Haenszel test [150], as applied to the $2 \times 2 \times 4$ contingency table in Table 5.6.[10] The Mantel-Haenszel test views a $2 \times 2 \times k$ contingency table as k independent hypergeometric variables, and it takes as its test statistic the total of the k counts in the upper left corners of the k tables, or $12 + 8 + 5 + 5 = 30$. The Mantel-Haenszel test, when applied in a randomized experiment, is a randomization test; indeed, for $k = 1$ it is Fisher's test for a 2×2 table. Because the hypergeometric distribution entails fixed marginal totals for each of the k tables, it does not matter which corner—here, the upper left corner—is used to define the test statistic, as any corner determines the entire table. The sensitivity analysis [233] compares the same test statistic to the convolution of extended hypergeometric random variables with parameter Γ'.

The stratified comparison in Table 5.6 is somewhat less sensitive to unmeasured bias than the unstratified comparison in Table 5.4. Table 5.7 compares the unstratified and stratified crosscut analyses; then, it combines the stratified crosscut analysis with the unchanged smoker/control analysis. In Table 5.7, the unstratified crosscut test yields a P-value bound of 0.044 at $\Gamma' = 1.6$, as before, but the stratified crosscut test yields a bound of 0.041 at $\Gamma' = 2$.

Using the stratified crosscut test, the joint analysis of both factors is insensitive to larger biases than the analysis in Table 5.5. In Table 5.7, the combined P-value is 0.030 at $(\Gamma, \Gamma') = (4.7, 2.4)$.

Why is the stratified crosscut test insensitive to larger biases than the unstratified crosscut test? Does this always happen? It does not. In §5.2, an adjustment for age led to increased sensitivity to unmeasured biases, whereas in Table 5.7 an adjustment for age and gender led to increased insensitivity to unmeasured biases. Can this be understood? It can. Many considerations affect the sensitivity to unmeasured biases [198, 223, Part III]. If bias due to an observed covariate has strengthened an

---

[10] In R, use the mh function in the `sensitivity2x2xk` package.

Table 5.6 *Stratified crosscut counts for smoking and periodontal disease. Cutting at the outer 20%, the counts relate the pair difference, smoker-minus-control, in periodontal disease to the number of cigarettes smoked per day by the smoker in a matched pair*

Cigarettes	Periodontal Disease		Total
	Female, $30 \leq Age \leq 55$		
	≤ -3.7	≥ 16.8	Total
≤ 5.6	12	2	14
≥ 20	5	13	18
Total	17	15	32
	Male, $30 \leq Age \leq 55$		
	≤ -1.7	≥ 42.7	Total
≤ 7	8	7	15
≥ 20	12	18	30
Total	20	25	45
	Female, $55 < Age \leq 80$		
	≤ 0.0	≥ 38.8	Total
≤ 5	5	0	5
≥ 20	3	5	8
Total	8	5	13
	Male, $55 < Age \leq 80$		
	$\leq -.9$	≥ 76.0	Total
≤ 5	5	2	7
≥ 20	3	5	8
Total	8	7	15

Table 5.7 *Stratified crosscut analysis for smoking and periodontal disease, and its combination with the unchanged smoker/control comparison that used the U-statistic. Combined P-values use the truncated product with truncation point 0.1. For comparison, the unstratified crosscut analysis from Table 5.5 is also included in the first column*

	Factor 2: Dose Cigarettes Per Day		Combined with Factor 1: Smoker/Control	
Γ'	Unstratified	Stratified	$\Gamma = 4.35$	$\Gamma = 4.7$
1.6	0.044	0.011	0.004	0.006
2	0.122	0.041	0.011	0.019
2.4	0.233	0.098	0.018	0.030

association between treatment and outcome, as appears to be the case in Figures 4.5 and 5.1, then adjustment for that covariate may weaken the observed association so that it can be explained by somewhat smaller biases. However, the opposite could have happened: bias from an observed covariate could have masked the association between treatment and outcome, so that adjustment for the observed covariate makes the association stronger, and hence insensitive to larger unmeasured biases. Additionally, adjustments for observed covariates can also remove sampling noise, and this too can result in insensitivity to larger unmeasured biases [200]. Finally, the magnitude of an effect may change with the level of an observed covariate—that is, there may be effect modification—and this too has consequences for sensitivity to unmeasured biases [112, 113, 136, 137]. Several of the odds ratios in Table 5.6 are quite large compared to Table 5.4; for instance, for younger women, the odds ratio is $15.6 = (12 \times 13)/(5 \times 2)$, much larger than 3.6 in Table 5.4.

5.4   Factors that Do Not Concur

5.4.1   Failure to Concur Comes in Two Forms

In an observational study, a null hypothesis of no treatment effect cannot be tested in isolation. Rather, the null hypothesis always entails both a claim about the treatment effect and a claim about the unmeasured biases that are present. In this chapter, the null hypothesis asserted that there is no treatment effect, and the biases affecting the two factors are at most (Γ, Γ'). Then, the magnitude, (Γ, Γ'), of unmeasured bias was varied to display the sensitivity of inferences to assumptions about unmeasured biases.

There are two very different ways two evidence factors may fail to concur: they may disagree, or one factor may fail to support the other. To speak simply about this, imagine that a treatment is of benefit if it reduces a particular outcome, and it is harmful if it increases that outcome. In §4.2, exposure to antineoplastic drugs is harmful if it increases DNA damage, as measured by the comet assay. Two factors manipulate the level of exposure: (i) working or not working with such drugs, (ii) the presence or absence of a ventilated hood for those who work with the drugs.

Two factors disagree if one factor is confident that there is benefit while the other is confident that there is harm. This should be a source of concern. In §4.2, the two factors agree, but they would have disagreed if working with antineoplastic drugs appeared harmful, but the absence of ventilation appeared beneficial. Such a dissonant finding would create a puzzle, an inconsistency, that would block any straightforward claim about the effects of the treatment: a compelling explanation would be required before setting aside such a glaring inconsistency.[11] Two factors disagree if each factor rejects the null hypothesis of no treatment effect at level α in the presence of a bias of (Γ, Γ'), but one factor rejects H_0 in the direction of benefit, while the other rejects H_0 in the direction of harm. Such a dissonant finding suggests the biases in treatment assignment are larger than the specified (Γ, Γ') for at least one of the factors [184, 186, 300]. For this reason, outright disagreement is a source of concern.

Factor two fails to support factor one if factor one rejects the null hypothesis at level α, but factor two does not. Failure to reject H_0 is not evidence that H_0 is true; rather, it is better described as failure to provide material evidence that H_0 is false.

---

[11] And yet, Aristotle writes, in Irwin's translation: "The solution of a puzzle is a discovery" [121, p. 120, 1146b5]. Irwin's glossary (p. axia) indicates that "puzzle" is Aristotle's "aporia," so that, consistent with Irwin's commentary [120], this might alternatively be expressed: "The resolution of an inconsistency is a discovery." Compare this with resolving an inconsistency in a crossword puzzle, such as Figure 3.2, by recognizing that one tentative entry is actually mistaken.

Here, the second factor does not contradict the first, but it fails to strengthen it. This may be a disappointment, but it is not, by itself, grounds for concern.

5.4.2 Benzene and Chromosome Aberrations Among Shoe Workers

Recall the study in §4.5 by Tunca and Egeli [275] of chromosome aberrations in lymphocytes among shoe workers exposed to benzene. In Figure 4.13, the first factor indicated higher levels of chromosome aberrations among shoe workers than among unexposed controls, while the second factor showed no relationship with years of exposure to benzene. In thinking about the relationship between chromosome aberrations and years of exposure to benzene, one needs to remember that some lymphocytes live for long periods, but many others are short-lived [272]. Possibly, damage to the chromosomes of a short-lived cell reflects only recent exposure to toxins.

Consider the second evidence factor, the association in the right panel of Figure 4.13. In a one-sided test of no association against positive association in the right panel of Figure 4.13, the P-value from Kendall's correlation is 0.386. The P-value from the crosscut test is also large, 0.590, at $\Gamma' = 1$. The truncated product of P-values does not distinguish these P-values when truncating at $\kappa = 0.1$. Indeed, as $\Gamma' \to \infty$, the upper bound on the P-value from the second factor in Figure 4.13 goes to 1, but with truncation at $\kappa = 0.1$, the P-bound for the pooled analysis based on the truncated product remains unchanged: all P-values above $\kappa = 0.1$ are essentially the same.

Still, the left panel of Figure 4.13, the first evidence factor, is not easily ignored. Using five-year age strata together with the Hodges-Lehmann aligned rank test [103, 140, 157], yields an upper bound on the one-sided P-value of 0.003627 at $\Gamma = 10$; see Ref. [221]. In a matched pair, a bias of $\Gamma = 10$ is about the same as an unobserved covariate that increases the odds of being a shoe worker by 20-fold and also increases the odds of a positive pair difference in chromosome aberrations by 20-fold [231, 234, Table 9.1]. Combining the two P-values, 0.003627 and 0.590, using the truncated product, truncating at 0.1, yields a combined P-value of 0.0138. So, the hypothesis of no effect is rejected at level $\alpha = 0.05$ for $(\Gamma, \Gamma') = (10, 1)$, and closed testing attributes the rejection to the first factor, with no support from the second. At $(\Gamma, \Gamma') = (10, \infty)$, the combined P-value is still 0.0138, owing to truncation at $\kappa = 0.1$. A price was paid for testing two hypotheses—at $(\Gamma, \Gamma') = (10, 1)$ or $(\Gamma, \Gamma') = (10, \infty)$, the P-value from the truncated product is 0.0138, rather than 0.003627 from the first factor alone—however, this price is not exorbitant, so the combined evidence from both factors is fairly strong.

Similar issues arise when testing hypotheses other than no effect, and when inverting such tests to obtain confidence intervals. The two factors may or may not concur about other hypotheses. These issues are discussed further in §6.2.

5.5 Summary: Strengthen Evidence of Cause and Effect

Two examples illustrated simple analyses with two evidence factors. In each example, the combined analysis using both factors was insensitive to larger unmeasured biases than were separate analyses for one factor or the other. In each example, an infinite bias affecting one factor would not invalidate the conclusion: both factors would have to be biased to a nontrivial degree and in different ways to invalidate the conclusion.

The simple analyses in the current chapter had several distinguishing features that made them simple.

- There were two factors, not three or more factors, as in §4.3. Closed testing with three factors is a bit more elaborate, though in most other respects a third factor entails only obvious alterations to the analysis with two factors. Inference with three or more evidence factors is discussed in §6.1.

- In the current chapter, the hypothesis of no treatment effect has been the focus of attention. Confidence intervals are often essential. In many contexts, "no effect" is only one important hypothesis among other important hypotheses. Figure 4.11 gives the striking appearance of an absence of harm from raising the minimum wage—a striking absence of effect—and the pressing question is whether or not that appearance is firmly established or potentially misleading. For this, confidence intervals or equivalence intervals are needed; see §6.2.

- No analysis was considered besides the analysis of the two evidence factors. At times, there is an equally important analysis that cannot be a factor in a pair of evidence factors. Typically, such an analysis draws some information from both factors. The incorporation of such an analysis is discussed in §6.3.

Chapter 6 considers planned analyses that are no longer simple in these specific ways.

5.6 Using R

5.6.1 Antineoplastic Drugs and DNA Damage

Some of the analyses from §5.2 are reproduced here; see also §4.7. The data [131] in §5.2 are available in the evident package as antineoplastic. The analysis uses the sen2sample function [225] in the senstrat package [221] package. Specifically, some of the results in Table 5.2 are reproduced. Consider, first, $\Gamma = 50$ for the first factor and $\Gamma' = 3$ for the second factor.

```
library(evident)
data(antineoplastic)
attach(antineoplastic)
library(senstrat)
sen2sample(rank(tailmoment),z1,gamma=50)
$pval
[1] 0.02864
sen2sample(rank(tailmoment[f2]),z2[f2],gamma=3)
$pval
[1] 0.03693
```

Table 5.2 combines the two *P*-values for the two factors using the truncated product of *P*-values [305] truncating at $\kappa = 0.1$. The `truncatedP` function is in the `sensitivitymv` package. At $\Gamma = 50$ for the first factor and $\Gamma' = 3$ for the second factor, the combined *P*-value in Table 5.2 is 0.005, computed as follows.

```
library(senstivitymv)
truncatedP(c(0.02864,0.03693),trunc=0.1)
0.00533757
```

Repeating this calculation at $\Gamma = 125$ for the first factor and $\Gamma' = 4$ for the second factor, the combined *P*-value in Table 5.2 is 0.022:

```
sen2sample(rank(tailmoment),z1,gamma=125)
$pval
[1] 0.09375
sen2sample(rank(tailmoment[f2]),z2[f2],gamma=4)
$pval
[1] 0.07398
truncatedP(c(0.09375,0.07398),trunc=0.1)
0.02195759
```

5.6.2 Periodontal Disease and Smoking

The calculations that follow illustrate some of the analyses in §5.3.

```
library(evident)
data(periodontal)
attach(periodontal)
library(DOS2)
y=pcteither[z==1]-pcteither[z==0]
```

Using Wilcoxon's signed rank statistic, rejection of the hypothesis of no effect is insensitive to a bias of $\Gamma = 2.75$:

```
senWilcox(y,gamma=2.75,conf.int=TRUE)
$pval
[1] 0.04652
```

As discussed in §2.4, Wilcoxon's statistic tends to exaggerate the degree of sensitivity to unmeasured bias, whereas other statistics do not. As anticipated by its design sensitivity [208], the U-statistic $(8,7,8)$ reports greater insensitivity to unmeasured bias. Specifically, using this statistic, rejection of the hypothesis of no effect is insensitive to a bias of $\Gamma = 4.35$, not $\Gamma = 2.75$:

```
senU(y,gamma=4.35,m=8,m1=7,m2=8)
```

```
$pval
[1] 0.04851
```

Where Wilcoxon's statistic thinks no effect is almost plausible at $\Gamma = 2.75$, the U-statistic thinks that the P-value must be small and the effect far from zero if the bias is at most $\Gamma = 2.75$:

```
senU(y,gamma=2.75,m=8,m1=7,m2=8,conf.int=TRUE)
$pval
8.252912e-05
$estimate
low   high
8.961 Inf
$ci
low   high
5.403 Inf
```

The crosscut analysis in Figure 5.2 is insensitive to a bias of $\Gamma' = 1.6$:

```
x=cigsperday[z==1]
crosscut(x,y,ct=.2,gamma=1.6)
$output$pval
0.0443
```

Table 5.5 combines the two P-values, from the U-statistic and from the crosscut statistic, using the truncated product of P-values [305] truncating at 0.1. At $\Gamma = 4.35$ for the U-statistic and $\Gamma' = 1.6$ for the crosscut test, the combined P-value in Table 5.5 is 0.009:

```
library(sensitivitymv)
truncatedP(c(0.04850672,0.04433723),trunc=.1)
 0.009326983
```

At $\Gamma = 4.7$ for the U-statistic and $\Gamma' = 1.9$ for the crosscut test, the two P-value bounds are found as:

```
senU(y,gamma=4.7,m=8,m1=7,m2=8)
$pval
[1] 0.09419
crosscut(x,y,ct=.2,gamma=1.9)
$output$pval
0.09899
```

which combine to

```
library(sensitivitymv)
truncatedP(c(0.09419,0.09899),trunc=.1)
 0.02676
```

5.7 Exercises

Exercise 5.1. *This exercise continues Exercises 4.2 and 4.3 concerning recent hand-gun purchases and risk of suicide [86]. Apply Fisher's one-sided test to Tables 4.2 and 4.3, looking for a positive association between recent purchase of a handgun and death by suicide rather than death by another cause. Obtain two one-sided P-values and combine them using the truncated product of P-values. (In R, use* fisher.test *in the* stats *package and* truncatedP *in the* sensitivitymv *package.)*

Exercise 5.2. *Repeat Exercise 5.1, but do a one-sided test in the opposite direction. Use the Bonferroni inequality to combine the two combined one-sided P-values from the truncated product into a two-sided P-value. In principle, could the two factors reject the hypothesis of no effect in opposite directions? Should we regard the two factors as providing mutual support if they reject in opposite directions?*

Exercise 5.3. *Repeat Exercise 5.1, but do a sensitivity analysis for each factor. (In R, replace* fisher.test *by* mh *in the* sensitivity2x2xk *package.)*

Exercise 5.4. *Do Exercise 11.1 in Chapter 11 to verify that the analyses you did in Exercises 5.1 - 5.3 are valid.*

Exercise 5.5. *This exercise continues Exercise 4.1 concerning DNA damage from chromium exposure at a tannery [306]. Compare controls to workers in the tannery as one factor, and workers in the tannery department to workers in the finishing department as a second factor. For instance, consider using the* senmw *and* senmwCI *functions in the* sensitivitymv *package. Such an analysis is done in Ref. [217, §4.3].*[12] *See also Refs. [209] and [223, §20.2], where the choice of test statistic is shown to affect the reported sensitivity to unmeasured bias in this example.*

Exercise 5.6. *Do Exercise 11.2 in Chapter 11 to verify that the analysis you did in Exercise 5.5 is valid.*

---

[12]The tannery data is a dataframe in which each row is a block of three people, and this structure is used in the sensitivitymw package. If the data are a dataframe in which each row is one person, then the similar functions senm and senmCI in the sensitivitymult package will be more convenient.

Planned Analyses with Evidence Factors

Abstract

The simple evidence factor analyses in Chapter 5 may be a component in some larger analysis. As several hypotheses are tested, attention must be paid to controlling the probability of falsely rejecting at least one true hypothesis. Several cases are considered. First, there may be more than two evidence factors. Second, confidence sets or confidence intervals are often needed. Third, there may be useful analyses that do not fit within an evidence factor analysis.

6.1 Closed Testing with Three Factors

6.1.1 Three Factors in the Study of Lead in Children's Blood

Recall the study in §4.3 by Morton et al. [159] of fathers exposed to lead at work and the blood lead levels of their children. That study had three factors in Figure 4.8: (i) children of workers versus matched control children, (ii) the level of exposure of the exposed father, (iii) the hygiene upon leaving work of the subset of fathers with high exposure. Exposed fathers worked at a battery plant where lead was used in manufacture, while the parents of control children did not work in the factory. Control children were matched to exposed children for age and neighborhood of residence, with particular attention to sources of lead in the neighborhood. Figure 4.8 looked at exposed-minus-control pair differences in blood lead levels of children. In factor (i), most differences were positive. In factor (ii), the differences tended to be larger if the father had higher exposure. In factor (iii), if the father had high exposure, the child's lead level was higher if the father had poor hygiene.

How is the situation different with three factors, rather than the two factors in Chapter 5? Most aspects are analogous. The most noticeable change is that closed testing [151] with three null hypotheses is a bit more complex.

As formulated here, in §4.3 the three hypotheses are: (i) H_Γ asserting no treatment effect and a bias in the treatment control comparison of at most Γ, (ii) $H_{\Gamma'}'$ asserting no treatment effect and a bias in the high exposure versus other of at most Γ', (iii) $H_{\Gamma''}''$ asserting no treatment effect and a bias in the poor hygiene versus other of at most Γ''.

Obviously, one could formulate these hypotheses differently. In Figure 4.8, for example, $H_{\Gamma''}''$ does not distinguish 3 fathers with high exposure and good hygiene from 3 additional fathers with high exposure and moderate hygiene. The hypothesis might be formulated to make this distinction, despite the very small size of these two subgroups.

Suppose that H_Γ is tested using Wilcoxon's signed rank test applied to the 33 pairs in Factor 1 of Figure 4.8. Suppose that $H_{\Gamma'}'$ and $H_{\Gamma''}''$ are each tested using Wilcoxon's rank sum statistic to compare two subsets of the 33 pairs. Again, there are alternative tests and formulations, but the goal at the present moment is to illustrate closed testing with three hypotheses in a simple case.

6.1.2   Three Null Hypotheses in Closed Testing

A conjunction of several hypotheses is a new hypothesis that asserts that all of the component hypotheses are simultaneously true. The hypothesis $H_\Gamma \wedge H_{\Gamma'}'$ asserts that H_Γ and $H_{\Gamma'}'$ are both true. Also, the conjunction $H_\Gamma \wedge H_{\Gamma'}' \wedge H_{\Gamma''}''$ asserts that both $H_{\Gamma''}''$ and $H_\Gamma \wedge H_{\Gamma'}'$ are true, and so on. The implications under discussion are solely those that follow from logical conjunction—the logical "and" denoted $\wedge$. Sometimes hypotheses have additional, non-logical implications by virtue of what the hypotheses mean. For instance, the hypothesis that the moon can fit in a quart milk container is false, but it implies that the moon can fit in a gallon milk container; however, purely logical conjunction is not involved in this implication.[1] Implications that are not purely logical are important in hypothesis testing [18, 253]; however, such additional implications are not part of the aspect of closed testing currently under discussion.

Conjunction Hypotheses A conjunction of several component hypotheses is a new hypothesis that asserts all of the component hypotheses are true.

With three component hypotheses, H_Γ, $H_{\Gamma'}'$ and $H_{\Gamma''}''$, there are $2^3 - 1 = 7$ nontrivial hypotheses formed by conjunction, namely $H_\Gamma \wedge H_{\Gamma'}' \wedge H_{\Gamma''}''$, $H_\Gamma \wedge H_{\Gamma'}'$, $H_\Gamma \wedge H_{\Gamma''}''$, $H_{\Gamma'}' \wedge H_{\Gamma''}''$, H_Γ, $H_{\Gamma'}'$, and $H_{\Gamma''}''$. As noted, there are various purely logical implications among some of these hypotheses, implications that depend upon conjunction $\wedge$, not upon the meaning of the hypotheses. There is a valid P-value testing each of the hypotheses separately, so that, for instance, there is a P-value testing $H_{\Gamma'}' \wedge H_{\Gamma''}''$ and

---

[1] Shaffer [253] discusses a consequential statistical example arising in a one-way analysis of variance with three treatment groups having expectations μ_1, μ_2, μ_3. The three hypotheses $H_{12} : \mu_1 = \mu_2$, $H_{13} : \mu_1 = \mu_3$ and $H_{23} : \mu_2 = \mu_3$ are related by virtue of what they mean. All three hypotheses could be true. All three hypotheses could be false. Any one hypothesis, say H_{12}, could be true. However, there cannot be precisely two true hypotheses among these three hypotheses, because of what these hypotheses mean. You have to look inside the hypotheses to see what they assert to recognize this. If H_{12} and H_{13} are both true, then H_{23} must be true, because things that are equal to the same thing are equal to each other. If $H^* : \mu_1 = \mu_2 = \mu_3$ is false, then there is at most one true hypothesis among H_{12}, H_{13}, H_{23}. In light of this, Shaffer [253] proposes a method that is always more powerful than the Holm [111] procedure for testing H_{12}, H_{13}, H_{23}. The Holm procedure uses the Bonferroni inequality in closed testing, and it loses to Shaffer's procedure because it ignores what the hypotheses mean.

that P-value is less than or equal to α with probability at most α if $H'_{\Gamma'} \wedge H''_{\Gamma''}$ is true, for each $0 \leq \alpha \leq 1$.

With three component hypotheses, H_Γ, $H'_{\Gamma'}$ and $H''_{\Gamma''}$, closed testing [151] says: reject a conjunction hypothesis at level α if and only if the P-values for that hypothesis and all hypotheses that imply it are $\leq \alpha$. For example, one hypothesis implies $H'_{\Gamma'} \wedge H''_{\Gamma''}$, namely $H_\Gamma \wedge H'_{\Gamma'} \wedge H''_{\Gamma''}$. Therefore, reject $H'_{\Gamma'} \wedge H''_{\Gamma''}$ at level α if two P-values are $\leq \alpha$, namely the P-value for $H'_{\Gamma'} \wedge H''_{\Gamma''}$ and the P-value for $H_\Gamma \wedge H'_{\Gamma'} \wedge H''_{\Gamma''}$. To reject H_Γ, list the hypotheses that imply it—namely $H_\Gamma \wedge H'_{\Gamma'} \wedge H''_{\Gamma''}$, $H_\Gamma \wedge H'_{\Gamma'}$, $H_\Gamma \wedge H''_{\Gamma''}$ and of course trivially H_Γ, and check that all four P-values are $\leq \alpha$.

> **Closed Testing of Three or More Hypotheses** Closed testing of three or more hypotheses requires a few additional steps, but it follows the same logic as testing two hypotheses. With two hypotheses, there is one conjunction hypothesis, but with three or more hypotheses, there are several conjunction hypotheses.

The basic claim [151] about closed testing is that it strongly controls the family-wise error rate at α, despite doing many tests at level α. Formally, no matter which of the component hypotheses, H_Γ, $H'_{\Gamma'}$, and $H''_{\Gamma''}$, are true, the probability of falsely rejecting at least one true hypothesis is at most α.[2]

With evidence factors, the P-values for H_Γ, $H'_{\Gamma'}$, and $H''_{\Gamma''}$ may be combined using the truncated product method [305] to produce P-values for the seven conjunction hypotheses. For instance, the P-value for $H'_{\Gamma'} \wedge H''_{\Gamma''}$ is based on the truncated product of the two P-values for $H'_{\Gamma'}$ and $H''_{\Gamma''}$. In the current chapter, P-values combine with truncation point $\kappa = 0.1$; see [112, Tables 2–3].

6.1.3 Lead in Children from their Fathers' Exposures

Table 6.1 shows the combination of three factors in Figure 4.8 by closed testing and the truncated product of P-values.

The first row of Table 6.1 is the randomization test of no effect, with $\Gamma = \Gamma' = \Gamma''$. All seven P-values for the $2^3 - 1 = 7$ conjunction hypotheses are all less than or equal to 0.05, so all hypotheses of no effect are rejected at level $\alpha = 0.05$ if randomization tests are used.

The same conclusion is reached in the second row of Table 6.1, where potential biases may be substantial with $\Gamma = 4.3$, $\Gamma' = 1.75$, $\Gamma'' = 1.1$.

In the final row of Table 6.1, the biases are larger, $\Gamma = 5$, $\Gamma' = 2.4$, $\Gamma'' = 2.0$, but closed testing rejects at $\alpha = 0.05$ only two hypotheses, $H_\Gamma \wedge H'_{\Gamma'} \wedge H''_{\Gamma''}$ and $H_\Gamma \wedge H'_{\Gamma'}$.

---

[2]The proof of this is remarkably simple [151]. We do not know which hypotheses are true and which are false, but despite our ignorance, let H^* be the conjunction of all of the true hypotheses. For instance, if $H'_{\Gamma'}$ and $H''_{\Gamma''}$ were true but H_Γ were false, then $H^* = H'_{\Gamma'} \wedge H''_{\Gamma''}$. The key point is that the existence of H^* is all-important, and our ignorance of the identity of H^* is of no importance; no matter what H^* is, we have done the right thing. Although we have computed many P-values, only one P-value actually matters, the one for H^*. By the rules of closed testing, to reject at least one true hypothesis, the P-value for H^* must be $\leq \alpha$, and the chance that this occurs is at most α.

No component hypothesis—H_Γ, $H'_{\Gamma'}$ and $H''_{\Gamma''}$—is rejected. A bias of $\Gamma = 5, \Gamma' = 2.4$, $\Gamma'' = 2.0$ is too small to lead to acceptance of the hypothesis of no effect, but the evidence in support of rejection requires at least two factors.

The third and fourth row of Table 6.1 are intermediate situations. In the third row, every conjunction involving two or more hypotheses is rejected at $\alpha = 0.05$ by closed testing, as is H_Γ. In the fourth row, every conjunction involving two or more hypotheses is rejected, but no component—H_Γ, $H'_{\Gamma'}$ and $H''_{\Gamma''}$—is rejected.

There are two important points. About the lead data, in the final row of Table 6.1, the three factors together reject no effect in the presence of much larger biases than any one factor can resist. In general, a few more steps are required with three factors, but the analysis is analogous to the situation with two factors in Chapter 5.

Table 6.1 *Three evidence factors in the lead data, combined using closed testing and the truncated product with truncation 0.1*

Γ	Γ'	Γ''	H	H'	H''	$H \wedge H'$	$H \wedge H''$	$H' \wedge H''$	$H \wedge H' \wedge H''$
1.0	1.0	1.0	0.000	0.010	0.040	0.000	0.000	0.002	0.000
4.3	1.75	1.1	0.049	0.049	0.048	0.010	0.010	0.010	0.003
4.3	2.4	1.7	0.049	0.099	0.099	0.017	0.017	0.028	0.007
5.0	2.4	1.7	0.074	0.099	0.099	0.023	0.023	0.028	0.010
5.0	2.4	2.0	0.074	0.099	0.125	0.023	0.143	0.188	0.045

6.1.4   Closed Testing with Any Number of Hypotheses

Closed testing with more than three null hypotheses is essentially the same [151]. Let $H_1,\ldots,H_L$ be L component hypotheses. Form all $2^L - 1$ nontrivial conjunctions of the component hypotheses. Reject a conjunction hypothesis at level α if and only if that hypothesis and all conjunctions that imply it have P-values $\leq \alpha$. No matter which of the component hypotheses are true, the probability of falsely rejecting at least one true hypothesis is at most α.[3]

6.2   Confidence Intervals for Magnitudes of Effect

6.2.1   Hypotheses About Magnitudes of the Treatment Effect

Chapter 5 focused on testing the hypothesis of no treatment effect in the presence of biases of various magnitudes. This approach extends immediately to testing any hypothesized value, ϕ_0, for the $N \times (|G| - 1)$ treatment effects in §1.8. Any such hypothesis, if true, produces an adjusted response for which Fisher's hypothesis of no effect is true. This hypothesis about adjusted responses yields three additional hypotheses: (i) the null hypothesis, H_Γ, of no effect for factor 1 in the presence of a bias of at most Γ, (ii) the null hypothesis $H'_{\Gamma'}$ for no effect for factor 2 in the presence

---

[3]The proof is the same [151]. Let H^* be the conjunction of all of the true hypotheses. By the rules of closed testing, to reject at least one true hypothesis, the P-value for H^* must be $\leq \alpha$, and the chance that this occurs is at most α.

of a bias of at most Γ', and (iii) their conjunction, $H_\Gamma \wedge H_{\Gamma'}'$. In turn, upper bounds on P-values for these hypotheses are determined, $\overline{P}_\Gamma$, $\overline{P}_{\Gamma'}'$, and $\overline{P}_{\wedge,\Gamma,\Gamma'}$. Closed testing is then applied.

In the case of the Card and Krueger's [34] minimum wage study in §4.4, consider the effect of raising the minimum wage in New Jersey by $0.80 from $4.25 to $5.05. Whether in New Jersey or Pennsylvania, restaurant j had a starting wage $s_j \geq \$4.25$ before the wage increase, because $4.25 was the Federal minimum wage applicable to all US states. So, the wage increase in New Jersey forced the starting wage in New Jersey to increase by $\max(0, 5.05 - s_j)$, while not forcing an increase in the starting wage in Pennsylvania. Presumably, if $s_j = 5.04$ so $\max(0, 5.05 - s_j) = 0.01$ or one cent, then we expect a smaller impact than if $s_j = 4.25$ so $\max(0, 5.05 - s_j) = 0.80$.[4] The quantity $\max(0, 5.05 - s_j)/(5.05 - 4.25)$ is zero for a restaurant whose starting wage was above $5.05 before the increase, is 1 for a restaurant whose starting wage was $4.25 before the increase, and is 0.6034 for the average of the 132 New Jersey restaurants in Figure 4.10.

A simple model says that the change in employment, after-minus-before, is r_{Cj} in Pennsylvania, or $r_{Cj} + \beta \max(0, 5.05 - s_j)/(5.05 - 4.25)$ in New Jersey, so the change in employment is proportional to the mandated change in starting wages. Card and Krueger [34, Equation (1b)] used a closely related model. Stigler [263] argued that an increase in the minimum wage reduces employment, that $\beta < 0$. Under this parametric hypothesis, a fast food restaurant forced to increase wages by the full $0.80 would lose β employees as a consequence, so $H_0 : \beta = -1$ is the loss of one employee for a restaurant forced to increase wages by the full amount, $0.80. As 0.6034 is the mean of $\max(0, 5.05 - s_j)/(5.05 - 4.25)$ for the 132 New Jersey restaurants in Figure 4.10, the value $H_0 : \beta = -1/0.6034 = -1.657$ corresponds with a loss of one employee on average per restaurant. Each hypothesized value of β_0 for β defines a value of the $N \times (|G| - 1)$ matrix ϕ_0 of treatment effects.

Table 6.2 tests the hypothesis $H_0 : \beta = -1.657$ against two alternatives, $\beta > -1.657$ and $\beta < -1.657$. Table 6.2 considers a randomization inference, with $\Gamma = \Gamma' = 1$ and the possibility of a nontrivial unobserved bias, $\Gamma = \Gamma' = 1.25$. In a matched pair, a bias of $\Gamma = 1.25$ corresponds with an unobserved covariate that doubles the odds of treatment and doubles the odds of a positive pair difference in responses [231, 234, Table 9.1]. If $\beta > -1.657$, then the job loss is less than one employee per restaurant, on average, whereas if $\beta < -1.657$ then the job less is greater than one employee per restaurant, on average. The two factors in Figure 4.12 are the two factors in Table 6.2. The first factor compares New Jersey and Pennsylvania. The second factor compares restaurants in New Jersey with a high starting wage before the increase—i.e., restaurants not required to make substantial changes in wages—to restaurants with a low starting wage before the increase—i.e., restaurants required

---

[4]Could this be false? It could. Perhaps the Burger King, j, in a poor neighborhood in Trenton, NJ has $s_j = 4.25$, while the Burger King j' in wealthy Princeton, NJ has $s_{j'} = 5.05$, so before the wage increase, some workers take the bus from Trenton to Princeton to earn an extra $0.80. After the increase in the minimum wage, this arrangement is less attractive, so perhaps the Burger King in Princeton loses employees or must increase its starting wage.

to make a substantial increase in wages. The two factors are combined using the truncated product of P-values, truncating at $\kappa = 0.1$.

Table 6.2 *In the minimum wage example, testing the hypothesis $H_0 : \beta = -1.657$ against two alternative hypotheses, H_A, allowing for no bias or for $\Gamma = \Gamma' = 1.25$. Tabulated values are upper bounds on one-sided P-values*

Alternative Hypothesis	Factor 1 PA versus NJ	Factor 2 in NJ High versus Low	Pooled by the Truncated Product
	Randomization Inference, $\Gamma = \Gamma' = 1$		
$H_A : \beta < -1.657$	0.9968	0.6753	1.0000
$H_A : \beta > -1.657$	0.0032	0.3247	0.0126
	Nontrivial Bias, $\Gamma = \Gamma' = 1.25$		
$H_A : \beta < -1.657$	0.9997	0.8566	1.0000
$H_A : \beta > -1.657$	0.0214	0.5596	0.0486

In Table 6.2, the randomization test with $\Gamma = \Gamma' = 1$ rejects $H_0 : \beta = -1.657$ in favor of $H_A : \beta > -1.657$, suggesting that the decline in employment, if any, was not as large as one employee per restaurant on average. However, before considering Table 6.2 in detail, issues involving two-sided tests require brief discussion.

Concerning the minimum wage, the direction of the effect is a matter of dispute. In this case, one option is a two-sided test. A two-sided test is viewed as two one-sided tests with a Bonferroni correction for testing twice [49, 252], thereby permitting rejection of H_0 to be interpreted as having established a direction of departure from H_0. The two evidence factors for each one-sided test are pooled using the truncated product *before* the Bonferroni correction is applied, because we do not want the two factors to seem to concur if, in fact, they reject H_0 in opposite directions. The smaller of the two pooled P-values is compared to $\alpha/2$ for a two-sided level-α test. An alternative to the two-sided test is discussed later in §6.2.

In Table 6.2, there is no indication that $\beta < -1.657$, as $\overline{P}_\Gamma$, $\overline{P}'_{\Gamma'}$, and $\overline{P}_{\wedge,\Gamma,\Gamma'}$ are all large, even in a randomization test. The hypothesis $H_0 : \beta = -1.657$ is rejected in favor of $\beta > -1.657$ with $\overline{P}_{\wedge,\Gamma,\Gamma'} \leq 0.05$ in a one-sided test with $\Gamma = \Gamma' = 1.25$, but not in a two-sided test which requires $\overline{P}_{\wedge,\Gamma,\Gamma'} \leq 0.025$; however, the two-sided randomization test does reject H_0 in favor of $\beta > -1.657$.

A two-sided, 0.05-level randomization test also rejects $H_0 : \beta = -1$ and $H_0 : \beta = -0.5$ in favor of larger values, but cannot reject $H_0 : \beta = 0$.

The test in Table 6.2 uses the permutation distribution of an m-statistic [153, 204], the quantity that Huber [115] equates to zero in forming an m-estimate. These are convenient statistics when faced with matched pairs and matched triples, as here. The mean is a particular m-statistic, but the statistic used here trims outliers for robustness and inliers for increased design sensitivity [212].[5]

---

[5]In R, this is implemented by the senm and senmCI functions of the sensitivitymult package with trim=3 and inner=0.5. The permutation distribution of the mean is obtained with trim=Inf and inner=0.The familiar m-statistics used here are not weighted, but if the matched-set size is small, say matched triples, then weighted m-statistics have larger design sensitivities $\tilde{\Gamma}$ under simple models

6.2.2 Duality of Tests and Confidence Intervals with Evidence Factors

The hypothesis $H_0 : \beta = \beta_0$ is true for at most one real number β_0. As a consequence, if we test $H_0 : \beta = \beta_0$ at level α for every real number β_0, then we test at most one true hypothesis and face a probability of at most α of rejecting a true hypothesis. As a logical consequence, if $H_0 : \beta = \beta_0$ is true for some β_0, then that true value is rejected with probability at most α, so the random set of β_0's not rejected at level α—that is, the $1 - \alpha$ confidence set—fails to contain the true β_0 with probability at most α. The $1 - \alpha$ confidence interval is the shortest interval that contains the confidence set. Because the confidence interval is either the same as the confidence set or a larger, more inclusive set, the stochastic confidence interval also covers the true fixed parameter, if it exists, with probability $1 - \alpha$. This is the familiar duality of hypothesis tests and confidence intervals [141, Chapter 3].

In the minimum wage example, a two-sided, 0.05-level randomization test based on $\bar{P}_{\wedge, \Gamma, \Gamma'}$ rejects $H_0 : \beta = \beta_0$ for $\beta_0 < -0.49$ and for $\beta_0 > 6.8$, so the two-sided 95% confidence interval is $[-0.49, 6.8]$. In this interval, the grave harm predicted by Stigler [263] is not evident. An unmeasured bias of $\Gamma = \Gamma' = 1.25$ expands the confidence interval substantially in both directions to $[-3.1, 9.4]$, though of course the null hypothesis of no effect, $H_0 : \beta = 0$, remains plausible.

6.2.3 A Test for Effect and for One-sided Equivalence

Dispute about the direction of an effect need not result in a preference for a two-sided test [13]. Instead, there can be a test for the harm predicted by critics of the minimum wage, together with a one-sided equivalence interval attempting to establish the claim of advocates of the minimum wage, namely that whatever harm occurs is not large. Although critics and advocates of the minimum wage disagree about the minimum wage, neither has an interest in producing unnecessarily long confidence intervals.

Bauer and Kieser [13] observe that the logic of inverting hypothesis tests to obtain confidence intervals does not require that every possible value β_0 of β be tested against the same alternative. One-sided tests may be performed for all β_0, but the direction of the one-sided test may change as the value of β_0 changes. Critics of the minimum wage assert that it is harmful to employment, that is, critics want to test $H_0 : \beta = 0$ versus the alternative that $\beta < 0$, in their attempt to establish that $\beta < 0$. Advocates of the minimum wage are concerned to show that if β is below zero, then it is not far below zero, by testing $H_0 : \beta = \beta_0$ versus the alternative that $\beta > \beta_0$ for each $\beta_0 < 0$. The resulting interval has one of two forms, either $[\beta_0, 0)$ or $[\beta_0, 0]$, where the half-open interval signifies that $H_0 : \beta = 0$ has been rejected in favor of $\beta < 0$, while the closed interval signifies that $H_0 : \beta = 0$ has not been rejected. Interval $[\beta_0, 0]$ with β_0 near 0 says: there may be no harm, and if there is harm then it is not substantial. Interval $[\beta_0, 0)$ with β_0 near 0 says: there is harm, but

---

[214, 217]. Weighted m-statistics are implemented in the R package sensitivitymw. The weighting that increases design sensitivity diminishes the importance of matched sets with nearly constant responses. The importance of weighting decreases as the size of the matched set increases. Weighting is most useful in matched sets of sizes 3, 4, and 5.

it is not substantial. Interval $[\beta_0, 0)$ with β_0 far below 0 says: there is harm, and it may be substantial. Interval $[\beta_0, 0]$ with β_0 far below 0 says: the data say little about whether there is harm and whether any harm is substantial or not. These are the issues in dispute, and they do not require the longer confidence intervals produced by two-sided tests.

The calculations are analogous to those in Table 6.2, except that each null hypothesis $H_0 : \beta = \beta_0$ is tested in one direction only, the direction depending upon the value of β_0, with $H_0 : \beta = \beta_0$ rejected if $\overline{P}_{\wedge,\Gamma,\Gamma'} \leq 0.05$; rather than testing in both directions and requiring $\overline{P}_{\wedge,\Gamma,\Gamma'} \leq 0.025$ for one of those directions. The 95% interval from a randomization test is $[0, 0]$; that is, every negative value of β_0 is rejected in the positive direction, and 0 is not rejected in the negative direction. The 95% interval in the presence of a bias of $\Gamma = \Gamma' = 1.25$ is $[-1.6, 0]$, so $H_0 : \beta = 0$ is not rejected, and a decline of one employee per restaurant on average is barely outside the interval at -1.657, the value discussed earlier.

The inference just performed is a one-sided test for effect together with a one-sided interval for near-equivalence [13]. The three-sided test of Goeman, Solari, and Stijnen [85] does a two-sided test of $H_0 : \theta = 0$, possibly establishing the sign of θ, together with a two-sided equivalence interval, possibly establishing that θ is not large, or not small, or near 0. Their equivalence interval will typically be shorter than a two-sided confidence interval. For a related problem, see Finner [66, 178].

6.3   Evidence Factors Plus an Incompatible Comparison

6.3.1   Some Interesting Comparisons Cannot Be Factors

In Kopjar and Garaj-Vrhovac's study [131] in §4.2 of the potential DNA damage from handling antineoplastic drugs, the ventilated hood was intended to reduce harm from exposure, to mitigate the effects of the treatment under study. One might plausibly argue that an analysis should examine the unmitigated effects of the treatment, by comparing controls and workers protected only by gloves. If handling cancer drugs damages DNA, then this should be most apparent when little is done to mitigate harm. This comparison is not one of the two comparisons in the evidence factor analysis in §5.2, nor could it replace one of the analyses in §5.2 while still producing two evidence factors. This statement is made precise in Theorem 9 of Chapter 11, but consider it informally here. To see the big picture quickly, skip the two optional subsections of §6.3 that are marked with an asterisk (*).

With three treatment groups, say A, B, and C, there are 3 comparisons of two groups: A versus B, A versus C, and B versus C. There are also three comparisons of one group with the union of the other two: A versus $B \cup C$, B versus $A \cup C$, and C versus $A \cup B$. Two evidence factors may be formed by pairing these in three ways. One pair of evidence factors is C versus $A \cup B$ and A versus B. A second pair is B versus $A \cup C$ and A versus C. The final pair is A versus $B \cup C$ and B versus C. The structure of two evidence factors is lost if there are three comparisons: (i) C versus $A \cup B$, (ii) A versus B, and (iii) A versus C; yet, these comparisons may be of interest. A solution is to make an adjustment to the analysis, described in the next subsection, so that there is an evidence factor analysis involving (i) and (ii) and an additional but separate analysis involving (iii). A small price is paid for the additional analysis, but the price may be worth paying.

In parallel, in the smoking and periodontal disease example in §4.1 and §5.3, a test statistic cannot be a part of an evidence factor analysis if it uses information from both panel (a) and panel (b) of Figure 4.2. Consider, for example, a smoker-minus-control signed rank statistic applied only to the subset of pairs that contain a heavy smoker, say at least 10 cigarettes per day. That statistic does not describe panel (a) exclusively, but nor does it describe panel (b) exclusively, so it cannot be one factor in an analysis with two essentially independent factors. Again, the precise meaning of this is in Theorem 9 of Chapter 11. Similarly, a signed rank statistic [190, 196, 277] that gives more weight to pairs in which the smoker smoked more cannot be one factor of a two-factor analysis of Figure 4.2. Yet, as will be seen later in this section, such an analysis may be a useful addition.

6.3.2   An Incompatible Primary Analysis

If the incompatible analysis is viewed as having overriding importance, then it can be the primary analysis. In this case, the evidence factor analysis is a secondary analysis, performed contingently if the primary analysis rejects its null hypothesis. This contingent structure for testing strongly controls the family-wise error rate [12, 56, 84, 130, 205].

The contingent structure of testing-in-order has advantages and disadvantages. One advantage is that there is no loss of power in the primary analysis due to corrections for multiple testing. Sometimes, there is another advantage: early tests in an ordered sequence of tests may reduce the magnitude of the multiple testing problem in later tests in the sequence, so the correction for multiple testing in later tests is less severe; see Refs. [84], [205, Proposition 3] and [223, Chapter 23]. The disadvantage is that failure to reject the primary null hypothesis stops all testing.

A primary analysis that focused on control versus treatment at high-dose would have been unsuccessful in the benzene example, because dose exhibited little or no relationship with the outcome. In the benzene example in §4.5 and §5.4, there was strong evidence of an effect from one factor—treatment versus control—but no evidence from the other—dose of treatment. This finding might have been hidden from view if the evidence factor analysis were contingent upon the outcome of a primary analysis. An alternative is to add an incompatible comparison to an evidence factor analysis in such a way that the family-wise error rate is strongly controlled in all analyses.

6.3.3   Adding an Incompatible Comparison

There are three hypotheses, H_Γ, $H_{\Gamma'}'$, $H_{\Gamma''}''$, where H_Γ and $H_{\Gamma'}'$ are compatible as evidence factors, but $H_{\Gamma''}''$ is incompatible. In §4.2 and §5.2, $H_{\Gamma''}''$ is the incompatible comparison of controls and health-care workers protected only by gloves. In §4.1 and §5.3, $H_{\Gamma''}''$ is the incompatible comparison that uses information from both panel

(a) and panel (b) of Figure 4.2. Here, hypothesis H_Γ says that there is no treatment effect and the bias in the first comparison is at most Γ, and similarly for $H'_{\Gamma'}$ and $H''_{\Gamma''}$.

These three null hypotheses, H_Γ, $H'_{\Gamma'}$, $H''_{\Gamma''}$ have valid individual upper bounds on P-values, $\overline{P}_\Gamma$, $\overline{P}'_{\Gamma'}$, $\overline{P}''_{\Gamma''}$, such that $\left(\overline{P}_\Gamma, \overline{P}'_{\Gamma'}\right)$ are jointly stochastically larger than uniform if $H_\Gamma \wedge H'_{\Gamma'}$ is true. So, let $\overline{P}_{\wedge,\Gamma,\Gamma'}$ be a valid bound on the P-value for testing the conjunction, $H_\Gamma \wedge H'_{\Gamma'}$, such as the P-value obtained by combining $\left(\overline{P}_\Gamma, \overline{P}'_{\Gamma'}\right)$, perhaps using the truncated product of P-values. The combined analysis is as follows.

1. If $\overline{P}''_{\Gamma''} \leq \alpha/2$, then reject $H''_{\Gamma''}$ and set $\lambda = \alpha$. Otherwise, set $\lambda = \alpha/2$.

2. If $\overline{P}_{\wedge,\Gamma,\Gamma'} > \lambda$, then stop testing and reject no additional hypotheses.

3. If $\overline{P}_{\wedge,\Gamma,\Gamma'} \leq \lambda$, then: (i) reject $H_\Gamma \wedge H'_{\Gamma'}$, (ii) reject H_Γ if $\overline{P}_\Gamma \leq \lambda$, (iii) reject $H'_{\Gamma'}$ if $\overline{P}'_{\Gamma'} \leq \lambda$.

4. If $\lambda = \alpha/2$ and $H_\Gamma \wedge H'_{\Gamma'}$, H_Γ and $H'_{\Gamma'}$ were all rejected in Step 3, then reject $H''_{\Gamma''}$ if $\overline{P}''_{\Gamma''} \leq \alpha$.

Steps 1–4 are based on general principles [30, 72, 111, 151, 286, 287], but this particular case is much simpler than the full scope of the general principles. A heuristic says that a bit of α is spent each time some hypothesis is tested but not rejected, and steps 1–4 spend neither more nor less than α. The heuristic is not, in any sense, a proof, but it helps to understand the steps. Step 1 tests $H''_{\Gamma''}$, expending $\alpha/2$ if $H''_{\Gamma''}$ is not rejected, but otherwise retains all of α for further testing. Step 2 always tests $H_\Gamma \wedge H'_{\Gamma'}$, sometimes at level α, sometimes at level $\alpha/2$, depending upon what happened at step 1. If neither $H''_{\Gamma''}$ nor $H_\Gamma \wedge H'_{\Gamma'}$ is rejected, then all of α has been expended, and testing stops in Step 2. If $H_\Gamma \wedge H'_{\Gamma'}$ is false, then the pair of hypotheses, H_Γ and $H'_{\Gamma'}$, includes at most one true hypothesis, so we may test both at level λ without spending 2λ on two true hypotheses. If $H_\Gamma \wedge H'_{\Gamma'}$, H_Γ and $H'_{\Gamma'}$ were all rejected at $\lambda = \alpha/2$ in step 3 because $H''_{\Gamma''}$ was not rejected in step 1, then $\alpha/2$ remains unspent in step 4, so it is recycled [30] in a second attempt to reject $H''_{\Gamma''}$, but now at level α. That is the intuition, but intuition does not demonstrate anything. A direct, simple but multistep proof follows as optional reading.

6.3.4 *Proof that Steps 1–4 Control the Family-wise Error Rate*

It is easy to prove that steps 1–4 falsely reject at least one true hypothesis with probability at most α. Saying the same thing in a technical phrase, steps 1–4 strongly control the family-wise error rate at level α: no matter which of the logically consistent hypotheses, H_Γ, $H'_{\Gamma'}$, $H''_{\Gamma''}$, $H_\Gamma \wedge H'_{\Gamma'}$, is true or false, the probability that steps 1–4 make at least one false rejection is at most α. Table 6.3.4 is the proof. There are eight situations, depending upon which of the hypotheses, H_Γ, $H'_{\Gamma'}$, $H''_{\Gamma''}$, are true, where the truth of the conjunction, $H_\Gamma \wedge H'_{\Gamma'}$, is logically determined by its components. In each row of Table 6.3.4, there is a barrier event, a choke point: that event

Table 6.3 *Proof that Steps 1–4 falsely reject at least one true hypothesis with probability at most α. A barrier event is an event that must occur if a false rejection occurs. T=true, F=false. The bound is an upper bound on the probability of the barrier event*

Situation	H_Γ	$H'_{\Gamma'}$	$H_\Gamma \wedge H'_{\Gamma'}$	$H''_{\Gamma''}$	Barrier Event	Bound
1	T	T	T	T	$\overline{P}''_{\Gamma''} \le \alpha/2$ or $\overline{P}_{\wedge,\Gamma,\Gamma'} \le \alpha/2$	α
2	T	F	F	T	$\overline{P}''_{\Gamma''} \le \alpha/2$ or $\overline{P}_\Gamma \le \alpha/2$	α
3	F	T	F	T	$\overline{P}''_{\Gamma''} \le \alpha/2$ or $\overline{P}'_{\Gamma'} \le \alpha/2$	α
4	F	F	F	T	$\overline{P}''_{\Gamma''} \le \alpha$	α
5	T	T	T	F	$\overline{P}_{\wedge,\Gamma,\Gamma'} \le \alpha$	α
6	T	F	F	F	$\overline{P}_\Gamma \le \alpha$	α
7	F	T	F	F	$\overline{P}'_{\Gamma'} \le \alpha$	α
8	F	F	F	F	NA	0

must occur if at least one true hypothesis in that row is to be rejected. The proof consists in showing that, in every row, the probability of the barrier event is at most α. Although, as investigators, we do not know which row we are in, we do know that our row has probability at most α of a false rejection, simply because every row has that property.

In Table 6.3.4, start at the bottom. In situation 8, there are no true hypotheses, so the probability of rejecting a true hypothesis is zero. In situation 7, $H'_{\Gamma'}$ is the only true hypothesis, so a false rejection occurs if and only if $H'_{\Gamma'}$ is rejected. The barrier event occurs in Step 3(iii) where rejection of $H'_{\Gamma'}$ requires $\overline{P}'_{\Gamma'} \le \lambda$, where λ is either α or $\alpha/2$; however, in either case, rejection of $H'_{\Gamma'}$ requires $\overline{P}'_{\Gamma'} \le \alpha$, and the chance of this is at most α because $\overline{P}'_{\Gamma'}$ is a valid P-value testing $H'_{\Gamma'}$. Situation 6 is essentially the same, but with H_Γ replacing $H'_{\Gamma'}$. In situation 5, at least one false rejection occurs if and only if $\overline{P}_{\wedge,\Gamma,\Gamma'} \le \lambda \le \alpha$ in Step 3, and the probability of this is at most α because $\overline{P}_{\wedge,\Gamma,\Gamma'}$ is a valid P-value testing $H_\Gamma \wedge H'_{\Gamma'}$.

In situation 4, only $H''_{\Gamma''}$ is true, so at least one true hypothesis is rejected if and only if $H''_{\Gamma''}$ is rejected. This can happen in two places, in Step 1 or in Step 4, but in either case it must happen that $\overline{P}''_{\Gamma''} \le \alpha$, and the chance of this is at most α because $H''_{\Gamma''}$ is true.

Situation 3 requires just a little more thought, because of the possibility of rejecting $H''_{\Gamma''}$ in either Step 1 or Step 4. In situation 3, only $H'_{\Gamma'}$ and $H''_{\Gamma''}$ are true, so at least one false rejection occurs if and only if at least one of these two hypotheses is rejected. Because the P-values are valid and $H'_{\Gamma'}$ and $H''_{\Gamma''}$ are true, $\Pr\left(\overline{P}'_{\Gamma'} \leq \alpha/2\right) \leq \alpha/2$ and $\Pr\left(\overline{P}''_{\Gamma''} \leq \alpha/2\right) \leq \alpha/2$. The Bonferroni inequality implies that the probability that $\overline{P}''_{\Gamma''} \leq \alpha/2$ or $\overline{P}'_{\Gamma'} \leq \alpha/2$ is at most $\alpha/2 + \alpha/2 = \alpha$. Let B be the event $\overline{P}''_{\Gamma''} \leq \alpha/2$ or $\overline{P}'_{\Gamma'} \leq \alpha/2$, so $\Pr(B) \leq \alpha$. Let E be the event that either $H'_{\Gamma'}$ or $H''_{\Gamma''}$ or both are rejected. So, to complete situation 3, we need to verify that B is a barrier event; i.e., E can occur only if B occurs. In Steps 1–4, there are only three ways E may occur, and each of them implies that B occurs. (i) If $\overline{P}''_{\Gamma''} \leq \alpha/2$ occurs, then $H''_{\Gamma''}$ is rejected in Step 1, and E does occur. (ii) If $\overline{P}''_{\Gamma''} > \alpha/2$ and $\overline{P}'_{\Gamma'} \leq \alpha/2$, then $\lambda = \alpha/2$ and $H'_{\Gamma'}$ may be rejected in Step 3(iii), so E may occur. (iii) If $\alpha \geq \overline{P}''_{\Gamma''} > \alpha/2$ and $\overline{P}'_{\Gamma'} \leq \alpha/2$, then $\lambda = \alpha/2$, so $H'_{\Gamma'}$ may be rejected in Step 3(iii) and $H''_{\Gamma''}$ may be rejected in Step 4. So E occurs only if B occurs, and $\Pr(E) \leq \Pr(B) \leq \alpha$; so, situation 3 is complete. Situation 2 is essentially the same, with H_Γ replacing $H'_{\Gamma'}$. Indeed, situation 1 is essentially the same, with $H_\Gamma \wedge H'_{\Gamma'}$ replacing $H'_{\Gamma'}$.

6.3.5   *Design Sensitivity as a Guide to Additional Analyses*

Different test statistics applied to the same data vary in their reports of the degree of insensitivity to unmeasured biases. The patterns seen in data are anticipated by theory, for instance, by design sensitivity and Bahadur efficiency of a sensitivity analysis; see §2.4 and Refs. [206, 208, 215, 223, Part III]. Wilcoxon's ranks tend to exaggerate sensitivity to unmeasured bias: the U-statistic [208] and other statistics [206, 210] have larger design sensitivity for matched pair differences that have Normal or logistic or t distributions. If larger effects occur at higher doses—a big if—then giving larger weights to pairs with higher doses tends to increase insensitivity to unmeasured biases, but setting low dose pairs aside often does better still [198, 223, §18.4]. Similarly, if larger effects occur in certain subpopulations defined by observed covariates—if there is effect modification—then emphasizing these subpopulations may also increase insensitivity to unmeasured biases [112]. Because we may not know, before examining the data, whether larger effects occur at higher doses, whether larger effects are present in certain subpopulations, adaptive methods may be preferred. Adaptive methods let the data decide. Adaptive methods are guided by the data in the choice of statistic, but they correctly allow for repeated use of the data, so that the adaptive test has the correct overall level and adaptive confidence intervals have the correct overall coverage [113, 136, 137, 210, 211, 222].

Some Test Statistics Are Better than Others In randomized controlled trials, some test statistics are better than others: With the same amount of data from the same source, a better test statistic has more power, that is, a higher probability of rejecting some false null hypothesis. The same thing happens in sensitivity analyses in observational studies: With the same amount of data from the same source, a better test statistic more often correctly reports insensitivity to larger unmeasured biases.

The facts just mentioned are illustrated in Table 6.4 for the data from §4.1 and §5.3 concerning smoking and periodontal disease. The 441 smoker-minus-control pair differences in periodontal disease are analyzed using eight test statistics. Three test statistics (W) use Wilcoxon's ranks, while three other test statistics use the U-statistic [208] with $(m, \underline{m}, \overline{m}) = (8, 7, 8)$. Two statistics use all 441 pairs without weights. Two statistics weight pairs by doses [190, 196, 277], where: dose 3 signifies a pair in which the smoker smoked at least 10 cigarettes per day and both members of the pair were at least 40 years of age, dose 2 signifies either the smoker smoked at least 10 cigarettes per day or both members of the pair were at least 40 years of age, but not both, and dose 1 signifies that neither of these conditions occurred. Two statistics use only the 191 pairs, of 441 pairs, with dose 3. The final two test statistics are adaptive: they use the data to pick a test statistic. The so-called d-statistic, focuses on subsets of pairs with demonstrated insensitivity to bias [222]. The final statistic, tt, uses two of the statistics in earlier columns, in this case the unweighted U-statistic and the high-dose U-statistic, and uses the joint distribution of the two statistics to correct for testing one hypothesis twice [211]. Adaptive statistics pay a price to empirically avoid a poor choice of test statistic. Adaptive procedures often pay a diminishing price with increasing sample size, so in large samples they may come in second best to knowing, a priori, which test statistic will report the greatest insensitivity to bias [210, 211]. Indeed, this is the pattern in Table 6.4: the two adaptive procedure are slightly behind the test statistic that reports greatest insensitivity to unmeasured bias, but both adaptive tests are better than a poor a priori choice of test statistic.

The various statistics in Table 6.4 offer very different impressions of the degree of insensitivity to unmeasured bias. Wilcoxon's statistic applied to all 441 pairs without weights is insensitive to a bias of $\Gamma = 2.75$ while the U-statistic applied to the 191 high-dose pairs is insensitive to a bias of $\Gamma = 5.5$. Generally, the U-statistic outperforms Wilcoxon's statistic in Table 6.4, focusing on high-dose pairs outperforms dose weighting, which in turn outperforms ignoring the doses. Second best to knowing which procedure to use are the two adaptive tests. The d-statistic [222] is agnostic about whether larger effects will be seen at higher doses, at older ages, or in pairs with larger absolute pair differences, and lets the data decide. The d-statistic procedure is insensitive to a bias of $\Gamma = 4.9$. Implicitly, the d-statistic considered 4095 possible test statistics. In contrast, testing twice (tt) in the final column of Table 6.4 uses two statistics from previous columns, and is insensitive to a bias of $\Gamma = 5.0$.

Table 6.4 *Sensitivity analysis for the periodontal data, using eight statistics. W=Wilcoxon ranks, U=U-statistic ranks, m = 8, $\underline{m}$ = 7, $\overline{m}$ = 8. In each column, the largest P-value ≤ 0.05 before rounding for display is in* **bold**

	Statistic							
	Unweighted		Dose-weighted		High-dose Only		Adaptive	
Γ	W	U	W	U	W	U	d-statistic	tt
1.0	0.000	0.000	0.000	0.000	0.000	0.000	0.000	0.000
2.75	**0.047**	0.000	0.013	0.000	0.001	0.000	0.000	0.000
2.8	0.061	0.000	0.018	0.000	0.001	0.000	0.000	0.000
2.95	0.126	0.000	**0.042**	0.000	0.003	0.000	0.000	0.001
3.0	0.154	0.000	0.054	0.000	0.003	0.001	0.001	0.001
3.8	0.777	0.012	0.516	0.007	**0.047**	0.004	0.003	0.008
4.0	0.875	0.021	0.654	0.013	0.073	0.007	0.005	0.011
4.3	0.955	**0.044**	0.816	0.027	0.127	0.011	0.014	0.018
4.4	0.969	0.054	0.855	0.034	0.149	0.013	0.017	0.021
4.5	0.980	0.066	0.888	**0.041**	0.173	0.015	0.024	0.024
4.6	0.986	0.079	0.915	0.050	0.198	0.017	0.027	0.028
4.7	0.991	0.094	0.936	0.060	0.225	0.020	0.031	0.032
4.8	0.994	0.111	0.952	0.072	0.253	0.022	0.043	0.036
4.9	0.996	0.129	0.965	0.084	0.282	0.025	**0.048**	0.040
5.0	0.998	0.149	0.975	0.098	0.312	0.028	0.053	**0.045**
5.5	1.000	0.267	0.996	0.185	0.468	**0.048**	0.090	0.073

Adaptive inference is briefly described in the following optional subsection.

6.3.6 *Brief Remarks About Adaptive Inference

The incompatible analysis may be adaptive. An adaptive inference may consider using information from both factors, but ultimately decide to focus on only one factor. Because it considered both factors before deciding, it cannot be a factor in a pair of evidence factors. For a detailed textbook discussion and several examples of adaptive inference and design sensitivity, see Ref. [223, §19.3].

There are several principles that produce adaptive statistics seeking to locate effects insensitive to unmeasured biases. This is a large topic, but a brief sketch follows.

Adaptive Inference Lets the Data Pick the Test Statistic Theory guides us away from some statistics, like Wilcoxon's statistic, that exaggerate the degree of sensitivity to unmeasured biases. Some other choices are more difficult to make, because the best choice of test statistic depends upon aspects of the process that produced the data. For these difficult choices, adaptive inference lets the data decide.

A simple approach uses the joint distribution of several test statistics to correct for testing one hypothesis several times [137, 206, 210, 233]. The tt method in Table 6.4 is of this form, in this case using two component statistics.[6] Often, several tests of the same hypothesis using the same data are highly correlated, so the correction for multiple testing is quite small compared to the correction derived from the Bonferroni inequality. This approach often has certain optimal properties: (i) it often has design sensitivity equal to the largest design sensitivity of the component tests [206, 210], and (ii) the sensitivity analysis often has Bahadur efficiency equal to the largest Bahadur efficiency of the component tests [20, 215]. These optimal large-sample properties, together with simulations confirming their relevance in finite samples, support a preference for this approach to adaptive inference. As is always true, there are some details; however, the intuition here is straightforward. If a sensitivity analysis is performed with its parameter, Γ, set below the design sensitivity, $\widetilde{\Gamma}$, then the upper bound on the P-value tends to zero as the sample size increases. This is true, in particular, of the component statistic with the largest design sensitivity, say $\widetilde{\Gamma}_{max}$. Eventually, with a sufficiently large sample size, the P-value for the statistic with the largest $\widetilde{\Gamma}$ is sufficiently small that it overcomes the correction for multiple testing, so the combined procedure also produces a P-value that tends to zero for $\Gamma < \widetilde{\Gamma}_{max}$. This fact is used to demonstrate (i), so now consider (ii). If $\Gamma < \widetilde{\Gamma}_{max}$, some of the component test statistics have P-value bounds that decline to zero as the sample size increases, and the Bahadur slope is a measure of the rate of that decline. If one component statistic has a larger Bahadur slope than the others, then its P-value bound tends to zero faster than the others, so in large enough samples it is all but certain to be the winning choice, and the correction for an all but certain choice is negligible [20]. In finite samples, with a few component statistics, simulations suggest that it is slightly better to know the best statistic a priori than to deduce it from data, but it is vastly better to deduce it from data than to guess wrong [137, 206].

A second approach selects one test statistic from several or many test statistics using information that all of the test statistics will discard [113, 136]. In the situation that has been studied most extensively, there are treated-minus-control matched pair differences in outcomes, Y_i, and the several test statistics all condition on $|Y_i|$. The test statistic is chosen based on the behavior of $|Y_i|$. Motivation for this strategy is provided by a general theorem of Kumar Jogdeo [123, Theorem 2.2]; see Ref. [113, §2.4]. On the positive side, this approach pays no price for its double-use of the data, no price for its adaptation to the distribution of $|Y_i|$. On the negative side, this approach may fail to identify the statistic with the largest design sensitivity, $\widetilde{\Gamma}_{max}$, even with infinite quantities of data. A wise or lucky choice of test statistic may outperform this approach even with infinite data. In the situation that has been studied most extensively, CART is used to predict $|Y_i|$ from covariates, cutting the population into a tree, typically a shallow tree, possibly a stump. Simulations suggest that the method can discover substantial effect modification, and otherwise the

---

[6]Three R packages that implement these methods are testtwice for matched pairs [211], sensitivity2x2xk for contingency tables [233], and submax for effect modification [137].

method does the single analysis—i.e., the stump analysis—that one would have done anyway [113]. The method can miss opportunities when there is only slight effect modification [137], and it can be misled by complex patterns of effect modification that CART cannot recognize from $|Y_i|$.

A final approach sacrifices some useful information to locate inferences that are insensitive to unmeasured bias; then, it uses the information that remains [222]. This approach builds a statistic with demonstrated insensitivity to bias—a d-statistic—using the data at hand. In the case of treated-minus-control pair differences, Y_i, it examines the frequency of positive differences, $Y_i > 0$, in subsets of data, checks that this frequency exceeds what is expected from a bias of Γ, and then performs an exact conditional test given the information it has used. At $\Gamma = 4.9$, bias alone can produce $Y_i > 0$ with probability $\Gamma/(1+\Gamma) = 4.9/5.9 = 0.83$, so only subsets with a higher frequency of $Y_i > 0$ are used in the analysis. In Table 6.4, at $\Gamma = 4.9$, the statistic decided to focus on pairs in which the smoker smoked at least 10 cigarettes per day and with a large absolute difference in periodontal disease, $|Y_i|$; however, it largely ignored age. Implicitly, in Table 6.4, the d-statistic was chosen from 4095 candidate statistics constructed in a combinatorial fashion. This contrasts with the tt procedure in Table 6.4: it selected from two candidate statistics, not from 4095 candidate statistics.

Although the third of the three approaches, the exact d-statistic, performed well in Table 6.4 with 441 matched pairs, it may be better suited to larger sample sizes, perhaps thousands of pairs. The first of the three approaches, tt in Table 6.4, [137, 206, 210, 233] may be the best approach with a few hundred pairs; see [223, §19.3].

6.3.7 Smoking and Periodontal Disease: Adding an Incompatible Comparison

An investigator might guess that periodontal disease will be most severe in heavier smokers who are not very young, so that, guided by an understanding of design sensitivity, the investigator might bet everything on the U-statistic applied to the 191 older, high-dose pairs. As it turns out, that is a good bet in Table 6.4, because age and cigarettes per day seem to matter, and the sample size is not extremely small. The same bet would have been unsuccessful in the benzene example in §4.5, because the ostensible effect was not larger with longer durations of exposure, and restricting attention to treated individuals with long durations would have diminished a modest sample size. At some cost but perhaps with greater safety, the investigator in the study of periodontal disease might have used the adaptive d-statistic, whose performance was second to the best guess in Table 6.4.

A key point is that some of the statistics in Table 6.4 cannot be used as evidence factors because they merge information from panels (a) and (b) of Figure 4.2. This is stated precisely in Theorem 9 of Chapter 11. Nonetheless, one could do an incompatible analysis with any one of the statistics in Table 6.4, using the procedure described in Steps 1–4. The combined analysis in Steps 1–4 has a probability of at most α of rejecting at least one true hypothesis.

> **Some Statistics Cannot Be Part of Evidence Factors** Some statistics use information from both factors in a manner that prevents these statistics from being part of an evidence factor analysis. Steps 1–4 permit incorporation of such incompatible statistics.

Set $\alpha = 0.05$ in Steps 1–4. If the incompatible analysis used the U-statistic applied to the 191 older, high-dose pairs, then that analysis would have $\overline{P}_{\Gamma''}'' \leq 0.025 = \alpha/2$ in Step 1 for $\Gamma'' \leq 4.9$ in Table 6.4. So, for $\Gamma'' \leq 4.9$, Steps 1–4 would repeat, without change, the evidence factor analysis using $\overline{P}_\Gamma$, $\overline{P}_{\Gamma'}'$, and $\overline{P}_{\wedge,\Gamma,\Gamma'}$, exactly as it was performed in §5.2, with exactly the same conclusions. In this example, the addition of an incompatible analysis has slightly strengthened the conclusion in §5.2. To the conclusions of that analysis, we may add that an analysis focused on older, high-dose pairs is insensitive to biases of magnitude $\Gamma'' \leq 4.9$, these being a bit larger than the biases in Table 5.6.

If the incompatible, adaptive d-statistic in Table 6.4 were used instead, then $\overline{P}_{\Gamma''}'' \leq 0.025 = \alpha/2$ in Step 1 for $\Gamma'' \leq 4.5$ in Table 6.4. This incompatible analysis is insensitive to somewhat larger biases than Factor 1 on its own in Table 5.5, but arguably it does little to strengthen Table 5.6.

6.4   Summary: Planned Analyses Can Accomplish More

Where Chapter 5 considered testing the hypothesis of no effect with two evidence factors, the current chapter has considered the role of such simple analyses in a more comprehensive analysis.

Three or more evidence factors were considered in §6.1. In most respects, the situation with three or more factors is analogous to the situation with two factors, but the use of closed testing to examine component hypotheses involves additional steps.

Confidence sets and intervals for treatment effects involve inverting tests for no effect, by the familiar duality of tests and confidence intervals [141, Chapter 3]. Confidence sets were discussed in §6.2. One subtle issue is that, in a two-sided test or a two-sided confidence interval, two evidence factors should be regarded as concurring only if they reject the null hypothesis in the same direction. Closely related to confidence intervals are: (i) equivalence intervals that may attempt to demonstrate that a treatment effect is small by rejecting all large effects [13], and (ii) three-sided tests that attempt to determine the sign while limiting the magnitude of an effect [85].

Some comparisons are of interest but cannot be a factor in a pair of evidence factors. For instance, an interesting analysis may incorporate information from both factors. Alternatively, theory based on design sensitivity may suggest that a particular comparison is likely to be insensitive to large unmeasured biases, so it is attractive to include that comparison, even if it cannot be a factor in a pair of evidence factors. Incorporation of such comparisons was the topic of §6.3.

6.5   Using R

6.5.1   Adaptive Inference for Periodontal Disease and Smoking

An adaptive inference allows the data to pick the test statistic with a view to reporting greater insensitivity to unmeasured bias. Because it tests the hypothesis of no effect several times, it must correct for multiple testing. The last two columns of Table 6.4 performed adaptive inferences for the periodontal data, and compared these to conventional or non-adaptive inferences in earlier columns. A few of these calculations are reproduced here. Before doing any analysis, several packages must be loaded and several variables must be defined. The variables subdivide pairs by age and by the number of cigarettes smoked by the smoker in a pair. See the discussion of Table 6.4.

```
library(evident)
data(periodontal)
attach(periodontal)
library(dstat)
library(DOS2)
x=cigsperday[z==1]
y=pcteither[z==1]-pcteither[z==0]
age40=(age[z==1]>=40)&(age[z==0]>=40)
u=(x>=10)&age40
ten=(x>=10)
tenf=factor(1*ten,levels=0:1,labels = c("<10",">=10"))
age40f=factor(1*age40,levels=0:1,labels=c("no","both"))
f=tenf:age40f
```

The calculations that follow reproduce a few of the conventional, non-adaptive analyses. The vector u picks out the subset of "high-dose only" pairs in Table 6.4 who smoked at least 10 cigarettes per day and were at least 40 years old. The computations immediately below compare the unweighted U-statistic to the "high-dose only" U-statistic. Alas, it would be hard to know a priori that the "high-dose only" U-statistic would report greater insensitivity to unmeasured bias than the unweighted U-statistic; for instance, doses were unhelpful in the benzene example in §4.5 and §5.4.

```
senU(y,m=8,m1=7,m2=8,gamma=4.4)
$pval
[1] 0.0539

senU(y[u],m=8,m1=7,m2=8,gamma=4.4)
$pval
[1] 0.0129

senU(y[u],m=8,m1=7,m2=8,gamma=5.5)
$pval
```

[1] 0.0476

The analysis that follows reproduces one of the results in the last column of Table 6.4, in which the data decide whether or not to focus on the "high-dose only" pairs. Instead of guessing, the adaptive test does both analyses and makes a small correction for testing twice [210, 211]. Because the two test statistics have correlation 0.772 under the null hypothesis of no effect, H_0, the correction for testing twice is very small compared with the familiar correction using the Bonferroni inequality. The deviate, 1.905, is larger for the "high-dose only" pairs, so it is the basis for rejecting H_0 at the 0.05 level in the presence of a bias of at most $\Gamma = 5$. Testing twice is implemented by the testtwice package.

```
library(testtwice)
u878=multrnk(y,m1=7,m2=8,m=8)
u878h=rep(0, length(u878))
u878h[u]=multrnk(y[u],m1=7,m2=8,m=8)

tt(y,cbind(u878,u878h),gamma=5)
$pval
[1] 0.04499
$dev
 u878    u878h
1.042    1.905
$cor
        u878    u878h
u878   1.000  0.772
u878h  0.772  1.000
```

The final analysis uses a d-statistic [222] and reproduces one of the results in the next-to-last column of Table 6.4. The statistic splits the pairs into 12 groups based on (i) age below or at least 40 years, (ii) fewer than or at least 10 cigarettes per day, and (iii) thirds of the absolute pair difference in periodontal disease, $12 = 2 \times 2 \times 3$. There are $4095 = 2^{12} - 1$ nontrivial statistics that may be formed by including or excluding each of these groups of pairs, and the d-statistic considered all of them. The full output for this analysis is more extensive than is shown here, and it indicates which groups contribute to the test. Here, the test emphasizes pairs with large absolute differences in periodontal disease and a smoker who smokes at least 10 cigarettes per day. The package dstat implements d-statistics.

```
dstat(y,f=f,gamma=4.9,fscore=c(1,2,2,3))
$pval
[1] 0.0480
```

6.6 Exercises

Exercise 6.1. *This exercise continues Exercise 5.3 in Chapter 5 concerning recent handgun purchases and risk of suicide [86]. The comparison of a handgun purchase within one year and no handgun purchase within three years (columns 1 and 3 of Table 4.1) is incompatible with the evidence factor analysis in Exercise 5.3. Use the four-step procedure in §6.3 to include this analysis in the evidence factor analysis.*

Exercise 6.2. *This exercise continues Exercise 5.5 in Chapter 5 concerning DNA damage from chromium exposure at a tannery [306]. The comparison of controls and workers in the tannery department of the tannery is incompatible with the evidence factor analysis in Exercise 5.5. Use the four-step procedure in §6.3 to include this analysis in the evidence factor analysis.*

Part III

Theory of Evidence Factors

Chapter 7

Dependent *P*-Values

Abstract

A single *P*-value is valid if it is stochastically larger than the uniform distribution when its null hypothesis is true. What is the analogous concept for a vector of possibly dependent *P*-values? A vector **P** is stochastically larger than uniform if **P** is stochastically larger than **P′** where **P′** has the same dimension as **P**, but **P′** has independent coordinates with uniform distributions. A dependent vector **P** of *P*-values may be stochastically larger than uniform, and this is shown to be true of certain sequences of conditional tests that gradually use more information.

7.1 Dependent *P*-values Larger Than Uniform

In the periodontal data in §4.1, smokers were compared to matched nonsmokers in Panel (a) of Figure 4.2, and pair differences in periodontal disease were connected to the number of cigarettes smoked by the smoker in Panel (b) of Figure 4.2. Are Panels (a) and (b) unrelated pieces of information? In §4.1, there were conflicting intuitions about Figure 4.2. On the one hand, Panel (a) of Figure 4.2 could be obtained from Panel (b) by projecting the points to the left, onto the vertical axis. The boxplot simply describes those projections. So, in that sense, Panel (a) is perfectly dependent upon Panel (b). On the other hand, Panel (a) provided no information about whether the amount smoked by the smoker predicted the difference in periodontal disease. In that sense, Panel (a) seemed to provide no information relevant to the question addressed by Panel (b).

The question addressed in this chapter is: How can it be that Panel (a) is perfectly dependent upon Panel (b), yet Panels (a) and (b) will provide two *P*-values that we can treat as if they were independent? The answer is given, in part, by Propositions 2 and 3 of this chapter, which are from Ref. [209]. The aspect that is addressed by these two propositions is based on the fact that the *P*-value we use for Panel (b) conditions on all of the information in Panel (a). The other aspect addressed later, in Theorem 9 of Chapter 11, is that conditioning on Panel (a) does not change our interpretation of Panel (b). The second aspect remains a bit vague in this chapter, but it is sharpened in later chapters. If Panel (b) had merely repeated the boxplot in Panel (a), then Proposition 2 would still be true, but it would be vacuous: Panel (b) would provide no information given Panel (a). There is something special about the relationship between Panels (a) and (b) such that the interpretation we would place on Panel (b) having seen Panel (a) is the same as the interpretation we would place on Panel (b) had we not seen Panel (a), so the conditioning in Proposition 2 is not draining Panel (b) of its meaning. The simpler, first part of this two-part story is discussed in this chapter, specifically in the conceptual Proposition 2 and its more practical form, Proposition 3.

Section 7.2 repeats some standard ideas from §5.1, but with a bit more technical detail. Section 7.3 contains this chapter's main results, as motivated above. Section 7.4 again repeats and expands upon some material from §5.1 about combining P-values, but again with a bit more technical detail. Please forgive the repetition in §7.2 and §7.4, but I wanted Part II to be self-contained yet limited in technical detail.

7.2 Jointly Larger Than Uniform

7.2.1 One P-value

A real random variable A is stochastically larger than another random variable B if $\Pr(A \leq k) \leq \Pr(B \leq k)$ for every k. Equivalently, A is stochastically larger than B if $\Pr(A \geq k) \geq \Pr(B \geq k)$ for every k. The random variable B has the uniform distribution on the unit interval $[0,1]$ if $\Pr(B \leq \alpha) = \alpha$ for $0 \leq \alpha \leq 1$. So, A is stochastically larger than the uniform distribution on $[0,1]$ if $\Pr(A \leq \alpha) \leq \alpha$ for $0 \leq \alpha \leq 1$.

By definition, a single valid P-value, P, associated with a test of a null hypothesis H_0 has the property $\Pr(P \leq \alpha) \leq \alpha$ for all $0 \leq \alpha \leq 1$ if H_0 is true: it is stochastically larger the uniform.

What is the analogous concept for J possibly related P-values?

7.2.2 Stochastic Order for Random Vectors

For a J-dimensional vector, write $\mathbf{y} \leq \mathbf{y}'$ if $y_1 \leq y'_1, \ldots, y_J \leq y'_J$. A real-valued function $f(\mathbf{y})$ is monotone increasing if $f(\mathbf{y}) \leq f(\mathbf{y}')$ whenever $\mathbf{y} \leq \mathbf{y}'$. In parallel, $f(\mathbf{y})$ is monotone decreasing if $f(\mathbf{y}) \geq f(\mathbf{y}')$ whenever $\mathbf{y} \leq \mathbf{y}'$, or equivalently if $-f(\mathbf{y})$ is monotone increasing.

Definition 1. *One J-dimensional random vector $\mathbf{A}$ is stochastically larger than another $\mathbf{B}$ if $\mathrm{E}\{f(\mathbf{A})\} \geq \mathrm{E}\{f(\mathbf{B})\}$ for every monotone increasing function $f(\cdot)$ for which the expectations exist.*

Definition 1 may be reinterpreted in terms of stochastic order for a single random variable that is an increasing function of the random vectors, $\mathbf{A}$ and $\mathbf{B}$. Specifically, consider the binary indicator $\chi(\cdot)$ of an event, so $\chi\{f(\mathbf{A}) \geq k\} = 1$ if $f(\mathbf{A}) \geq k$ and is zero otherwise. Then $\chi\{f(\cdot) \geq k\}$ is bounded and monotone increasing whenever $f(\cdot)$ is monotone increasing. From Definition 1, if $\mathbf{A}$ is stochastically larger than $\mathbf{B}$, then $\Pr\{f(\mathbf{A}) \geq k\} = \mathrm{E}[\chi\{f(\mathbf{A}) \geq k\}] \geq \mathrm{E}[\chi\{f(\mathbf{B}) \geq k\}] = \Pr\{f(\mathbf{B}) \geq k\}$ for every k for every monotone increasing $f(\cdot)$. In words, if $\mathbf{A}$ is stochastically larger than **B**, then $f(\mathbf{A})$ is stochastically larger than $f(\mathbf{B})$ for every monotone increasing function $f(\cdot)$.

Definition 1 refers to the distributions of **A** and **B** separately, not about their joint behavior. Even if **A** and **B** have a joint distribution, **A** can be stochastically larger than **B**, yet the event $f(\mathbf{A}) < f(\mathbf{B})$ can have positive probability for a monotone increasing function $f(\cdot)$. Nonetheless, Lemma 1 is true [254, Theorem 6.B.1] and is often useful. In Lemma 1, $\left(\widetilde{\mathbf{A}}, \widetilde{\mathbf{B}}\right)$ is called a coupling.

Lemma 1. *If* **A** *is stochastically larger than* **B**, *then we may construct a joint distribution* $\left(\widetilde{\mathbf{A}}, \widetilde{\mathbf{B}}\right)$ *such that: (i)* **A** *and* $\widetilde{\mathbf{A}}$ *have the same distribution, (ii)* **B** *and* $\widetilde{\mathbf{B}}$ *have the same distribution, and (iii)*

$$1 = \Pr\left\{ f\left(\widetilde{\mathbf{A}}\right) \geq f\left(\widetilde{\mathbf{B}}\right) \right\} \tag{7.1}$$

for every monotone increasing $f(\cdot)$.

7.2.3 Several P-values

A J-dimensional vector of P-values, $\mathbf{P} = (P_1, \ldots, P_J)^T$, takes a value in the J-dimensional unit cube, $[0,1]^J = [0,1] \times \cdots \times [0,1]$.

Definition 2. *A* J-*dimensional random vector* $\mathbf{P} = (P_1, \ldots, P_J)^T$ *taking values in* $[0,1]^J$ *is stochastically larger than uniform if* $\mathbf{P}$ *is stochastically larger than* $\mathbf{P}'$ *where*

$$\Pr\left(P_1' \leq \alpha_1, P_2' \leq \alpha_2, \ldots, P_J' \leq \alpha_J\right) = \alpha_1 \times \alpha_2 \times \cdots \alpha_J \text{ for all } (\alpha_1, \ldots, \alpha_J)^T \in [0,1]^J. \tag{7.2}$$

In Definition 2, $\mathbf{P}'$ has the distribution of J independent uniform random variables, $P_1', \ldots, P_J'$.

Definition 2 often arises in the literature on adaptive design of randomized clinical trials [27, 283]. In some adaptive randomized clinical trials, the first half of the trial is completed yielding a valid P-value, P_1, testing the null hypothesis H_0 of no treatment effect. On the basis of the first half, the second half of the trial is redesigned, and the second half yields a second valid P-value, P_2, also testing H_0. With appropriate care in the design of an adaptive clinical trial, the pair of P-values, (P_1, P_2), is stochastically larger than uniform when H_0 is true, and the two P-values are combined to produce a new valid P-value for the trial as a whole.

If $\mathbf{P}$ is stochastically larger than uniform, then

$$\Pr(P_1 \leq \alpha_1, P_2 \leq \alpha_2, \ldots, P_J \leq \alpha_J) \leq \alpha_1 \times \alpha_2 \times \cdots \alpha_J, \tag{7.3}$$

because $\mathrm{E}\left[\chi\left\{P_1 \leq \alpha_1, \ldots, P_J \leq \alpha_J\right\}\right] \leq \mathrm{E}\left[\chi\left\{P_1' \leq \alpha_1, \ldots, P_J' \leq \alpha_J\right\}\right] = \alpha_1 \times \alpha_2 \times \cdots \alpha_J$ in (7.2). If each P_j were stochastically larger than the uniform distribution on

[0, 1] and if the coordinates of **P** were independent, then (7.3) would be true. However, **P** can be stochastically larger than uniform yet have dependent coordinates, as will be seen in the next section. Also, some or all coordinates of **P** may be discrete— i.e., have finite or countable support—yet **P** can be stochastically larger than uniform.

Geometrically, $[0, \alpha_1] \times \cdots \times [0, \alpha_J]$ defines a "lower-left" rectangle contained in the unit cube $[0, 1]^J$. Condition (7.3) says **P** is less likely to fall in every such rectangle than is a J-dimensional vector of independent uniform random variables.

7.3 Creating Jointly Valid, Possibly Dependent *P*-values

The current section describes an elementary way in which dependent *P*-values **P** can be stochastically larger than uniform.

> **Conditional Tests**   A sequence of conditional tests may produce a dependent vector of *P*-values that is stochastically larger than uniform if each test conditions on the information used by earlier tests in the sequence.

Suppose that we have J random quantities, $V_1, \ldots, V_J$. For instance, $V_1, \ldots, V_J$ might be J random variables or J random matrices. We will do J hypothesis tests, gradually using more V_j's, conditioning at each step on the information we previously used. Specifically, on the basis of these J quantities, we will do J hypothesis tests, yielding *P*-values, $P_1, \ldots, P_J$. The jth *P*-value, P_j, is a function of the first j quantities, $(V_1, \ldots, V_j)$, and it is a valid *P*-value conditionally given $(V_1, \ldots, V_{j-1})$ in the sense that $\Pr\left(P_j \leq \alpha \mid V_1, \ldots, V_{j-1}\right) \leq \alpha$ for all $0 \leq \alpha \leq 1$ when its null hypothesis is true.[1] In general, *P*-values built in this way are dependent because, for instance, they are all functions of V_1. Does this dependence matter? I will answer this question twice, once in a simple form in Proposition 2; then, a second time in a form that is more useful in practice in Proposition 3. Proposition 2 is a special case of Proposition 3, so only the latter is proved.

Proposition 2. *Suppose that: (i) $V_1, \ldots, V_J$ are random quantities, (ii) P_j is a function of the first j quantities, $(V_1, \ldots, V_j)$, and (iii) $\Pr\left(P_j \leq \alpha \mid V_1, \ldots, V_{j-1}\right) \leq \alpha$ for all $0 \leq \alpha \leq 1$, for $j = 1, \ldots, J$. Then $\mathbf{P} = (P_1, \ldots, P_J)^T$ is stochastically larger than the uniform distribution on $[0, 1]^J$.*

In practice, it is often important to ask: How strong is the remaining evidence if certain evidence is temporarily set aside? How strong is the evidence from P_1 and P_3 if P_2 is set aside? Is all of the evidence of a treatment effect from P_2? Or would there still be strong evidence of an effect from P_1 and P_3, setting P_2 aside? Generally, how strong is the evidence from P_j, $j \in \mathscr{J} \subseteq \{1, 2, \ldots, J\}$, if the evidence

---

[1] Strictly speaking, we should say $\Pr\left(P_j \leq \alpha \mid V_1, \ldots, V_{j-1}\right) \leq \alpha$ for almost all $V_1, \ldots, V_{j-1}$; however, I will not speak that strictly in this book.

from P_ℓ, $\ell \in \{1,2,\ldots,J\} - \mathcal{J}$ is set aside? The subtlety in this question is that, P_j, $j \in \mathcal{J}$, generally depends upon all of $(V_1,\ldots,V_J)$, including perhaps V_ℓ with $\ell \in \{1,2,\ldots,j\} - \mathcal{J}$. For instance, if we ask about the evidence from P_1 and P_3 if P_2 is set aside, then P_3 may still depend upon V_2. Does this matter? As seen in Proposition 3, what matters is that P_j is a valid *P*-value given $(V_1,\ldots,V_{j-1})$ for $j \in \mathcal{J}$; however, it does not matter whether P_ℓ is a valid *P*-value given $(V_1,\ldots,V_\ell)$ for $\ell \in \{1,2,\ldots,j\} - \mathcal{J}$. Proposition 3 is from Ref. [209, §2].

Proposition 3. *Suppose that: (i) $V_1, \ldots, V_J$ are random quantities, (ii) P_j is a function of the first j quantities, $(V_1,\ldots,V_j)$, and (iii) $\mathrm{Pr}\left(P_j \le \alpha \,\middle|\, V_1,\ldots,V_{j-1}\right) \le \alpha$ for all $0 \le \alpha \le 1$, for $j \in \mathcal{J} \subseteq \{1,2,\ldots,J\}$. Then P_j, $j \in \mathcal{J}$, are stochastically larger than the uniform distribution on $[0,1]^{|\mathcal{J}|}$.*

Proof. Let $\mathbf{P}'$ be a vector of $|\mathcal{J}|$ independent uniform random variables, and let $\mathbf{P}$ be the $|\mathcal{J}|$-dimensional vector of P_j, $j \in \mathcal{J}$; so the task is to show that $\mathbf{P}$ is stochastically larger than $\mathbf{P}'$. Pick constants $(\alpha_1,\ldots,\alpha_J)^T \in [0,1]^J$. For any random quantities $\mathbf{A}$ and $\mathbf{B}$ such that $\mathbf{B}$ is a function of $\mathbf{A}$,

$$\mathrm{Pr}\left(P_j \le \alpha_j \,\middle|\, \mathbf{B}\right) = \mathrm{E}\left\{\mathrm{Pr}\left(P_j \le \alpha_j \,\middle|\, \mathbf{A},\mathbf{B}\right) \,\middle|\, \mathbf{B}\right\} = \mathrm{E}\left\{\mathrm{Pr}\left(P_j \le \alpha_j \,\middle|\, \mathbf{A}\right) \,\middle|\, \mathbf{B}\right\}. \quad (7.4)$$

Take $\mathbf{A} = (V_1,\ldots,V_{j-1})$ in (7.4), so that $\mathrm{Pr}\left(P_j \le \alpha_j \,\middle|\, \mathbf{A}\right) \le \alpha_j$ for $j \in \mathcal{J}$ by assumption (iii). Define $\mathcal{I}_j = \{k \in \mathcal{J} : k \le j-1\}$, where it is possible that $\mathcal{I}_j = \emptyset$. If $\mathcal{I}_j \neq \emptyset$, for $k \in \mathcal{I}_j$, take $B_k = P_k$ and define $\mathbf{B}$ in (7.4) to be the vector of dimension $|\mathcal{I}_j|$ containing the B_k, $k \in \mathcal{I}_j$; otherwise, if $\mathcal{I}_j = \emptyset$ then omit conditioning on $\mathbf{B}$ or equivalently take $\mathbf{B}$ to be a constant. By assumption (ii), $\mathbf{B}$ is a function of $\mathbf{A}$. So, in (7.4), $\mathrm{Pr}\left(P_j \le \alpha_j \,\middle|\, \mathbf{B}\right) = \mathrm{E}\left\{\mathrm{Pr}\left(P_j \le \alpha_j \,\middle|\, \mathbf{A}\right) \,\middle|\, \mathbf{B}\right\} \le \mathrm{E}\left(\alpha_j \,\middle|\, \mathbf{B}\right) = \alpha_j$ for $j \in \mathcal{J}$. Using the fact that $\mathbf{P}'$ has independent uniform coordinates, it follows that for each $j \in \mathcal{J}$, and for each fixed $\mathbf{p} \in [0,1]^{|\mathcal{I}_j|}$

$$
\begin{aligned}
\mathrm{Pr}\left(P_j \le \alpha_j \,\middle|\, P_k = p_k, k \in \mathcal{I}_j\right) &= \mathrm{Pr}\left(P_j \le \alpha_j \,\middle|\, \mathbf{B} = \mathbf{p}\right) \le \alpha_j \quad (7.5) \\
&= \mathrm{Pr}\left(P_j' \le \alpha_j\right) \\
&= \mathrm{Pr}\left(P_j' \le \alpha_j \,\middle|\, P_k' = p_k, k \in \mathcal{I}_j\right).
\end{aligned}
$$

The conclusion now follows from Cohen and Sackrowitz [42, Theorem 2.5], where their condition (1.3) is (7.5), and their condition (1.7) holds trivially for $\mathbf{P}'$ with its independent coordinates. In place of [42, Theorem 2.5], one may use the similar textbook result [254, Theorem 6.B.3], again because $\mathbf{P}'$ has independent coordinates. □

7.4   Combining Jointly Valid, Possibly Dependent P-values

7.4.1   General Issues

A collection, P_j, $j \in \mathscr{J} \subseteq \{1, 2, \ldots, J\}$, of P-values may be used to jointly test aspects of a single joint null hypothesis, H_0. Were H_0 true, all of the aspects would be true, and a valid collection, P_j, $j \in \mathscr{J}$, of P-values would be stochastically larger than the uniform distribution in the sense of Definition 2. Write **P** for the $|\mathscr{J}|$-dimensional vector containing the P_j, $j \in \mathscr{J}$, write $\mathbf{P}'$ for a $|\mathscr{J}|$-dimensional vector of independent uniform random variables, and write **p** for an element of the $|\mathscr{J}|$-dimensional unit cube, $\mathbf{p} \in [0, 1]^{|\mathscr{J}|}$.

Various real-valued functions $f(\cdot)$ on $[0, 1]^{|\mathscr{J}|}$ are used to combine evidence from several P-values testing aspects of a single joint hypothesis, H_0. Typically, these functions are monotone increasing, so that, like the P-values that $f(\cdot)$ summarizes, $f(\mathbf{p})$ becomes smaller, signifying stronger evidence against H_0, as the coordinates of **p** become smaller. Typically, a new joint P-value, say $P_{\mathscr{J}}$, is computed using $f(\mathbf{P})$. For this purpose, it makes no difference whether the combining function is $f(\cdot)$ or $g\{f(\cdot)\}$ for any strictly increasing function $g(\cdot)$, so $f(\cdot)$ and $g\{f(\cdot)\}$ are regarded as essentially the same method of combining P-values.

To be valid, the joint P-value, $P_{\mathscr{J}}$, would have to be a valid P-value in the usual sense that if the joint hypothesis H_0 were true, then $\Pr\left(P_{\mathscr{J}} \leq \alpha\right) \leq \alpha$ for all $0 \leq \alpha \leq 1$. Proposition 4 simply states that if **P** is larger than uniform when H_0 is true, then an increasing combination function $f(\cdot)$ yields a valid P-value.

Proposition 4. *Let* $\Psi(k) = \Pr\{f(\mathbf{P}') \leq k\}$, *where* $f(\cdot)$ *is monotone increasing and* $\mathbf{P}'$ *is a* $|\mathscr{J}|$-*dimensional vector of independent uniform random variables. If* **P** *is larger than uniform, then (i)* $\Pr\{f(\mathbf{P}) \leq k\} \leq \Psi(k)$, *for each* k, *and (ii)* $\Pr\left(P_{\mathscr{J}} \leq \alpha\right) \leq \alpha$ *for all* $0 \leq \alpha \leq 1$ *where* $P_{\mathscr{J}} = \Psi\{f(\mathbf{P})\}$.

Proof. Part (i) is immediate from Definition 2. For (ii), use the coupling in Lemma 1. Because $\Psi(k)$ is the distribution of both $\mathbf{P}'$ and $\widetilde{\mathbf{P}}'$ in Lemma 1,

$$\Pr\left[\Psi\left\{f\left(\widetilde{\mathbf{P}}'\right)\right\} \leq \alpha\right] = \Pr\left[\Psi\{f(\mathbf{P}')\} \leq \alpha\right] \leq \alpha.$$

Now, $\Psi\{f(\cdot)\}$ is monotone increasing (because both $f(\cdot)$ and $\Psi(\cdot)$ are monotone increasing); so,

$$\Psi\left\{f\left(\widetilde{\mathbf{P}}\right)\right\} \geq \Psi\left\{f\left(\widetilde{\mathbf{P}}'\right)\right\}.$$

Therefore,

$$\Pr\left(P_{\mathscr{J}} \leq \alpha\right) = \Pr\left[\Psi\{f(\mathbf{P})\} \leq \alpha\right] = \Pr\left[\Psi\left\{f\left(\widetilde{\mathbf{P}}\right)\right\} \leq \alpha\right] \leq \alpha.$$

$\square$

7.4.2   Fisher's Product of P-values

The familiar and venerable method of combining independent P-values, P_j, $j \in \mathscr{J}$, to test H_0 is due to Sir Ronald Fisher [67]. There are two essentially equivalent forms:

$$f(\mathbf{P}) = \prod_{j \in \mathscr{J}} P_j \quad \text{or} \quad g\{f(\mathbf{P})\} = -2 \sum_{j \in \mathscr{J}} \log(P_j) \text{ where } g(a) = -2\log(a). \quad (7.6)$$

Form $g\{f(\mathbf{P})\}$ is attractive in the limited sense that $g\{f(\mathbf{P}')\}$ has the chi-square distribution with $2\,|\mathscr{J}|$ degrees of freedom when $\mathbf{P}'$ is a vector of $|\mathscr{J}|$ independent uniform random variables.

Despite being familiar, Fisher's method is not well-suited to use in sensitivity analyses in observational studies; specifically, it often has low power [112, §3.5]. Sensitivity analyses combine upper bounds on several P-values, and these are larger than uniform under appropriate conditions; however, some of the upper bounds may be close to 1, while Fisher's method is paying for uniformly distributed P-values. More powerful methods focus on small P-values, rather than all P-values, often using truncated products of P-values.

7.4.3   Truncated Products of P-values

The truncated product of P-values was briefly discussed in §5.1 and Table 5.1. Let κ be a fixed number, $0 < \kappa \le 1$, and $\chi(E)$ be the binary indicator of event E, so $\chi(P_j \le \kappa) = 1$ if $P_j \le \kappa$ and $\chi(P_j \le \kappa) = 0$ otherwise. Zaykin, Zhivotovsky, Westfall, and Weir [305] combine P-values using the truncated product,

$$f(\mathbf{P}) = \prod_{j \in \mathscr{J}} P_j^{\chi(P_j \le \kappa)}, \quad (7.7)$$

so (7.7) is the product of just those P-values that are at most κ. Of course, (7.7) is not itself a P-value, but it is a statistic, and a P-value may be derived from it. Taking $\kappa = 1$ in (7.7) yields Fisher's method in (7.6). For $\kappa = 0.1$, the truncated product statistic is the product of those P-values that are at most 0.1; that is, the product of those P-values that are either below or not far above the conventional 0.05 level. The truncated product in (7.7) is never smaller than Fisher's $\prod_{j \in \mathscr{J}} P_j$ in (7.6); so, the null distributions of (7.6) and (7.7) are quite different, as is evident in Table 5.1. When truncating two independent uniform random variables at $\kappa = 0.1$, the truncated product in (7.7) has probability $(1 - 0.1)^2 = 0.81$ of being equal to 1, while Fisher's product (7.6) equals 1 with probability zero. When used in sensitivity analyses, where some upper bounds on P-values may be much larger than uniform, the truncated product (7.7) often has higher power than does Fisher's method [112, §3.5].

Zaykin et al. [305] use a calculus argument to derive the distribution $\Psi(k) = \Pr\{f(\mathbf{P}') \le k\}$ when $\mathbf{P}'$ consists of $|\mathscr{J}|$ independent uniform random variables. An alternative derivation of the same distribution uses its representation as a binomial mixture of gamma distributions [112, expression (6)].[2]

---

[2]The distribution of the truncated product may be computed in R using the `truncatedP` or

7.4.4   Rank-truncated Product of P-values

An alternative to the truncated product is due to Dudbridge and Koeleman [59]. They propose two methods, an alternative to (7.7) and a generalization that includes both this alternative and (7.7) as special cases. The alternative is the rank-truncated product defined to be the product of the K smallest P-values, where $K \leq |\mathcal{J}|$, so this is $\min_{j \in \mathcal{J}} P_j$ for $K = 1$ and it is Fisher's method for $K = |\mathcal{J}|$. The generalization is the product of the K smallest P-values if at least K P-values are less than or equal to κ; otherwise, if fewer than K P-values are less than or equal to κ, then it is the product of all of the P-values that are less than or equal to κ.

The exercises consider various simple ways to combine independent P-values.

7.5   Summary: Dependent *P*-values Jointly Larger Than Uniform

Proposition 3 in this chapter is the first of two technical steps in building evidence factors from repeated analyses of the same data. The second of the two technical steps is Theorem 9 of Chapter 11.

7.6   Exercises

Exercise 7.1. *For $f(\mathbf{P}) = \min_{j \in \mathcal{J}} P_j$, determine $\Psi(k) = \Pr\{f(\mathbf{P}') \leq k\}$ in Proposition 4, where $\mathbf{P}'$ consists of $|\mathcal{J}|$ independent uniform random variables.*

Exercise 7.2. *For $f(\mathbf{P}) = \max_{j \in \mathcal{J}} P_j$, determine $\Psi(k) = \Pr\{f(\mathbf{P}') \leq k\}$ in Proposition 4, where $\mathbf{P}'$ consists of $|\mathcal{J}|$ independent uniform random variables.*

Exercise 7.3. *Let $P_{(1)} \leq P_{(2)} \leq \cdots \leq P_{(|\mathcal{J}|)}$ be the order statistics of $\mathbf{P}$. Fix ℓ with $1 \leq \ell \leq |\mathcal{J}|$. For $f(\mathbf{P}) = P_{(\ell)}$, determine $\Psi(k) = \Pr\{f(\mathbf{P}') \leq k\}$ in Proposition 4 where $\mathbf{P}'$ consists of $|\mathcal{J}|$ independent uniform random variables.*

Exercise 7.4. *Continuing Exercise 7.3, with $|\mathcal{J}| = 3$ factors and $f(\mathbf{P}) = P_{(2)}$: What value of $P_{(2)}$ is just significant at the 0.05 level in the combined test?*

---

truncatedPbg functions in the sensitivitymv package. Setting $\kappa = 1$ in these functions yields Fisher's method. Use of these functions is illustrated in Ref. [217].

Chapter 8

Treatment Assignments as Permutations

Abstract

A study design has N treatment positions, and a treatment assignment for N individuals places one individual in each treatment position. So, each treatment assignment is a permutation of N individuals into N treatment positions, and such a permutation may be represented in a familiar form as an $N \times N$ permutation matrix. Although there are $N!$ permutations of N individuals, most study designs restrict the allowed treatment assignments to be fewer than $N!$. When individuals are permuted, they carry with them their personal attributes, such as observed and unobserved covariates and potential outcomes under alternative treatments; however, the treatments they receive are determined by their ultimate position in the study design, and the treatments they receive determine which potential outcome they will exhibit. Though very simple, this description of treatment assignments as permutations is the most general formulation of the notion of a fixed study design with many alternative treatment assignments. This is the first of several chapters that assemble the components from which evidence factors are built. In particular, we will discover again and again that permutation matrices that assign treatments can be written uniquely as the product of two permutation matrices of different types. In later chapters, this representation of a treatment assignment as the product of two or more terms will become the basis for evidence factors.

8.1 Formalizing Intuition about Unrelated Pieces of Evidence

This chapter is the first of several chapters that formalize the intuition we had in Chapter 4 that certain pieces of evidence from the same data are, in some sense, unrelated, despite being statistically dependent. For instance, the evidence we derived from Panels (a) and (b) of Figure 4.2 seemed to be unrelated, even though Panel (a) can be derived from Panel (b) by projecting points horizontally to the left to the vertical axis. Proposition 2 in Chapter 7 was a small step on the path of formalizing intuition: perhaps we are thinking about the additional contribution of Panel (b) conditionally given the information in Panel (a). This is only a small step because our intuitive interpretation of Panel (b) seems to be the same whether or not we say we are conditioning on Panel (a). We would view Panel (b) in the same way, whether or not we had first viewed Panel (a). That perspective is the perspective of independence, not of conditional independence. Had Panel (b) duplicated Panel (a), then Panel (b) would provide information on its own, but would provide no additional information conditionally given the information in Panel (a), so we would not have two evidence factors, and Proposition 2 would be true but vacuous. When is Proposition 2 vacuous and when is it useful? So, at this stage, our intuition about Panels (a) and (b) of Figure 4.2 has elements that have not yet been formalized, elements that remain puzzling.

Why should we care whether our intuition about Panels (a) and (b) of Figure 4.2 has been formalized? First, we may be misinterpreting Figure 4.2 in the absence of a rigorous argument in support of claims made about it. Second, and more importantly, without a formal development, we do not know the scope of such arguments, when they are valid, when they are invalid. Are evidence factors something peculiar and rare? Or, are we surrounded by them, but unable to recognize their presence? The examples in Chapter 4 seemed to have certain symmetries, but their symmetries were different; moreover, in Chapter 5, Table 5.6 abandoned one symmetry in favor of another. Is there any order to this? Third, as we push into related topics that are intrinsically formal, such as formal statistical inferences, we do not know whether and how we can integrate extant formalities with current intuitions about situations like Figure 4.2.

Could our intuitions about Figure 4.2 and the other examples in Chapters 4–6 simply be mistaken in their entirety? Actually, we already know how to formalize certain bits and pieces, specifically the parts having to do with certain rank tests, under the null hypothesis, in randomized experiments with untied responses. Focus on this case for one moment. Intuitively, a rank correlation, like Kendall's correlation, applied to Panel (b) of Figure 4.2 cares not at all about the marginal distributions of the two variables being correlated,[1] so it cares not at all about Panel (a), and this implies independence of a rank correlation in Panel (b) and a signed rank statistic in Panel (a); see Ref. [207]. More familiar still is the independence of the successive rank sum statistics in §4.2; specifically, this fact traces back to a result of Alfred Renyi that has been extended several times [3, 60, 152].

Still, the bits and pieces that have been formalized seem too specialized, for several reasons. First, rank tests and their associated confidence intervals and estimates are often reasonable [110, 140], but it seems odd and unnatural to be required to use them in the examples in Chapter 4. Second, many rank tests do not yield the desired exact independence: in §5.2, Wilcoxon's test does, but the Hodges-Lehmann [103] test does not. It is well known that ranking within small blocks often yields inefficient tests [140, 165], and Hodges and Lehmann [103] proposed their aligned ranks to restore efficiency with small blocks. The restriction to particular rank tests, excluding for example the Hodges and Lehmann test, is not without consequences for test performance. Third, the results about exact independence require continuous distributions free of ties; yet, this again seems odd and unnatural. Should we actually worry about a few ties? Are evidence factors unavailable for discrete data recorded in contingency tables? Fourth and most important: We are interested in evidence factors for the light they may shed on unmeasured biases from nonrandomized treatment as-

---

[1] In the absence of ties, rank correlations depend only upon the copula [247]. In contrast, for discrete distributions, joint distributions are often constrained in their dependence by their marginal distributions.

signment. A theory applicable only with randomized treatment assignment is missing key elements.

In Theorem 9 in Chapter 11, it will turn out that we do not need any of the following elements: (i) rank tests, (ii) continuous distributions free of ties, (iii) randomized treatment assignment. Exact independence of factors will not be achieved. However, in randomization tests under the null hypothesis, the vector of P-values from several factors will be stochastically larger than the uniform distribution on a multi-dimensional cube. In sensitivity analyses, under the null hypothesis, the vector of upper bounds on P-values will be stochastically larger than the uniform distribution. This is all we need to act as if the factors came from independent studies, perhaps affected by different unmeasured biases.

The path to Theorem 9 is a long, scenic, gentle slope, hopefully a pleasant stroll through familiar terrain populated by elementary matrix algebra and elementary combinatorics. To complete this stroll, we must stop thinking about factoring the distribution of outcomes, and start thinking about factoring the distribution of treatment assignments. For two evidence factors, we must represent treatment assignments as a set of permutation matrices that factors uniquely into two sets of permutation matrices. In Figure 4.2, one set of permutation matrices will permute treatments within pairs, while the other permutes intact pairs among doses of smoking. These factorizations of treatment assignments occur in many ways, and each way may be compounded with itself, or with other ways, to produce additional factors. Many factorizations occur naturally in simple study designs. In the room where you sit, you are surrounded by evidence factors, but perhaps you have not noticed them.

Chapter 12 and some of the exercises in earlier chapters will observe that many of the structures encountered in Chapters 8–11 occur all the time in the theory of finite groups.[2] However, you may skip the exercises and ignore Chapter 12, yet understand evidence factors in their entirety from Chapters 8–11.

8.2 Individuals, Strata, and Treatment Positions

There are S strata, $s = 1, \ldots, S$, defined by observed covariates, and n_s individuals, $i = 1, \ldots, n_s$, in stratum s, with $N = n_1 + n_2 + \cdots + n_S$ individuals in total. For instance, strata might be defined so that people in the same stratum have the same age and gender. An individual's stratum is an aspect of the individual, determined by the person's observed covariates, so an individual's stratum does not change if the individual is assigned to a different treatment.

Individuals are often people, but strictly speaking they need not be people. Strictly speaking, an individual is an opportunity to apply or withhold a treatment,[3]

---

[2]If a group of permutation matrices has a subgroup, then each group element may be written uniquely as the product of an element of the subgroup and an element of a system of distinct representatives of the cosets of that subgroup. From this, the structure required for two evidence factors is obtained. See Chapter 12.

[3]Sometimes, the neutral word "unit" is used instead of "individual." The word "unit" emphasizes that units need not be people. The word "individual" emphasizes the typical case, and by doing so it can make somewhat technical sentences seem less obscure. I have opted for the word "individual" in this book.

so if each person receives a single treatment, then an individual is a person. Sometimes a treatment cannot be applied to a single person — perhaps, whole schools must be assigned to treatment or control — and in this case an individual is a school, not a person. Instead, an individual might be an eye, so each person contributes two eyes, two individuals. One eye might be assigned to treatment, the other to control, and in this case a person is a stratum s containing that person's $n_s = 2$ eyes.

The study design also involves N treatment positions. A treatment assignment places the N individuals into the N treatment positions, thereby assigning each individual to a particular treatment position. Regarding the treatment positions as fixed, a treatment assignment permutes the N individuals so that each one has a home in a different treatment position.[4] Write **n** for the column vector $(1, 2, \ldots, N)^T$ of identifiers of the N individuals, so a treatment assignment is a permutation of the coordinates of **n**. If no restrictions were placed upon the treatment assignments, then there would be $N! = N \times (N-1) \times \cdots \times 2 \times 1$ possible treatment assignments, because there are $N!$ ways to rearrange the coordinates of **n**. Often, there are restrictions.

This one notation covers a number of situations. First, the situation without strata is the same as the situation in which all N individuals fall in a single stratum, $S = 1$ and $N = n_1$, so that situation does not require separate notation. This situation arose in §4.2 in the unstratified comparison of DNA damage in health-care workers handling antineoplastic drugs, with $N = 59$. In contrast, in the same example in §4.2, but with $S = 3$ age strata, stratum 20–29 years had $n_1 = 20$ individuals, stratum 30-39 years had $n_2 = 19$ individuals, and stratum 40-55 years had $n_3 = 20$ individuals. Second, in treatment-control matched pairs, S is even, there are $S/2$ pairs, with $n_s = 2$ for $s = 1, \ldots, S$. Third, suppose that each stratum s contains $n_s = 3$ individuals. Then there might be three treatments, as in §4.4, each applied once in each stratum — a so-called complete block design — or there might be just treatment/control, with one treated individual and two controls in each stratum — so-called 1-to-2 matched sets.

Often there are restrictions on the treatment assignments, so that not all $N!$ assignments are considered. For instance, we may wish to compare individuals in stratum s to other individuals in stratum s, because individuals in the same stratum are similar in terms of observed covariates; so, we may restrict attention to permutations of **n** that permute individuals within but not across strata. In this case, there are at most $n_1! \times n_2! \times \cdots \times n_S!$ treatment assignments, rather than $N!$ treatment assignments.

If we permuted individuals within but not across $S = N/2$ matched pairs, there would be 2^S possible treatment assignments, as $n_s! = 2! = 2$ for each s. If S doses of treatment varied among pairs, with one untreated control and one individual treated at a particular dose, then there would be $S!$ assignments of pairs to doses, together with 2^S treatment/control assignments within pairs, making $S! \times 2^S$ permutations that do not alter the pairing of individuals. This is the situation in the periodontal data in §4.1.

It is useful to distinguish strata and blocks, despite their similarity.[5] Strata are attributes of individuals, while blocks are attributes of study designs. Strata are at-

---

[4]We could, instead, regard the people as having fixed positions, permuting the treatment — it makes no difference.

[5]Alas, the term "block" has several interrelated but distinct meanings in different fields that overlap

tributes of individuals not yet assigned to treatment positions. Blocks are collections of treatment positions not yet inhabited by individuals. Stratum s is an attribute of the n_s individuals who inhabit stratum s; change their treatment assignments and their stratum does not change. In contrast, a block is an attribute of the study design. For instance, the first block may have positions for two individuals, one untreated control and one individual treated at a particular dose. A treatment assignment might assign a particular stratum or pair containing two individuals to this first block, then assign one of these two individuals to control, the other to treatment at the specified dose. The distinction between strata and blocks is especially important when different blocks are treated in different ways. For instance, the distinction is important if different blocks may have different doses of treatment. The distinction is also important when different blocks house different treatments, say block 1 houses treatments A, B, and C, while block 2 houses treatments A, B, and D, as occurs in so-called incomplete block designs. A stratum of size 3 assigned to the first block will have different options for treatment than if it were assigned to the second block. A stratum containing n_s individuals can only be assigned to a block containing n_s treatment positions, even if both stratum and block sizes may vary.

How else might the permutations be restricted? Although N treatment positions are needed to house N individuals, there may be fewer than N distinct treatments. For instance, suppose there were a single stratum, $S = 1$ with $N = n_1$, with m_1 treated individuals and $n_1 - m_1$ untreated controls. Treated individuals, in this case, are all treated in the same way, and controls are treated in the same way. Then, there are $n_1!$ ways to assign n_1 individuals to n_1 positions, but there are really only $\binom{n_1}{m_1} = n_1! / \{m_1! \times (n_1 - m_1)!\}$ practically distinct ways to assign treatment/control, so we might wish to restrict attention to $\binom{n_1}{m_1}$ permutations, rather than $n_1!$ permutations. It is sometimes convenient to restrict attention to permutations that represent practically distinct treatment assignments.

8.3 Permutation Matrices

Definition 3. *An $N \times N$ permutation matrix is an $N \times N$ matrix of 0's and 1's with precisely one 1 in each row and column.*

For instance,

$$\mathbf{g} = \begin{bmatrix} 0 & 0 & 0 & 1 \\ 0 & 0 & 1 & 0 \\ 1 & 0 & 0 & 0 \\ 0 & 1 & 0 & 0 \end{bmatrix} \tag{8.1}$$

is a 4×4 matrix that permutes $\mathbf{n} = (1, 2, 3, 4)^T$ to $\mathbf{gn} = (4, 3, 1, 2)^T$.

A treatment assignment is a permutation of the N individuals in $\mathbf{n}$ into N treatment positions. Each treatment assignment may be represented by a permutation matrix.

---

with this book. In this book, the term block has one meaning: a collection of treatment positions in a study design.

The treatment assignment **g** in (8.1) assigns individual 4 to treatment position 1, individual 3 to treatment position 2, individual 1 to treatment position 3, and individual 2 to treatment position 4. If individuals 1 and 2 were paired — if they were in the same first stratum $s = 1$ with $n_1 = 2$ individuals — and if individuals 3 and 4 were paired in stratum $s = 2$, then **g** would have: (i) left the pairing intact, (ii) interchanged the two pairs, so pair $s = 2$ occupies the first two treatment positions, and (iii) switched the order of the two people in pair $s = 2$ while leaving the two people in pair $s = 1$ in their original order. Although the number of 4×4 permutation matrices is $4! = 4 \times 3 \times 2 \times 1 = 24$, only $2! \times 2^2 = 8$ such matrices are like **g** in (8.1) in that they leave the pairing intact.

8.4 Pick Matrices

A pick matrix is a special type of permutation matrix. Stated informally, for $1 \leq m \leq N$, an (N, m)-pick matrix selects m individuals from N individuals, without disturbing the order of these m individuals or the order of the complementary $N - m$ individuals. Later, pick matrices will represent, without redundancy, picking m individuals for treatment and $N - m$ individuals for control.

Definition 4. *An (N, m)-pick matrix is an $N \times N$ permutation matrix* $\mathbf{k} = [k_{ij}]$ *such that for $i = 1, \ldots, m - 1$ and $j = 1, \ldots, N$ it has*

$$k_{ij} \;\geq\; k_{i'j} \quad for \;\; 1 \leq i < i' \leq m, \; j = 1, \ldots, N,$$

$$k_{ij} \;\geq\; k_{i'j} \quad for \;\; m + 1 \leq i < i' \leq N, \; j = 1, \ldots, N.$$

For instance,

$$\mathbf{k} = \begin{bmatrix} 0 & 1 & 0 & 0 & 0 \\ 0 & 0 & 0 & 1 & 0 \\ 1 & 0 & 0 & 0 & 0 \\ 0 & 0 & 1 & 0 & 0 \\ 0 & 0 & 0 & 0 & 1 \end{bmatrix} \tag{8.2}$$

is a $(5, 2)$-pick matrix. In (8.2), **k** picks 2 of 5 individuals without disturbing the order of the 2 selected individuals or the 3 remaining individuals, by permuting $\mathbf{n} = (1, 2, 3, 4, 5)^T$ to $\mathbf{kn} = (2, 4, 1, 3, 5)^T$. That is, **k** in (8.2) picks individuals 2 and 4, leaving 2 before 4, rejects individuals 1, 3, and 5, leaving 1 before 3 and 3 before 5. Later, **k** in (8.2) will represent one of the $\binom{5}{2} = 10$ ways to select 2 of 5 individuals for treatment, assigning the remaining 3 individuals to control.

How many (N, m)-pick matrices are there? It is easy to see that the answer is $\binom{N}{m}$. There are $\binom{N}{m}$ ways to pick m columns from the N columns. Having selected m columns, put a 1 in the first row of the first selected column, a 1 in the second row of the second selected column and so on. Having done this, there is only one way to produce a permutation matrix filling in the remaining $N - m$ rows consistent with Definition 4.

> **Why Are Pick Matrices Useful?** Many different permutation matrices split N individuals into the same two groups of sizes m and $N-m$, because these permutation matrices also order the individuals within each group. In fact, $m! \times (N-m)!$ different permutation matrices produce the same split. A pick matrix is a single permutation that represents the entire collection of $m! \times (N-m)!$ permutation matrices that produce the same split, the same division into two groups.

8.5 Direct Sums of Permutation Matrices

Immediately from Definition 3, if $\mathbf{k}_1$ is an $N_1 \times N_1$ permutation matrix and $\mathbf{k}_2$ is an $N_2 \times N_2$ permutation matrix, then

$$\mathbf{k} = \begin{bmatrix} \mathbf{k}_1 & \mathbf{0} \\ \mathbf{0} & \mathbf{k}_2 \end{bmatrix} \tag{8.3}$$

is an $(N_1 + N_2) \times (N_1 + N_2)$ permutation matrix, called the direct sum of $\mathbf{k}_1$ and $\mathbf{k}_2$. In (8.3), $\mathbf{0}$ denotes a matrix of appropriate dimensions containing zeros, so the $\mathbf{0}$ in the upper right corner is $N_1 \times N_2$ while the $\mathbf{0}$ in the lower left corner is $N_2 \times N_1$.

Definition 5. *If $\mathbf{k}_\ell$ is an $N_\ell \times N_\ell$ permutation matrix for $\ell = 1, \ldots, L$, then their direct sum is the $\left(\sum_{\ell=1}^{L} N_\ell\right) \times \left(\sum_{\ell=1}^{L} N_\ell\right)$ permutation matrix*

$$\mathbf{k} = \begin{bmatrix} \mathbf{k}_1 & \mathbf{0} & \cdots & \mathbf{0} \\ \mathbf{0} & \mathbf{k}_2 & \cdots & \mathbf{0} \\ \vdots & \vdots & \ddots & \vdots \\ \mathbf{0} & \mathbf{0} & \cdots & \mathbf{k}_L \end{bmatrix}. \tag{8.4}$$

For instance, as in the age stratified analysis in §5.2, we might entertain only those treatment assignments that permute individuals within their own strata, leaving the strata in their original order. In this case, a treatment assignment is an $N \times N$ permutation matrix $\mathbf{k}$ of the form (8.4), where $N = n_1 + \cdots + n_S$, $L = S$, and $\mathbf{k}_s$ is an $n_s \times n_s$ permutation matrix. If we allowed every possible permutation in stratum s, then there would be $n_s!$ possible choices for $\mathbf{k}_s$. If we further allowed every possible $(\mathbf{k}_1, \ldots, \mathbf{k}_S)$ in (8.4), then there would be $n_1! \times \cdots \times n_S!$ treatment assignments of the form (8.4). In the simplest case, if we permute treatment/control without constraints within $S = N/2$ matched pairs, so $n_s = 2$ for each s, then each $\mathbf{k}_s$ is either

$$\mathbf{a} = \begin{bmatrix} 1 & 0 \\ 0 & 1 \end{bmatrix} \text{ or } \mathbf{b} = \begin{bmatrix} 0 & 1 \\ 1 & 0 \end{bmatrix}, \tag{8.5}$$

and there are $n_1! \times \cdots \times n_S! = 2! \times \cdots \times 2! = 2^S$ matrices of the form (8.4); that is, there are 2^S possible treatment assignments.

Are there study designs in which we impose constraints, so that the choice for $\mathbf{k}_1$ is constrained by the choices for $(\mathbf{k}_2, \ldots, \mathbf{k}_S)$? Indeed, there are. Suppose that there are S people, each with two eyes, making $N = 2S$ eyes in total in S matched pairs. One eye of each person will be given the treatment, the other eye will be given the control. In (8.5), $\mathbf{k}_s = \mathbf{a}$ means that the left eye of person s is treated and the right eye is control, while $\mathbf{k}_s = \mathbf{b}$ means that the right eye is treated and the left eye is control. An unconstrained choice of $\mathbf{k}$ in (8.4) is logically possible but could produce a very poor experimental design, say a design in which all S left eyes are treated and all S right eyes are control, so treatment/control is totally confounded with left/right. With an even number S of people, a crossover design insists that half of the people have $\mathbf{k}_s = \mathbf{a}$, or a treated left eye, and the remaining half have $\mathbf{k}_s = \mathbf{b}$, or a treated right eye; so, left/right is balanced rather than confounded with treatment/control. In the crossover study with S pairs of eyes, attention is restricted to $\binom{S}{S/2}$ treatment assignments of the form (8.4), not 2^S treatment assignments.

An important special case of (8.3) has $\mathbf{k}_1$ equal to the $N_1 \times N_1$ identity matrix, $\mathbf{I}$, so that

$$\mathbf{k} = \begin{bmatrix} \mathbf{I} & \mathbf{0} \\ \mathbf{0} & \mathbf{a} \end{bmatrix} \tag{8.6}$$

where $\mathbf{a}$ is an $N_2 \times N_2$ permutation matrix. A treatment assignment of the form (8.6) fixes the assignments of the first N_1 individuals while permuting the remaining N_2 individuals. Often, a complex treatment assignment may be decomposed into a sequence of steps, where each step has the simple form (8.6). One example is discussed in §8.6.

Why Are Direct Sums Useful? A direct sum of permutation matrices reassigns treatments within strata without destroying the strata.

8.6 Subpick Matrices

8.6.1 A Subpick Matrix Picks from What Remains

An (N,m)-pick matrix in §8.4 served to pick m individuals for treatment, assigning the remaining $N - m$ individuals to control. If there are $L \geq 3$ treatments rather than treatment/control, then we may assign treatments by picking m individuals from N individuals for treatment 1, picking m' individuals from the remaining $N - m$ individuals for treatment 2, and so on. At step ℓ of this process, we fixed the decisions already made in steps $1, \ldots, \ell - 1$, so step ℓ has the form (8.6) with N_1 individuals already assigned in steps $1, \ldots, \ell - 1$, and $N_2 = N - N_1$ individuals still available to be assigned to treatment ℓ. At each step, the matrix (8.6) is $N \times N$, but at successive steps N_1 increases and N_2 decreases.

Definition 6. *An (N,m,m')-subpick matrix is an $N \times N$ permutation matrix of the form*

$$\mathbf{h} = \begin{bmatrix} \mathbf{I} & \mathbf{0} \\ \mathbf{0} & \mathbf{a} \end{bmatrix}$$

where $\mathbf{I}$ is the $m \times m$ identity matrix and $\mathbf{a}$ is an $(N-m,m')$-pick matrix.

For instance, $\mathbf{h}$ in (8.7) is a $(5,2,1)$-subpick matrix.

$$\mathbf{h} = \begin{bmatrix} 1 & 0 & 0 & 0 & 0 \\ 0 & 1 & 0 & 0 & 0 \\ 0 & 0 & 0 & 0 & 1 \\ 0 & 0 & 1 & 0 & 0 \\ 0 & 0 & 0 & 1 & 0 \end{bmatrix} \tag{8.7}$$

Specifically, $\mathbf{h}$ in (8.7) is a 5×5 permutation matrix that is the direct sum of a 2×2 identity matrix and a $(5-2,1)$-pick matrix of size 3×3. By itself, the matrix $\mathbf{h}$ in (8.7) would act on individuals $\mathbf{n} = (1,2,3,4,5)^T$ by fixing individuals 1 and 2, and permuting individuals 3, 4, and 5, to obtain $\mathbf{hn} = (1,2,5,3,4)^T$. However, a subpick matrix with $m > 0$ is not typically applied on its own, but rather after m individuals have been assigned to earlier treatments.

> **Why Are Subpick Matrices Useful?** As with pick matrices, many different permutation matrices further subdivide $N - m$ individuals into two groups of sizes m' and $N - m - m'$ because they also order the individuals in the subdivided groups. A subpick matrix is a single representative of the collection of permutation matrices that produce the same subdivision.

8.6.2 Forming 3 Treatment Groups in 2 Steps, A Pick and a Subpick

Suppose that there are three treatments and five individuals. Suppose that $m = 2$ individuals are to be assigned to treatment 1, that $m' = 1$ individual is to be assigned to treatment 2, and $N - m - m' = 5 - 2 - 1 = 2$ individuals are to be assigned to treatment 3. Such a treatment assignment is obtained by multiplying a $(5,2,1)$-subpick matrix by a $(5,2)$-pick matrix: the pick matrix selects $m = 2$ individuals for treatment 1, the subpick matrix fixes those two people and selects from those remaining $m' = 1$ person for treatment 2. For instance, $\mathbf{k}$ in (8.2) is a $(5,2)$-pick matrix that picks individuals 2 and 4 for treatment group 1. Multiplying $\mathbf{h}$ in (8.7) by $\mathbf{k}$ in (8.2) yields

$$\mathbf{hkn} = \begin{bmatrix} 1 & 0 & 0 & 0 & 0 \\ 0 & 1 & 0 & 0 & 0 \\ 0 & 0 & 0 & 0 & 1 \\ 0 & 0 & 1 & 0 & 0 \\ 0 & 0 & 0 & 1 & 0 \end{bmatrix} \begin{bmatrix} 0 & 1 & 0 & 0 & 0 \\ 0 & 0 & 0 & 1 & 0 \\ 1 & 0 & 0 & 0 & 0 \\ 0 & 0 & 1 & 0 & 0 \\ 0 & 0 & 0 & 0 & 1 \end{bmatrix} \begin{bmatrix} 1 \\ 2 \\ 3 \\ 4 \\ 5 \end{bmatrix} \tag{8.8}$$

$$
= \begin{bmatrix} 1 & 0 & 0 & 0 & 0 \\ 0 & 1 & 0 & 0 & 0 \\ 0 & 0 & 0 & 0 & 1 \\ 0 & 0 & 1 & 0 & 0 \\ 0 & 0 & 0 & 1 & 0 \end{bmatrix} \begin{bmatrix} 2 \\ 4 \\ 1 \\ 3 \\ 5 \end{bmatrix} = \begin{bmatrix} 2 \\ 4 \\ 5 \\ 1 \\ 3 \end{bmatrix},
$$

Here, **k** picked individuals 2 and 4 for treatment 1, **h** respected that decision as final and picked individual 5 for treatment 2 from the remaining individuals 1, 3, 5, leaving individuals 1 and 3 for treatment group 3. Notice that **h**, **k**, and **hk** split $\mathbf{n} = (1,2,3,4,5)^T$ into groups, but within each group the original order of individuals is retained: group 1 has $(2,4)$, group 2 has (5), and group 3 has $(1,3)$.

Picks and Subpicks Work Together A division of N individuals into three treatment groups of size m, m', and $N - m - m'$ can be represented in precisely one way as the product of a pick and a subpick, even though many different permutation matrices produce this same division. A pick and a subpick jointly and uniquely represent the collection of $m! \times m'! \times (N - m - m')!$ permutation matrices that produce the same division into three treatment groups.

8.6.3   Forming L Treatment Groups in L − 1 Steps

Equation (8.8) multiplies one subpick matrix **h** by one pick matrix **k** to divide 5 individuals into 3 groups, but the same process may be applied iteratively, multiplying by additional subpick matrices to further divide individuals into additional groups. For instance, the $(5,3,1)$-subpick matrix

$$
\mathbf{a} = \begin{bmatrix} 1 & 0 & 0 & 0 & 0 \\ 0 & 1 & 0 & 0 & 0 \\ 0 & 0 & 1 & 0 & 0 \\ 0 & 0 & 0 & 0 & 1 \\ 0 & 0 & 0 & 1 & 0 \end{bmatrix}
$$

is a 5×5 permutation matrix that fixes the first three coordinates and picks one of the remaining two individuals for treatment 3, putting the final individual in group 4. Multiplying (8.8) by **a** yields $\mathbf{ahkn} = (2,4,5,3,1)^T$, so **h** respects **k**'s assignments, and **a** respects both **h** and **k**'s assignments. Clearly, any number N of individuals may be assigned to L groups by multiplying a pick matrix and $L - 2$ subpick matrices.

8.6.4   How Many Subpicks Are There?

From §8.4, the number of (N,m)-pick matrices is $\binom{N}{m}$, one for each way of picking m individuals for treatment 1 from N individuals. How many (N,m,m')-subpick matrices are there? From Definition 6, the number of (N,m,m')-subpick matrices equals the number of $(N-m,m')$-pick matrices, or $\binom{N-m}{m'}$, one for each way of picking m' individuals for treatment 2 from the remaining $N - m$ individuals.

There are

$$\frac{N!}{m!\,m'!\,(N-m-m')!} = \binom{N}{m}\binom{N-m}{m'}$$

ways to split N individuals into three groups, one of size m, the second of size m', the third of size $N - m - m'$, and that equals the number of ways to write a product, $\mathbf{hk}$, of an (N, m, m')-subpick matrix $\mathbf{h}$ and an (N, m)-pick matrix $\mathbf{k}$. Are all of these products, $\mathbf{hk}$, distinct matrices? One way to answer is to think about $\mathbf{h}$ and $\mathbf{k}$ as permutations, not as matrices. Can we check that they are distinct directly from the definitions of pick and subpick matrices? Indeed, we can. As seen in §8.4, an (N, m)-pick matrix $\mathbf{k}$ is uniquely determined by its first m rows. Moreover, for all (N, m, m')-subpick matrices, say $\mathbf{h}$ and $\mathbf{h}'$, the first m rows of $\mathbf{k}$ equal the first m rows of both $\mathbf{hk}$ and $\mathbf{h}'\mathbf{k}$, so $\mathbf{hk} \neq \mathbf{h}'\mathbf{k}'$ whenever $\mathbf{k} \neq \mathbf{k}'$. Because permutation matrices are nonsingular, $\mathbf{hk} \neq \mathbf{h}'\mathbf{k}$ if and only if $\mathbf{h} \neq \mathbf{h}'$. Therefore, the $\binom{N}{m}\binom{N-m}{m'}$ products, $\mathbf{hk}$, are distinct matrices.

8.7   Treatments with Doses

8.7.1   Doses of Treatment Within Treatment Groups

In §8.4, there were two treatments, perhaps treatment and control, perhaps treatment A and treatment B. Some treatments have varied doses; others do not. Smokers may currently smoke two cigarettes per day or two packs per day, so smoking is a treatment with doses. Nonsmokers all currently smoke zero cigarettes per day, so nonsmoking is a treatment that cannot be further subdivided by the amount currently smoked. Viewed in this way, treatment A has doses but treatment B does not. For instance, see the benzene example in §4.5.

If treatments A and B were two medications, then they might each have doses, and the dose of A might not be commensurate with the dose of B. To say that doses of different treatments may be incommensurate is simply to say that there is no reason to regard the same number of milligrams of aspirin or ibuprofen as equal doses.

Sometimes, the dose of smoking is recorded as packs-per-day multiplied by years-of-smoking, and in this case current nonsmokers would have doses of smoking that are nonzero if they had smoked in the past but quit; then, A and B would both have doses. Alternatively, doses may be viewed as multidimensional: two people who are the same in terms of current smoking may have different pasts. Two people who currently smoke a pack a day may have different histories of smoking, hence different cumulative pack-years. Two current nonsmokers may differ: one never smoked, the other smoked for a decade but quit.

Each of these possibilities refers to a different design with different evidence factors.

8.7.2   One Treatment Has Doses, the Other Does Not

Suppose first that treatment A has doses but treatment B does not. There are N individuals, of whom m individuals will be moved to the initial m positions in the design to receive treatment A. This movement will be produced by an (N, m)-pick matrix, as in §8.4. Each of those m positions has a dose of treatment A. To be definite, suppose that, in the design, the m treatment positions for treatment A are arranged in nondecreasing order, so position 1 has the lowest dose of A and position m has the highest dose. The m selected individuals are then permuted among the m treatment positions for A by a second permutation matrix; so, a treatment assignment is the product of two permutation matrices, one determining A or B, the other determining the dose of A. The second permutation matrix is a direct sum of the form

$$\mathbf{h} = \begin{bmatrix} \mathbf{h}_1 & \mathbf{0} \\ \mathbf{0} & \mathbf{I} \end{bmatrix} \tag{8.9}$$

where $\mathbf{h}_1$ is an $m \times m$ permutation matrix and $\mathbf{I}$ is an $(N-m) \times (N-m)$ identity matrix. There are $m!$ matrices of the form (8.9). Consider, for instance, $\mathbf{k}$ in (8.2) which picked $m = 2$ of $N = 5$ individuals for treatment A, specifically individuals 2 and 4. Then the permutation matrix

$$\mathbf{hk} = \begin{bmatrix} 0 & 1 & 0 & 0 & 0 \\ 1 & 0 & 0 & 0 & 0 \\ 0 & 0 & 1 & 0 & 0 \\ 0 & 0 & 0 & 1 & 0 \\ 0 & 0 & 0 & 0 & 1 \end{bmatrix} \begin{bmatrix} 0 & 1 & 0 & 0 & 0 \\ 0 & 0 & 0 & 1 & 0 \\ 1 & 0 & 0 & 0 & 0 \\ 0 & 0 & 1 & 0 & 0 \\ 0 & 0 & 0 & 0 & 1 \end{bmatrix}$$

acts on the individuals $\mathbf{n} = (1, 2, \ldots, N)^T$ to produce $\mathbf{hkn} = (4, 2, 1, 3, 5)^T$, so individuals 2 and 4 receive treatment A, individuals 1, 3, and 5 receive treatment B, but individual 2 receives the higher dose of treatment A.

There are $\binom{N}{m}$ ways to pick m of N individuals for treatment A, assigning the rest to treatment B. As discussed in §8.4, there are $\binom{N}{m}$ distinct (N, m)-pick matrices, $\mathbf{k}$. There are $m!$ ways to sort the m individuals selected for treatment A into the m positions in the design for treatment A, where each position has a dose. There are $m!$ permutation matrices of the form (8.9). So, there are $\binom{N}{m} m!$ treatment assignments, and each is uniquely represented as the product $\mathbf{hk}$ of an $\mathbf{h}$ of the form (8.9) and (N, m)-pick matrix $\mathbf{k}$. This factorization of the treatment assignment into $\mathbf{hk}$ will result in two evidence factors.

8.7.3 Two Treatments, Each with Doses

If both treatment A and treatment B have doses, then an (N, m)-pick matrix $\mathbf{k}$ divides individuals into group A and group B, a matrix of the form (8.9) assigns individuals in A to dose positions, and a matrix

$$\mathbf{h}' = \begin{bmatrix} \mathbf{I} & \mathbf{0} \\ \mathbf{0} & \mathbf{h}_2 \end{bmatrix}$$

assigns individuals in B to doses, where $\mathbf{I}$ is an $m \times m$ identity matrix and $\mathbf{h}_2$ is an $(N-m) \times (N-m)$ permutation matrix. The treatment assignment for individuals

$\mathbf{n} = (1, \dots, N)^T$ is $\mathbf{h'hkn}$. Note that, unlike most pairs of matrices, $\mathbf{h}$ and $\mathbf{h'}$ commute in the sense that $\mathbf{hh'} = \mathbf{h'h}$ as

$$\mathbf{hh'} = \begin{bmatrix} \mathbf{h}_1 & 0 \\ 0 & \mathbf{I} \end{bmatrix} \begin{bmatrix} \mathbf{I} & 0 \\ 0 & \mathbf{h}_2 \end{bmatrix} = \begin{bmatrix} \mathbf{h}_1 & 0 \\ 0 & \mathbf{h}_2 \end{bmatrix} \qquad (8.10)$$

$$= \begin{bmatrix} \mathbf{I} & 0 \\ 0 & \mathbf{h}_2 \end{bmatrix} \begin{bmatrix} \mathbf{h}_1 & 0 \\ 0 & \mathbf{I} \end{bmatrix} = \mathbf{h'h}.$$

With doses in both groups, there can be three evidence factors $\mathbf{h'hk}$ representing a comparison of A and B, a check for dose-response in A, and another check for dose-response in B. Do current smokers differ from nonsmokers? Do current heavy smokers differ from current light smokers? Do nonsmokers who quit smoking differ from nonsmokers who never smoked?

Alternatively, there could be two factors, a pick $\mathbf{k}$ and a direct sum of $\mathbf{h}_1$ and $\mathbf{h}_2$ in the middle of (8.10) which equals $\mathbf{hh'}$. Are smokers different from nonsmokers, A versus B? Among smokers and separately among nonsmokers, does pack-years of smoking predict the outcome?

8.7.4   Tied Doses

What if several doses are equal? What if some doses of treatment A are tied? Many smokers smoke one-pack-a-day. The dose "one-pack-a-day" will appear repeatedly in the design. As described here, many of the treatment positions for treatment A, smoking, have the same dose, one pack-a-day. The $m!$ matrices of the form (8.9) will distinguish doses of A that are not distinct. A statistical analysis should not distinguish treatments that are in fact identical. How should this issue be addressed? My sense is that this issue does need to be addressed, but a single method of addressing the issue should not be baked into the design at this stage. In many cases, it will suffice to use statistics that are unaffected by (or invariant to) swaps of treatment positions representing identical treatments, and commonly used statistics do that automatically.

In contrast, in some cases, we may seek additional evidence factors through additional subdivisions. This means that $\mathbf{h}$ in (8.9) would be replaced by a product of permutation matrices. Suppose that current smoking is recorded in three intervals of packs-per-day, namely $(0, 1)$, $[1, 2)$, and $[2, \infty)$. A pick matrix assigns individuals to nonsmokers and smokers. A subpick matrix splits smokers into heavy smokers with $[2, \infty)$ packs-per-day and other smokers. A second subpick matrix splits the remaining smokers, $(0, 1)$ or $[1, 2)$ packs per day. A different subpick matrix splits nonsmokers into never-smokers and quitters. Yet another subpick matrix splits heavy smokers into two groups defined by their median years-of-smoking, and so on.

8.8   Permuting Strata of the Same Size

Suppose that all S strata have the same size, $n_1 = n_2 = \cdots = n_S = n$, say, so that $N = Sn$. Also, the study design has S blocks of size n, so we might permute whole

S strata into their homes in the S blocks. Perhaps doses of treatment vary among blocks but not within them. For instance, matched pairs are strata of size $n_s = 2$ for $s = 1, \ldots, S$, and $N = 2S$. In the list of individuals, $\mathbf{n} = (1, \ldots, N)^T$, individuals 1 to n are in stratum $s = 1$, individuals $n + 1$ to $2n$ are in stratum $s = 2$, and so on. How could we permute whole strata without rearranging the individuals inside those strata? That is to say: However we decide to permute the S strata, inside stratum $s = 2$, the first individual should be $n + 1$ and the last individual should be $2n$, even if stratum $s = 2$ has been moved to become the last stratum. The matrix $\mathbf{h}$ in (8.11) is an $N \times N$ permutation matrix in the form of an $S \times S$ matrix of $n \times n$ matrices, where each $n \times n$ matrix is either the identity, $\mathbf{I}$, or the zero matrix $\mathbf{0}$, and each row and column contains exactly one identity matrix,

$$
\mathbf{h} = \begin{bmatrix} \mathbf{0} & \mathbf{I} & \cdots & \mathbf{0} \\ \mathbf{0} & \mathbf{0} & \cdots & \mathbf{I} \\ \vdots & \vdots & \ddots & \vdots \\ \mathbf{I} & \mathbf{0} & \cdots & \mathbf{0} \end{bmatrix}.
\tag{8.11}
$$

Then $\mathbf{hn}$ moves stratum 2 to the first position, stratum S to the second position, $\ldots$, and stratum 1 to the last position, but as it does this, the individuals inside a stratum retain their original ordering. There are $S!$ permutation matrices with the same form as (8.11); that is, $N \times N$ permutation matrices composed of $S \times S$ submatrices of size $n \times n$, where each submatrix is $\mathbf{I}$ or $\mathbf{0}$, with precisely one $\mathbf{I}$ in each row and column.

The form (8.11) may be described using a familiar concept from linear algebra, namely the Kronecker product. If $\mathbf{a}$ is an $S \times S$ matrix and $\mathbf{b}$ is an $n \times n$ matrix, then their Kronecker product, $\mathbf{a} \otimes \mathbf{b}$ is an $Sn \times Sn$ matrix consisting of an $S \times S$ matrix of $n \times n$ matrices, where the $n \times n$ matrix in row i and column j of the $S \times S$ matrix is $a_{ij} \mathbf{b}$. The $S!$ matrices of the form (8.11) are the $S!$ Kronecker products $\mathbf{a} \otimes \mathbf{I}$ as $\mathbf{a}$ ranges over the $S!$ permutation matrices of size $S \times S$.

8.9 Permuting Several Permutation Matrices

8.9.1 Treatments that Vary Within and Between Blocks

As in §8.8, suppose that all S strata have the same size, $n_1 = n_2 = \cdots = n_S = n$, say, so that $N = Sn$. Also, the study design has S blocks of size n. Whole strata of size n are assigned to blocks of size n. How can strata be permuted, individuals be permuted within strata, without altering which individuals are found together in the same stratum? Perhaps treatment/control varies within blocks. Perhaps the dose of treatment varies among the blocks, so permuting the strata to find homes within the blocks entails assigning a dose to each stratum.

Take $L = S$ in (8.4) and consider the product of $\mathbf{h}$ in (8.11) and $\mathbf{k}$ in (8.4):

$$
\mathbf{hk} = \begin{bmatrix} \mathbf{0} & \mathbf{I} & \cdots & \mathbf{0} \\ \mathbf{0} & \mathbf{0} & \cdots & \mathbf{I} \\ \vdots & \vdots & \ddots & \vdots \\ \mathbf{I} & \mathbf{0} & \cdots & \mathbf{0} \end{bmatrix} \begin{bmatrix} \mathbf{k}_1 & \mathbf{0} & \cdots & \mathbf{0} \\ \mathbf{0} & \mathbf{k}_2 & \cdots & \mathbf{0} \\ \vdots & \vdots & \ddots & \vdots \\ \mathbf{0} & \mathbf{0} & \cdots & \mathbf{k}_S \end{bmatrix}
\tag{8.12}
$$

$$
= \begin{bmatrix} \mathbf{0} & \mathbf{k}_2 & \cdots & \mathbf{0} \\ \mathbf{0} & \mathbf{0} & \cdots & \mathbf{k}_S \\ \vdots & \vdots & \ddots & \vdots \\ \mathbf{k}_1 & \mathbf{0} & \cdots & \mathbf{0} \end{bmatrix} ,
\tag{8.13}
$$

so stratum 2 is permuted by $\mathbf{k}_2$ and moved to be in the first block, stratum S is permuted by $\mathbf{k}_S$ and moved to be in the second block, and so on.

Suppose that we place no restrictions on the permutations beyond the structures in (8.4) and (8.11). Then we may permute within stratum s in $n!$ ways, and we may combine that permutation with any permutations in the other strata, so we may permute within all the strata in $(n!)^S$ ways; equivalently, there are $(n!)^S$ possible choices for the matrix $\mathbf{k}$ in (8.12). Also, there are $S!$ ways to permute the S strata; equivalently, there are $S!$ choices for the matrix $\mathbf{h}$ in (8.12). Permuting within strata and permuting the strata themselves may be done in $S!\,(n!)^S$ ways, and each way is represented in exactly one way as the product of a matrix of the form (8.4) and a matrix of the form (8.11) to yield a matrix of the form (8.13). In the case of S matched pairs, $n = 2$, there are $S!$ permutations of the pairs and 2^S permutations within pairs, making $S!\,2^S$ permutations in all.

8.9.2   Restricting the Assignments of Strata to Blocks

Individuals in the same stratum are similar to one another, but individuals in different strata might be quite different. If a treatment varies between blocks, it may not be reasonable to consider all $S!$ reassignments of strata to blocks. If the S strata are matched pairs, $n_s = 2$ for $s = 1, \ldots, S$, matched for age, gender, and many other covariates, then it might seem unreasonable to swap two blocks for a pair of men aged 82 and a pair of women aged 21. True, we are looking at the difference in outcomes between two men aged 82, and the difference in outcomes between two women aged 21, so we have controlled age and gender in one way; that is, by differencing outcomes for two similar individuals. Nonetheless, we might wish to control twice for age and gender, once by differencing within strata, and again by restricting permutations of strata so that only similar strata are interchanged. Instead of entertaining all $S!$ permutations of strata into blocks, we might restrict attention to swaps of pairs of the same gender in the same 10-year age category. We might interchange a pair of men aged 82 with a pair of men aged 86, but refuse to interchange a pair of men aged 82 with a pair of women aged 21. It is easy to impose such a restriction, in effect by stratifying the matched pairs into strata defined by gender and 10-year age categories. Something similar was done in Table 5.6 for the periodontal data, where pairs that were matched for age and gender were additionally only permuted within four categories of pairs defined by age and gender.

Specifically, we might restrict the matrix $\mathbf{h}$ in (8.11) and (8.12) so that it never swaps two strata that are very different. Suppose that we had collected the S strata into $L < S$ bundles of strata, where strata in the same bundle were similar, say sharing the same gender and 10-year age category. For notational convenience, we sort the strata by their bundles, so strata in the same bundle are contiguous, bundle 1, bundle

$2, \ldots$, bundle L. Then we wish to restrict $\mathbf{h}$ so that it permutes strata within but not between bundles. We do this by requiring $\mathbf{h}$ in (8.11) to have the form $\mathbf{a} \otimes \mathbf{I}$ where $\mathbf{a}$ is an $S \times S$ permutation matrix that is a direct sum of the form (8.4).

8.10 Doing Several Things at Once

The various structures in this chapter may be superimposed upon one another, producing a wide variety of study designs with evidence factors. Two are mentioned here as illustrations.

8.10.1 Strata with Three Treatments

In stratum s, m_s individuals are picked for treatment A, and from the remaining $n_s - m_s$ individuals, m_s' individuals are picked for treatment B, with the rest assigned to treatment C. In stratum s, this is produced by an (n_s, m_s)-pick matrix $\mathbf{a}_s$ and an $\left(n_s, m_s, m_s'\right)$-subpick matrix $\mathbf{b}_s$ whose product $\mathbf{b}_s \mathbf{a}_s$ determines treatment assignment in stratum s. Both $\mathbf{a}_s$ and $\mathbf{b}_s$ are of size $n_s \times n_s$. The direct sum (8.4) of these matrices determines the treatment assignment in all S strata as:

$$
\begin{bmatrix}
\mathbf{b}_1 \mathbf{a}_1 & \mathbf{0} & \cdots & \mathbf{0} \\
\mathbf{0} & \mathbf{b}_2 \mathbf{a}_2 & \cdots & \mathbf{0} \\
\vdots & \vdots & \ddots & \vdots \\
\mathbf{0} & \mathbf{0} & \cdots & \mathbf{b}_S \mathbf{a}_S
\end{bmatrix}
$$

$$
= \begin{bmatrix}
\mathbf{b}_1 & \mathbf{0} & \cdots & \mathbf{0} \\
\mathbf{0} & \mathbf{b}_2 & \cdots & \mathbf{0} \\
\vdots & \vdots & \ddots & \vdots \\
\mathbf{0} & \mathbf{0} & \cdots & \mathbf{b}_S
\end{bmatrix}
\begin{bmatrix}
\mathbf{a}_1 & \mathbf{0} & \cdots & \mathbf{0} \\
\mathbf{0} & \mathbf{a}_2 & \cdots & \mathbf{0} \\
\vdots & \vdots & \ddots & \vdots \\
\mathbf{0} & \mathbf{0} & \cdots & \mathbf{a}_S
\end{bmatrix}
= \mathbf{ba}, \text{ say.}
$$

Each treatment assignment is represented uniquely as the product of two permutation matrices, $\mathbf{b}$ and $\mathbf{a}$, where $\mathbf{a}$ is the direct sum of pick matrices, and $\mathbf{b}$ is the direct sum of subpick matrices. Correspondingly, the design will have two evidence factors. This structure was present in the age-stratified analysis in §5.2 of DNA damage among health-care workers handling antineoplastic drugs.

    If one or more of treatment groups A, B, and C have doses of their treatments, then there can be more than two evidence factors formed by also permuting doses within assigned groups, as in §8.7. If all three treatment groups have doses, there could be up to five evidence factors, formed from a direct sum of pick matrices, a direct sum of subpick matrices, and three direct sums of matrices analogous to (8.9).

8.10.2 Pairs and Triples with Three Treatments and Doses

Suppose that the S strata are of two sizes, $S = S_1 + S_2$, and there are S_1 pairs with $n_s = 2$ for $s = 1, \ldots, S_1$, and S_2 triples with $n_s = 3$ for $s = S_1 + 1, \ldots, S_1 + S_2$. The pairs contain treatment A and treatment B, while the triples contain treatments A, B, and C. Treatment A is applied at doses that vary among the pairs and among the triples, so permuting strata entails changing the dose of A.

Consider first the S_1 pairs. The pairs can be permuted among themselves, and the triples can be permuted among themselves, but pairs cannot be permuted with triples while keeping the strata intact. Taking $L = S_1$ in (8.4) and each $\mathbf{k}_s$ to be $\mathbf{a}$ or $\mathbf{b}$ in (8.5) $s = 1,\dots,S_1$, yields 2^{S_1} permutation matrices $\mathbf{c}$ of size $2S_1 \times 2S_1$ of the form (8.4), and each of these may be multiplied by a permutation matrix $\mathbf{d}$ of size $2S_1 \times 2S_1$ of the form (8.11), to obtain $\mathbf{cd}$ which permutes within pairs and then permutes the pairs. There are $S_1!$ such matrices $\mathbf{d}$ making $2^{S_1} S_1!$ permutations of the pairs, each represented in a unique way as a product $\mathbf{cd}$.

Within triple s, we may pick one individual for treatment C, then pick one of the remaining two individuals for treatment A. This decision is the product of a 3×3 pick matrix $\mathbf{e}_s$, of which there are 3, and a 3×3 subpick matrix $\mathbf{f}_s$, of which there are 2, so this decision may be made in $3 \times 2 = 6 = 3!$ ways. Taking the direct sum (8.4) of S_2 such products $\mathbf{f}_s \mathbf{e}_s$ yields a $3S_2 \times 3S_2$ permutation matrix, and each one is the product of the direct sum, say $\mathbf{f}$, of the $\mathbf{f}_s$ and the direct sum, say $\mathbf{e}$, of the $\mathbf{e}_s$,

$$
\mathbf{fe} =
\begin{bmatrix}
\mathbf{f}_1 & \mathbf{0} & \cdots & \mathbf{0} \\
\mathbf{0} & \mathbf{f}_2 & \cdots & \mathbf{0} \\
\vdots & \vdots & \ddots & \vdots \\
\mathbf{0} & \mathbf{0} & \cdots & \mathbf{f}_{S_2}
\end{bmatrix}
\begin{bmatrix}
\mathbf{e}_1 & \mathbf{0} & \cdots & \mathbf{0} \\
\mathbf{0} & \mathbf{e}_2 & \cdots & \mathbf{0} \\
\vdots & \vdots & \ddots & \vdots \\
\mathbf{0} & \mathbf{0} & \cdots & \mathbf{e}_{S_2}
\end{bmatrix}
\tag{8.14}
$$

$$
=
\begin{bmatrix}
\mathbf{f}_1\mathbf{e}_1 & \mathbf{0} & \cdots & \mathbf{0} \\
\mathbf{0} & \mathbf{f}_2\mathbf{e}_2 & \cdots & \mathbf{0} \\
\vdots & \vdots & \ddots & \vdots \\
\mathbf{0} & \mathbf{0} & \cdots & \mathbf{f}_{S_2}\mathbf{e}_{S_2}
\end{bmatrix}
$$

There are $(3!)^{S_2} = 6^{S_2} = 3^{S_2} \times 2^{S_2}$ matrices of the form (8.14), uniquely composed from 3^{S_2} choices for $\mathbf{e}$ and 2^{S_2} choices for $\mathbf{f}$. The S_2 triples are permuted among the doses for A for triples by matrices like (8.11), or more precisely by $3S_2 \times 3S_2$ permutation matrices $\mathbf{h} = \mathbf{m} \otimes \mathbf{I}$ where $\mathbf{m}$ is an $S_2 \times S_2$ permutation matrix and $\mathbf{I}$ is the 3×3 identity matrix. For the $\mathbf{h}$ in (8.11) the $3S_2 \times 3S_2$ permutation matrix is

$$
\mathbf{hfe} =
\begin{bmatrix}
\mathbf{0} & \mathbf{f}_2\mathbf{e}_2 & \cdots & \mathbf{0} \\
\mathbf{0} & \mathbf{0} & \cdots & \mathbf{f}_{S_2}\mathbf{e}_{S_2} \\
\vdots & \vdots & \ddots & \vdots \\
\mathbf{f}_1\mathbf{e}_1 & \mathbf{0} & \cdots & \mathbf{0}
\end{bmatrix}.
$$

There are $6^{S_2} S_2!$ such matrices and each one is uniquely represented as a product $\mathbf{hfe}$.

We obtain a treatment assignment for the entire design, pairs and triples together, by taking the direct sum (8.3) of $\mathbf{cd}$ and $\mathbf{hfe}$,

$$
\begin{bmatrix}
\mathbf{cd} & \mathbf{0} \\
\mathbf{0} & \mathbf{hfe}
\end{bmatrix}
=
\begin{bmatrix}
\mathbf{c} & \mathbf{0} \\
\mathbf{0} & \mathbf{h}
\end{bmatrix}
\begin{bmatrix}
\mathbf{d} & \mathbf{0} \\
\mathbf{0} & \mathbf{f}
\end{bmatrix}
\begin{bmatrix}
\mathbf{I} & \mathbf{0} \\
\mathbf{0} & \mathbf{e}
\end{bmatrix}.
\tag{8.15}
$$

In (8.15), the last matrix on the far right, with diagonal elements $\mathbf{I}$ and $\mathbf{e}$, does nothing to the pairs and picks one individual in each triple for treatment C. In (8.15), the matrix with diagonal elements $\mathbf{d}$ and $\mathbf{f}$ picks one of the two remaining individuals in each stratum for treatment A. Finally, in (8.15), the matrix with diagonal elements $\mathbf{c}$ and $\mathbf{h}$ permutes pairs and separately permutes triples to determine the dose of A in each stratum. Each of the $2^{S_1} S_1! \times 6^{S_2} S_2!$ treatment assignments is uniquely represented as a product of the form (8.15).

The design will have three evidence factors corresponding with the three factors on the right in (8.15). The factor involving treatment C will receive a nontrivial contribution only from the S_2 triples. Although pairs and triples both have doses of A, these doses will be permuted among pairs and among triples, but not from a pair to a triple.

8.11 Summary: A Treatment Assignment Is a Permutation

The current chapter has considered a fixed study design with N treatment positions. The study design may have blocks, multiple treatments, doses of some or all treatments. The N individuals are assigned to treatment by a permutation matrix that places individuals in treatment positions. We found repeatedly, in very different contexts, that it is often possible to write a treatment assignment uniquely as the product of several factors, a product of several permutation matrices with specific properties. These factorizations of treatment assignments into products of permutation matrices will, in later chapters, be the basis for evidence factors.

8.12 Complement: Split Matrices

A minor but practically useful variation on a theme of this chapter is considered in this complement to this chapter.[6]

An (N, m)-pick matrix in Definition 4 divides N individuals into m individuals in treatment group A and a remainder, and then an (N, m, m')-subpick matrix in Definition 6 leaves the A group fixed and subdivides the $N - m$ individuals in the remainder into a treatment group B of m' individuals and a remainder containing $N - m - m'$ individuals, where the remainder may be further subdivided by further subpick matrices. At each stage in these subdivisions, the original ordering of the individuals, $\mathbf{n} = (1, 2, \ldots, N)^T$, is unchanged inside new subdivisions, but of course is changed between new subdivisions. Individual 1 is the first individual in whichever treatment group contains individual 1, and individual N is the last individual in whichever treatment group contains individual N; however, individual N might be in group B and individual 1 might be in the remainder. This preservation of order within subdivisions is key in representing a permutation matrix in a unique way as a product of simpler permutation matrices. Subpick matrices are block diagonal matrices, with two nonzero diagonal blocks, the first of which is an identity matrix (8.7); so, they look nice, are easy to manipulate in a quick calculation like (8.8), and they capture the central idea of subdividing an undivided collection of individuals.

---

[6]See the Preface for a discussion of the role of "complements."

Split matrices embody the same idea, work in about the same way, but do not look quite so nice. Nonetheless, split matrices often reflect the subdivision needed in some practical application. Having divided N individuals into m individuals in A, m' individuals in B, and a remainder containing $N - m - m'$ individuals, our next thought might not be to subdivide the remainder, but to subdivide A, or subdivide B, or simultaneously subdivide each of A, B, and the remainder to form six rather than three collections of individuals. A split matrix subdivides some or all of previously intact collections of individuals, and does this without reordering the individuals in the newly refined subdivisions. Recall that the number of (N, m)-pick matrices is $\binom{N}{m}$, and one of these matrices is the $N \times N$ identity matrix. With three treatment groups of sizes m, m' and $N - m - m'$, a split matrix $\mathbf{s}$ is an $N \times N$ permutation matrix that is block diagonal,

$$\mathbf{s} = \begin{bmatrix} s_1 & 0 & 0 \\ 0 & s_2 & 0 \\ 0 & 0 & s_3 \end{bmatrix} \tag{8.16}$$

where s_1 is $m \times m$, s_2 is $m' \times m'$, s_3 is $(N - m - m') \times (N - m - m')$, and s_1, s_2, and s_3 are each pick matrices. If s_1 and s_2 are both identity matrices, then $\mathbf{s}$ is simply a subpick matrix dividing the remainder, exactly as in Definition 6. If s_2 and s_3 are both identity matrices, then $\mathbf{s}$ subdivides group A, fixing group B and the remainder. If none of the three blocks in $\mathbf{s}$ is an identity matrix, then $\mathbf{s}$ subdivides all three groups at once.

Split matrices subdivide existing groups, and can produce a tree-structure in which larger groups are subdivided as we move further from the root of the tree. One might compare the repeated divisions created by split matrices to the orthogonal rank contrasts proposed by Marden [152].

The matrix $\mathbf{s}$ in (8.16) may always be rewritten as

$$\mathbf{s} = \begin{bmatrix} s_1 & 0 & 0 \\ 0 & I & 0 \\ 0 & 0 & I \end{bmatrix} \begin{bmatrix} I & 0 & 0 \\ 0 & s_2 & 0 \\ 0 & 0 & I \end{bmatrix} \begin{bmatrix} I & 0 & 0 \\ 0 & I & 0 \\ 0 & 0 & s_3 \end{bmatrix},$$

where the factors commute and may be written in any order. So, subdividing three groups at once may be viewed as one factor or three, admittedly of different forms.

A split matrix need not have three blocks, as in (8.16); rather, it could have two blocks to divide two groups, or more than three blocks to divide more than three groups. Indeed, if (8.16) had a single block dividing the N undivided individuals, $\mathbf{n} = (1, 2, \ldots, N)^T$, then $\mathbf{s}$ would simply be a pick matrix. So, both pick and subpick matrices are special cases of split matrices.

8.13 Exercises

Exercise 8.1. *Show that the transpose of an $N \times N$ permutation matrix $\mathbf{g}$ is its inverse, $\mathbf{g}^{-1} = \mathbf{g}^T$, and hence that: (i) $\mathbf{g}^{-1}$ is also an $N \times N$ permutation matrix and (ii) permutation matrices are nonsingular.*

Exercise 8.2. *Show that the product of two $N \times N$ permutation matrices, $\mathbf{g}$ and $\mathbf{g}'$, is an $N \times N$ permutation matrix, $\mathbf{gg}'$.*

Exercise 8.3. List the $2! \times 2^2 = 8$ permutation matrices like $\mathbf{g}$ in (8.1) that preserve the pairing of the first two individuals and the last two individuals. How many matrices on your list do not change the order of the two pairs? How many matrices on your list preserve the original order of the two individuals inside both pairs, while perhaps reordering the pairs themselves? Is the identity matrix on your list? If you take the inverse of a matrix on your list, is this inverse also on your list? If you multiply two matrices on your list, is the product also on your list?

Exercise 8.4. Is the inverse of an (N,m)-pick matrix also an (N,m)-pick matrix? (Hint: The inverse is the transpose. What is $\mathbf{k}\mathbf{k}^T$ in (8.2)?)

Exercise 8.5. The form of the direct sum in (8.4) is a block diagonal matrix with blocks $(\mathbf{h}_1, \ldots, \mathbf{h}_L)$, where each $\mathbf{h}_\ell$ is an $N_\ell \times N_\ell$ permutation matrix. Show that the inverse of a matrix of the form (8.4) is a permutation matrix of the same form. (Hint: Take the transpose.) Show that the product of two permutation matrices of the form (8.4) is a permutation matrix of the same form.

Exercise 8.6. Matrix $\mathbf{k}$ in (8.6) has the form of a direct sum of an $N_1 \times N_1$ identity matrix and an $N_2 \times N_2$ permutation matrix. Show that $\mathbf{k}^{-1}$ has the same form. (Hint: Take the transpose, $\mathbf{k}^T$.) Show that if both $\mathbf{k}$ and $\mathbf{k}'$ have this form, then so does their product, $\mathbf{k}\mathbf{k}'$. Suppose $\mathbf{a}$ has the form (8.3) and $\mathbf{b}$ has the form (8.6). Show that $\mathbf{a}^{-1}\mathbf{b}\mathbf{a}$ has the form (8.6).

Exercise 8.7. Consider the form (8.11) and the $S!$ matrices of this form, namely $\mathbf{a} \otimes \mathbf{I}$ as $\mathbf{a}$ ranges over the $S!$ permutation matrices of size $S \times S$. Show that the inverse of a matrix $\mathbf{a} \otimes \mathbf{I}$ of this form is also of this form, and give an expression for $(\mathbf{a} \otimes \mathbf{I})^{-1}$ in terms of $\mathbf{a}$. (Hint: No, by now, you know the hint.) Show that the product of two matrices, $\mathbf{a} \otimes \mathbf{I}$ and $\mathbf{b} \otimes \mathbf{I}$, of this form is also of this form, and give an expression for the matrix product, $(\mathbf{a} \otimes \mathbf{I})(\mathbf{b} \otimes \mathbf{I})$, in terms of $\mathbf{a}$ and $\mathbf{b}$.

Exercise 8.8. There are $S! (n!)^S$ permutation matrices of the form (8.13). If $\mathbf{a}$ and $\mathbf{b}$ have the form (8.13), show that $\mathbf{a}^{-1}$ and $\mathbf{a}\mathbf{b}$ both have this same form. If $\mathbf{a}$ has the form (8.13), and $\mathbf{k}$ has the form (8.4) with $L = S$ and $n_1 = \cdots = n_S = n$, then show that $\mathbf{a}^{-1}\mathbf{k}\mathbf{a}$ has the form (8.4).

Exercise 8.9. In (8.8), propose a 5×5 split matrix (8.16) to premultiply $\mathbf{h}\mathbf{k}$ to subdivide the first treatment group into two parts, the first containing individual 4, the second containing individual 2.

Chapter 9

Sets of Treatment Assignments

Abstract

The previous chapter represented a single treatment assignment as one permutation matrix. It was observed that this one permutation matrix can often be represented as the product of several factors, where each factor is a permutation matrix. The current chapter considers sets of permutation matrices, and asks when this factorization is unique.

9.1 Sets of Permutation Matrices

Chapter 8 viewed a study design as N fixed treatment positions, together with a set G of allowed permutations of N individuals into treatment positions; that is, G is a set of $N \times N$ permutation matrices. The set G would contain all $N!$ permutation matrices if there were no restrictions on the assignment of individuals to treatment positions, but this is not common. As always, if A is any finite set, $|A|$ denotes the number of elements of A. For any set G of $N \times N$ permutation matrices, $|G| \leq N!$.

If we have $N = 4$ individuals, in $S = 2$ strata, each of size $n_s = 2$ — if we have two matched pairs, 1 paired with 2, 3 paired with 4 — then the set of $2^2 = 4$ permutations of treatments within pairs is the set

$$K = \{k_1, k_2, k_3, k_4\} \tag{9.1}$$

$$k_1 = \begin{bmatrix} 1 & 0 & 0 & 0 \\ 0 & 1 & 0 & 0 \\ 0 & 0 & 1 & 0 \\ 0 & 0 & 0 & 1 \end{bmatrix}, \quad k_2 = \begin{bmatrix} 0 & 1 & 0 & 0 \\ 1 & 0 & 0 & 0 \\ 0 & 0 & 1 & 0 \\ 0 & 0 & 0 & 1 \end{bmatrix}$$

$$k_3 = \begin{bmatrix} 1 & 0 & 0 & 0 \\ 0 & 1 & 0 & 0 \\ 0 & 0 & 0 & 1 \\ 0 & 0 & 1 & 0 \end{bmatrix}, \quad k_4 = \begin{bmatrix} 0 & 1 & 0 & 0 \\ 1 & 0 & 0 & 0 \\ 0 & 0 & 0 & 1 \\ 0 & 0 & 1 & 0 \end{bmatrix}.$$

Here, k_1 is the 4×4 identity matrix I, k_2 swaps the treatments in the first pair, k_3 swaps the treatments in the second pair, and k_4 swaps the treatments in both pairs. Each element of K is a direct sum (8.3) of two 2×2 submatrices from (8.5), and the set K exhausts the four possibilities. That is, K is the set of permutations within pairs, including of course the permutation $k_1 = I$ that leaves things as they are. If there were S pairs rather than 2 pairs, then the analogous set K would contain 2^S permutation matrices, each of size $2S \times 2S$.

The set,

$$H = \{\mathbf{h}_1, \mathbf{h}_2\} \tag{9.2}$$

$$\mathbf{h}_1 = \begin{bmatrix} 1 & 0 & 0 & 0 \\ 0 & 1 & 0 & 0 \\ 0 & 0 & 1 & 0 \\ 0 & 0 & 0 & 1 \end{bmatrix}, \quad \mathbf{h}_2 = \begin{bmatrix} 0 & 0 & 1 & 0 \\ 0 & 0 & 0 & 1 \\ 1 & 0 & 0 & 0 \\ 0 & 1 & 0 & 0 \end{bmatrix},$$

contains the 4×4 identity matrix $\mathbf{I} = \mathbf{h}_1$, and $\mathbf{h}_2$ which swaps the first and second pair without altering the order of the individuals within the two pairs. The set $H = \{\mathbf{h}_1, \mathbf{h}_2\}$ in (9.2) is the set of 4×4 matrices for two pairs of the general form (8.11). The matrices in H permute the two pairs in all 2! ways without reordering the two individuals inside each pair. With S pairs, the analogous set H contains $S!$ permutation matrices, each of size $2S \times 2S$.

Chapter 8 often spoke of permutation matrices that had a certain form or pattern, such as the (N, m)-pick matrices in Definition 4, or permutation matrices of the form (8.13). The set M of (N, m)-pick matrices contains $|M| = \binom{N}{m}$ matrices.

9.2   Products of Sets

9.2.1   Definition and Example

Given two sets of $N \times N$ permutation matrices, a new set of $N \times N$ permutation matrices may be formed from them by taking the product of their elements.

Definition 7. *If* H *and* K *are two nonempty sets of* $N \times N$ *permutation matrices, then their product* HK *is a set of* $N \times N$ *permutation matrices given by:*

$$HK = \{\mathbf{hk} : \mathbf{h} \in H, \mathbf{k} \in K\}.$$

If H *contains a single permutation matrix,* $H = \{\mathbf{h}\}$, *then write* $\mathbf{h}K$ *in place of* $\{\mathbf{h}\}K$. *If* K *contains a single permutation matrix,* $K = \{\mathbf{k}\}$, *then write* $H\mathbf{k}$ *in place of* $H\{\mathbf{k}\}$.

For instance, the product $G = HK$ of the set $H = \{\mathbf{h}_1, \mathbf{h}_2\}$ in (9.2) and the set $K = \{\mathbf{k}_1, \mathbf{k}_2, \mathbf{k}_3, \mathbf{k}_4\}$ in (9.1) is the set of eight $N \times N$ permutation matrices

$$\begin{aligned} G \;&=\; HK = \{\mathbf{h}_1\mathbf{k}_1, \mathbf{h}_1\mathbf{k}_2, \mathbf{h}_1\mathbf{k}_3, \mathbf{h}_1\mathbf{k}_4, \mathbf{h}_2\mathbf{k}_1, \mathbf{h}_2\mathbf{k}_2, \mathbf{h}_2\mathbf{k}_3, \mathbf{h}_2\mathbf{k}_4\} \\ &=\; \{\mathbf{k}_1, \mathbf{k}_2, \mathbf{k}_3, \mathbf{k}_4, \mathbf{h}_2\mathbf{k}_1, \mathbf{h}_2\mathbf{k}_2, \mathbf{h}_2\mathbf{k}_3, \mathbf{h}_2\mathbf{k}_4\} = K \cup \mathbf{h}_2 K, \end{aligned}$$

because $\mathbf{h}_1 = \mathbf{I}$, so $G = HK$ contains the four matrices in K in (9.1) plus the four matrices in $\mathbf{h}_2 K = \{\mathbf{h}_2\mathbf{k}_1, \mathbf{h}_2\mathbf{k}_2, \mathbf{h}_2\mathbf{k}_3, \mathbf{h}_2\mathbf{k}_4\}$, namely:

$$\mathbf{h}_2\mathbf{k}_1 = \begin{bmatrix} 0 & 0 & 1 & 0 \\ 0 & 0 & 0 & 1 \\ 1 & 0 & 0 & 0 \\ 0 & 1 & 0 & 0 \end{bmatrix}, \quad \mathbf{h}_2\mathbf{k}_2 = \begin{bmatrix} 0 & 0 & 1 & 0 \\ 0 & 0 & 0 & 1 \\ 0 & 1 & 0 & 0 \\ 1 & 0 & 0 & 0 \end{bmatrix},$$

$$h_2k_3 = \begin{bmatrix} 0 & 0 & 0 & 1 \\ 0 & 0 & 1 & 0 \\ 1 & 0 & 0 & 0 \\ 0 & 1 & 0 & 0 \end{bmatrix}, \quad h_2k_4 = \begin{bmatrix} 0 & 0 & 0 & 1 \\ 0 & 0 & 1 & 0 \\ 0 & 1 & 0 & 0 \\ 1 & 0 & 0 & 0 \end{bmatrix}.$$

For two matched pairs, the set product $G = HK$ of H in (9.2) and K in (9.1) is the set of $2^2 2! = 8$ permutation matrices of the form (8.13). The $|G| = 8$ permutations in $G = HK$ are the eight ways to permute two pairs without breaking up the pairs.

9.2.2 Are HK and KH Equal?

Matrices in general, and permutation matrices in particular, often do not commute; that is, for many h and k, $hk \neq kh$. For instance, in (9.1) and (9.2), $h_2k_2 \neq k_2h_2$ because

$$h_2k_2 = \begin{bmatrix} 0 & 0 & 1 & 0 \\ 0 & 0 & 0 & 1 \\ 1 & 0 & 0 & 0 \\ 0 & 1 & 0 & 0 \end{bmatrix} \begin{bmatrix} 0 & 1 & 0 & 0 \\ 1 & 0 & 0 & 0 \\ 0 & 0 & 1 & 0 \\ 0 & 0 & 0 & 1 \end{bmatrix} = \begin{bmatrix} 0 & 0 & 1 & 0 \\ 0 & 0 & 0 & 1 \\ 0 & 1 & 0 & 0 \\ 1 & 0 & 0 & 0 \end{bmatrix}$$

$$\neq \begin{bmatrix} 0 & 0 & 0 & 1 \\ 0 & 0 & 1 & 0 \\ 1 & 0 & 0 & 0 \\ 0 & 1 & 0 & 0 \end{bmatrix} \begin{bmatrix} 0 & 1 & 0 & 0 \\ 1 & 0 & 0 & 0 \\ 0 & 0 & 1 & 0 \\ 0 & 0 & 0 & 1 \end{bmatrix} = \begin{bmatrix} 0 & 0 & 1 & 0 \\ 0 & 0 & 0 & 1 \\ 1 & 0 & 0 & 0 \\ 0 & 1 & 0 & 0 \end{bmatrix} = k_2h_2;$$

however, $k_2h_2 = h_2k_3$. It follows that, in general, $AB \neq BA$ for sets A and B of $N \times N$ permutation matrices. For instance, $h_2k_2 \neq k_2h_2$ implies $Hk_2 \neq k_2H$ because $Hk_2 = \{k_2, h_2k_2\}$ and $k_2H = \{k_2, k_2h_2\}$ as $h_1 = I$. In general, $AB \neq BA$, but equality does hold in some interesting special cases; in particular, in (9.1) and (9.2), we do have $HK = KH$ even though the elements of H and K do not commute.

9.3 Unique Representation as a Product of Two Factors

9.3.1 Does $|AB| = |A| \times |B|$?

The product of the sizes, or cardinalities, of the sets H in (9.2) and K in (9.1) is $|H| \times |K| = 2 \times 4 = 8 = |HK|$, but it is *not* generally true that $|AB| = |A| \times |B|$ for sets A and B of $N \times N$ permutation matrices. For example, for H in (9.2): $HH = H$, so $|H| \times |H| = 2 \times 2 = 4 \neq 2 = |H| = |HH|$.

By definition, $|AB| = |\{ab : a \in A, b \in B\}| \leq |A| \times |B|$, but strict inequality is possible.

9.3.2 Unique Representation Can Be Demonstrated by Counting

In evidence factors, it will often be important to have a unique representation of a treatment assignment g as the product of two factors. Consider, for example, the set G containing the eight 4×4 permutation matrices g that assign treatment/control to individuals inside two pairs and that permute the pairs to assign a pair to a dose, so

$8 = |G|$. Each $\mathbf{g} \in G$ has one and only one representation as the product $\mathbf{g} = \mathbf{hk}$, where $\mathbf{k} \in K$ in (9.1) and $\mathbf{h} \in H$ in (9.2). When is such a representation unique? Lemma 5 is elementary but useful: it says that we can establish that a representation is unique, or not unique, without checking for equality of the matrix products one by one; rather, we can simply count them, and check that the total counts are correct.

Lemma 5. *If* A *and* B *are sets of* $N \times N$ *permutation matrices, then each* $\mathbf{g} \in$ AB *has a unique representation as* $\mathbf{g} = \mathbf{ab}$, $\mathbf{a} \in$ A, $\mathbf{b} \in$ B, *if and only if* $|AB| = |A| \times |B|$.

Proof. This is almost immediate from $|AB| = |\{\mathbf{ab} : \mathbf{a} \in A, \mathbf{b} \in B\}| \leq |A| \times |B|$. Suppose each $\mathbf{g} \in AB$ has only one representation as $\mathbf{g} = \mathbf{ab}$, $\mathbf{a} \in A$, $\mathbf{b} \in B$; then the $|A| \times |B|$ products $\mathbf{ab}$, $\mathbf{a} \in A$, $\mathbf{b} \in B$, are distinct permutation matrices and $|AB| = |A| \times |B|$. Conversely, suppose there is some $\mathbf{c} \in AB$ that can be written in at least two ways, $\mathbf{c} = \mathbf{ab}$ and $\mathbf{c} = \mathbf{a'b'}$ with $\mathbf{a}, \mathbf{a'} \in A$ and $\mathbf{b}, \mathbf{b'} \in B$, $\mathbf{a} \neq \mathbf{a'}$ or $\mathbf{b} \neq \mathbf{b'}$; then the $|AB| \leq (|A| \times |B|) - 1 < |A| \times |B|$. $\qquad\square$

9.3.3   Example: Picks and Subpicks

Suppose that there are three treatment groups to which N individuals will be assigned, and the first m treatment positions are for the first treatment group, the next m' positions are for the second treatment group, and the last $N - m - m'$ positions are for the third treatment group. Many different $N \times N$ permutation matrices produce the same split into three groups; specifically, $m! \, m'! \, (N - m - m')!$ different permutation matrices produce each possible split. These $m! \, m'! \, (N - m - m')!$ different permutation matrices not only divide individuals into three treatment groups, but also order the individuals within groups. We have no interest in the ordering of individuals within a treatment group. We would like one representation, not $m! \, m'! \, (N - m - m')$ different representations, of each assignment of individuals to treatment groups, and we would like to represent each such assignment uniquely as the product of two factors. Each treatment assignment is to be represented as the product of two decisions: (i) Who is picked for treatment one? (ii) How are the rest divided into treatment two and treatment three?

We can divide N individuals into three groups of sizes m, m' and $N - m - m'$ in

$$\frac{N!}{m! \, m'! \, (N - m - m')!} = \binom{N}{m}\binom{N-m}{m'}$$

ways. Let A be the set of (N, m)-pick matrices, and let B be the set of (N, m, m')-subpick matrices, so A and B are sets of $N \times N$ permutation matrices. As discussed in §8.6, each $\mathbf{a} \in A$ picks m individuals for the first treatment group, and each $\mathbf{b} \in B$ fixes these m individuals and picks for the second treatment group m' individuals from the remaining $N - m$ individuals. As discussed in §8.4, there are $|A| = \binom{N}{m}$ pick matrices and $|B| = \binom{N-m}{m'}$ subpick matrices, so by Lemma 5 the set AB is a unique representation of each assignment of individuals to three groups as the product of two assignments for the two decisions (i) and (ii) in the previous paragraph.

9.3.4 Example: Treatments Assigned Within Strata and Doses Assigned Between Strata

In §8.9, suppose S strata are triples, $n_1 = \cdots = n_S = 3$, and the S blocks each have two untreated control positions and one treated position at dose of treatment d_s, where the S doses are different. There are then $S! \, 3^S$ treatment assignments. Let A be the set of $S!$ Kronecker products $\mathbf{a} \otimes \mathbf{I}$ as $\mathbf{a}$ ranges over the $S!$ permutation matrices of size $S \times S$; see (8.11). Let B be the set that contains all 3^S direct sums (8.4) of $(3,1)$-pick matrices. The $S! \, 3^S$ products in AB are all distinct, so by Lemma 5 the set AB is a unique representation of the $S! \, 3^S$ treatment assignments as the products $\mathbf{ab}$, $\mathbf{a} \in A$, $\mathbf{b} \in B$, in the form (8.12).

9.3.5 Products of Several Sets

In §8.6, §8.7, and §8.10, a treatment assignment was represented as the product of more than two factors. No new issues are involved when additional factors are introduced.

Definition 8. *If A_ℓ is a nonempty set of $N \times N$ permutation matrices for $\ell = 1, \ldots L$, then their product is a set of $N \times N$ permutation matrices given by:*

$$A_1 A_2 \cdots A_L = \{\mathbf{a}_1 \mathbf{a}_2 \cdots \mathbf{a}_L : \mathbf{a}_1 \in A_1, \ldots, \mathbf{a}_L \in A_L\}.$$

Lemma 6. *If A_ℓ is a nonempty set of $N \times N$ permutation matrices for $\ell = 1, \ldots L$, then each $\mathbf{g} \in A_1 A_2 \cdots A_L$ has a unique representation as $\mathbf{a}_1 \mathbf{a}_2 \cdots \mathbf{a}_L$ with $\mathbf{a}_1 \in A_1, \ldots$, $\mathbf{a}_L \in A_L$ if and only if $|A_1 A_2 \cdots A_L| = |A_1| \times \cdots \times |A_L|$.*

9.4 *Closure

A nonempty set A of $N \times N$ permutation matrices may or may not be closed under various operations applied to A.

The set H in (9.2) is closed under the operation of taking matrix inverses, because $\mathbf{h}_1^{-1} = \mathbf{h}_1^T = \mathbf{h}_1 \in H$ and $\mathbf{h}_2^{-1} = \mathbf{h}_2^T = \mathbf{h}_2 \in H$. Write $A^{-1} = \{\mathbf{a}^{-1} : \mathbf{a} \in A\}$ and say that a nonempty A is closed under matrix inversion if $A^{-1} \subseteq A$. In particular, all of the following are closed under matrix inversion: $H^{-1} \subseteq H$ in (9.2), $K^{-1} \subseteq K$ in (9.1), $\{\mathbf{k}_1, \mathbf{k}_2\}^{-1} \subseteq \{\mathbf{k}_1, \mathbf{k}_2\}$, and $\{\mathbf{k}_2\}^{-1} \subseteq \{\mathbf{k}_2\}$. However, $\{\mathbf{a}\}^{-1} \not\subseteq \{\mathbf{a}\}$ if $\mathbf{a}$ is asymmetric; for instance, $\{\mathbf{k}\}^{-1} \not\subseteq \{\mathbf{k}\}$ for the single pick matrix $\mathbf{k}$ in (8.2).

The set H in (9.2) is closed under the operation of multiplying elements of H, because $\mathbf{h}_1 \mathbf{h}_1 = \mathbf{h}_1 \in H$, $\mathbf{h}_2 \mathbf{h}_2 = \mathbf{h}_1 \in H$, and $\mathbf{h}_1 \mathbf{h}_2 = \mathbf{h}_2 \mathbf{h}_1 = \mathbf{h}_2 \in H$. Say that a nonempty A is closed under multiplication if $AA \subseteq A$. Then $HH \subseteq H$ in (9.2), $KK \subseteq K$ in (9.1), $\{\mathbf{k}_1, \mathbf{k}_2\} \{\mathbf{k}_1, \mathbf{k}_2\} \subseteq \{\mathbf{k}_1, \mathbf{k}_2\}$; however, $\{\mathbf{k}_2\} \{\mathbf{k}_2\} \not\subseteq \{\mathbf{k}_2\}$ because $\mathbf{k}_2 \mathbf{k}_2 = \mathbf{I} \notin \{\mathbf{k}_2\}$.

If a nonempty A is closed under inversion and multiplication, then $\mathbf{I} \in A$, because A contains an element $\mathbf{a}$, so A contains $\mathbf{a}^{-1}$, so A contains $\mathbf{a} \mathbf{a}^{-1} = \mathbf{I}$.

A set of $N \times N$ permutation matrices that is closed under matrix multiplication and matrix inversion is called a group of $N \times N$ permutation matrices; see Chapter 12.

9.5   Summary: Factoring Sets of Treatment Assignments

In Chapter 8, a single $N \times N$ permutation matrix $\mathbf{g}$ was a single way of assigning treatments to the N individuals. Often, such a matrix $\mathbf{g}$ could be written in a unique way as the product of two or more simpler $N \times N$ permutation matrices, say $\mathbf{g} = \mathbf{hk}$, where $\mathbf{h}$ captured one aspect of treatment assignment and $\mathbf{k}$ captured another; for instance, $\mathbf{k}$ divides individuals into treatment group 1 and the remainder, while $\mathbf{h}$ divides the remainder into treatment groups 2 and 3. Ultimately, these factors, $\mathbf{h}$ and $\mathbf{k}$ in $\mathbf{g} = \mathbf{hk}$, are the factors in "evidence factors." Chapter 9 shifted the focus from an individual $N \times N$ permutation matrix $\mathbf{g}$ to a set G of $N \times N$ permutation matrices consisting of those treatments $\mathbf{g}$ that might occur in a particular study design. For instance, G might contain one $\mathbf{g}$ for each possible way of assigning N individuals to three treatment groups of specified sizes. Attention shifted from factoring a single treatment assignment, $\mathbf{g} = \mathbf{hk}$, to uniquely factoring the set of treatment assignments, G = HK where HK = $\{\mathbf{hk} : \mathbf{h} \in$ H$, \mathbf{k} \in$ K$\}$, where the factorization is unique if each $\mathbf{g} \in$ G has one and only one representation as $\mathbf{g} = \mathbf{hk}$ with $\mathbf{h} \in$ H, $\mathbf{k} \in$ K. Because the factorization is unique, as soon as we speak about a particular $\mathbf{g} \in$ G, its factors $\mathbf{g} = \mathbf{hk}$ are well-defined, and we can speak without ambiguity about the $\mathbf{h}$ and $\mathbf{k}$ that correspond with this particular $\mathbf{g} \in$ G.

9.6   Exercises

Exercise 9.1. *In §8.6, the division of N individuals into $L = 4$ treatment groups was represented as a product of three permutation matrices, a pick matrix and two subpick matrices. Count these matrices and apply Lemma 6 to show that this representation is unique.*

Exercise 9.2. *In (9.1), is $\{\mathbf{k}_3, \mathbf{k}_4\}^{-1} \subseteq \{\mathbf{k}_3, \mathbf{k}_4\}$? Is $\{\mathbf{k}_3, \mathbf{k}_4\} \{\mathbf{k}_3, \mathbf{k}_4\} \subseteq \{\mathbf{k}_3, \mathbf{k}_4\}$?*

Exercise 9.3. *A set of $N \times N$ permutation matrices A is closed under conjugation by a set of $N \times N$ permutation matrices B if $\mathbf{b}^{-1}\mathbf{ab} \in$ A for all $\mathbf{a} \in$ A and $\mathbf{b} \in$ B. Find such a pair of sets (A, B). (Hint: Review Exercise 8.6.) Find another such pair of sets (A, B). (Hint: Review Exercise 8.8.)*

Chapter 10

Probability Distributions for Treatment Assignments

Abstract

The previous chapter considered sets of treatment assignments represented as sets of
permutation matrices. The current chapter introduces probability distributions on those
sets. In a randomized experiment, the distribution of treatment assignments is known,
but in an observational study the distribution is unknown. Sensitivity analysis is defined
in terms of sets of probability distributions on a set of treatment assignments.

10.1   One Distribution

10.1.1   One Distribution **p** on G

Suppose that G is a set of $N \times N$ permutation matrices, so there are $|G|$ matrices **g** in
G. For ease in referring to the matrices **g** in G, it is convenient to number them, $\mathbf{g}_1$,
$\mathbf{g}_2, \ldots, \mathbf{g}_{|G|}$. A probability distribution on G is a vector

$$\mathbf{p} = \left(p_{\mathbf{g}_1}, \ldots, p_{\mathbf{g}_{|G|}} \right)^T$$

of dimension $|G|$ such that

$$p_{\mathbf{g}_j} \geq 0 \;\; \text{for} \;\; j = 1, \ldots, |G| \;\; \text{and} \;\; 1 = \sum_{j=1}^{|G|} p_{\mathbf{g}_j}.$$

If we pick a random $N \times N$ permutation matrix **G** from G with probability distribution
p, then $p_{\mathbf{g}_j} = \Pr(\mathbf{G} = \mathbf{g}_j)$. The uniform distribution on G is

$$\mathbf{p} = \left(\frac{1}{|G|}, \ldots, \frac{1}{|G|} \right)^T. \tag{10.1}$$

10.1.2   Randomized Treatment Assignment

For example, suppose that we have S matched pairs, and we will conduct a random-ized experiment, flipping a fair coin independently S times to assign one individual in each pair to treatment, the other to control. In the case of $S = 2$ pairs, the set G of 4×4 permutation matrices G is given as K in (9.1) with $|G| = 4$ permutation matri-ces, and randomized treatment assignment entails $\mathbf{p} = \left(\frac{1}{4}, \frac{1}{4}, \frac{1}{4}, \frac{1}{4}\right)^T$. For S pairs: G is a set of $2S \times 2S$ permutation matrices; G contains $|G| = 2^S$ matrices, and $p_{\mathbf{g}_j} = 2^{-S}$ for $j = 1, \ldots, 2^S$. In general, in a uniformly randomized experiment, each $\mathbf{g} \in$ G is given the same probability, $p_{\mathbf{g}_j} = \Pr(\mathbf{G} = \mathbf{g}_j) = |G|^{-1}$ for $j = 1, \ldots, |G|$. In a ran-domized experiment, we know the distribution $\mathbf{p}$ of treatment assignments, because we created $\mathbf{p}$ and used it to pick the treatment assignment $\mathbf{G} \in$ G for the experiment; so, there is no need to speculate about $\mathbf{p}$ in a randomized experiment—there is one $\mathbf{p}$ and we know $\mathbf{p}$.

Chapter 9 also considered another G for another study with S matched pairs, in which treatment/control was assigned within S pairs in 2^S ways, and pairs were assigned to doses of the treatment in $S!$ ways, so there are $|G| = S! \times 2^S$ elements in G, and each element is a $2S \times 2S$ permutation matrix. For $S = 2$, the set G is the set product G = HK, with K in (9.1) and H in (9.2), where $|G| = 2! \times 2^2 = 8 = 2 \times 4 = |H| \times |K|$. A study with this G could be randomized. Randomization for $S = 2$ with this G entails $\mathbf{p} = \left(\frac{1}{8}, \frac{1}{8}, \ldots, \frac{1}{8}\right)^T$; for general S it entails $p_{\mathbf{g}_j} = \left(S! \times 2^S\right)^{-1}$ for $j = 1, \ldots, S! \times 2^S$. Because the representation G = HK is unique, when we sample a $\mathbf{G} \in$ G, we have implicitly sampled a unique $\mathbf{H} \in$ H and $\mathbf{K} \in$ K such that $\mathbf{G} = \mathbf{HK}$, so $\mathbf{H}$ and $\mathbf{K}$ inherit distributions from the distribution of $\mathbf{G} \in$ G. Implicitly, the randomization distribution $\mathbf{p} = \left(\frac{1}{8}, \frac{1}{8}, \ldots, \frac{1}{8}\right)^T$ on G for $S = 2$ implies a marginal distribution for K in (9.1), and for each $\mathbf{k} \in$ K it implies a conditional distribution for $\mathbf{H} \in$ H given $\mathbf{K} = \mathbf{k} \in$ K. Can you see what those implied distributions are?

10.1.3   Testing Fisher's Hypothesis of No Effect

If Fisher's hypothesis H_0 of no effect were true, then changing the treatment assign-ment $\mathbf{g} \in$ G changes the positions individuals occupy in the design, but it does not alter their outcomes. For the purpose of testing H_0, we may write a test statistic $t(\cdot)$ concisely as a function $t(\mathbf{g})$ of the treatment assignment $\mathbf{g} \in$ G, suppressing its genuine dependence on other quantities that do not change as treatment assignments change.

Under Fisher's hypothesis H_0 of no treatment effect, the probability that $t(\mathbf{g}) \geq c$, or the upper tail probability, is simply the sum of $p_{\mathbf{g}}$ over all $\mathbf{g}$ such that $t(\mathbf{g}) \geq c$, namely

$$\Upsilon_{\mathbf{p}, G, t}(c) = \sum_{\mathbf{g} \in G: t(\mathbf{g}) \geq c} p_{\mathbf{g}}. \tag{10.2}$$

Therefore, $P = \Upsilon_{\mathbf{p}, G, t}\{t(\mathbf{G})\}$ is the one-sided P-value. In a randomized experiment,

p is known, so the computation of $\Upsilon_{\mathbf{p},G,t}(c)$ is straightforward in principle.[1] Fisher's hypothesis H_0 of no effect is rejected at level α if $P \leq \alpha$.

10.2 A Set of Distributions

10.2.1 A Set $\mathscr{P}$ of Distributions on G

A set $\mathscr{P}$ of distributions on G is simply a set of vectors **p**, where each **p** is a distribution on G.

In a randomized experiment, the true distribution **p** of treatment assignments is created by the investigator in the process of randomly assigning treatments; so, **p** is known to the investigator and there is no need to consider a set $\mathscr{P}$ containing other distributions on G. In an observational study, treatments are not assigned using random numbers generated by a computer, so the true distribution **p** of treatment assignments is not known. In an observational study, a set $\mathscr{P}$ of distributions on G can be used to express a controlled degree of uncertainty about the true distribution **p** of treatment assignments; see section 10.4 about sensitivity analysis.

10.2.2 Finite Sets $\mathscr{P}$

Here is one such set $\mathscr{P}$ of distributions on the two-element set H in (9.2):

$$\mathscr{P} = \left\{ \begin{bmatrix} \frac{1}{2} \\ \frac{1}{2} \end{bmatrix}, \begin{bmatrix} \frac{2}{3} \\ \frac{1}{3} \end{bmatrix}, \begin{bmatrix} \frac{1}{3} \\ \frac{2}{3} \end{bmatrix} \right\}. \tag{10.3}$$

In (10.3), $\mathscr{P}$ contains a coin flip, namely $\mathbf{p} = (p_{\mathbf{h}_1}, p_{\mathbf{h}_2})^T = \left(\frac{1}{2}, \frac{1}{2}\right)^T$, but it also contains two biased treatment assignments, namely $\mathbf{p} = \left(\frac{2}{3}, \frac{1}{3}\right)^T$ and $\mathbf{p} = \left(\frac{1}{3}, \frac{2}{3}\right)^T$. Although very simple, the set $\mathscr{P}$ in (10.3) has several interesting aspects. First, $\mathscr{P}$ in (10.3) includes uniform treatment assignment, but it also includes two moderately large departures from uniform assignment. Second, for all $\mathbf{p} \in \mathscr{P}$ in (10.3), the odds of $\mathbf{h}_1 \in \mathsf{H}$ rather than $\mathbf{h}_2 \in \mathsf{H}$ in (9.2) is never greater than 2-to-1 and never less than 1-to-2, hinting that the magnitude of departure from uniform assignment in $\mathscr{P}$ might in some way or other be characterized by an odds ratio. For instance, the set

$$\mathscr{P}' = \left\{ \begin{bmatrix} \frac{1}{2} \\ \frac{1}{2} \end{bmatrix}, \begin{bmatrix} \frac{3}{4} \\ \frac{1}{4} \end{bmatrix}, \begin{bmatrix} \frac{1}{4} \\ \frac{3}{4} \end{bmatrix} \right\} \tag{10.4}$$

seems to permit a larger departure from uniform treatment assignment, characterized by odds of at most 3-to-1 and at least 1-to-3. Third, $\mathscr{P}$ in (10.3) contains a distribution $\mathbf{p} = \left(\frac{2}{3}, \frac{1}{3}\right)^T$ that favors $\mathbf{h}_1 \in \mathsf{H}$ over $\mathbf{h}_2 \in \mathsf{H}$, and a distribution $\mathbf{p} = \left(\frac{1}{3}, \frac{2}{3}\right)^T$ that

---

[1] That is, computing the tail probability $\Upsilon_{\mathbf{p},G,t}(c)$ or the P-value $\Upsilon_{\mathbf{p},G,t}\{t(\mathbf{G})\}$ is simply a numerical computation. In practice, G is often a large set, so direct exact computation of $\Upsilon_{\mathbf{p},G,t}(c)$ is impractical, and large-sample approximations are used instead. The needed approximations exist for many situations, and they are not discussed in detail in this book. For inference in randomized experiments, one attractive introduction to such approximations is given by Lehmann [140].

favors $\mathbf{h}_2 \in H$ over $\mathbf{h}_1 \in H$; however, as a whole, the set $\mathscr{P}$ in (10.3) favors neither $\mathbf{h}_1 \in H$ nor $\mathbf{h}_2 \in H$. The biased distributions $\mathbf{p} \in \mathscr{P}$ in (10.3) are sometimes very asymmetrical, favoring $\mathbf{h}_1 \in H$ or $\mathbf{h}_2 \in H$, but the set $\mathscr{P}$ is symmetrical, favoring neither $\mathbf{h}_1$ nor $\mathbf{h}_2$. That is, $\mathscr{P}$ in (10.3) is a symmetrical set of objects, where some of the objects are asymmetrical. Stated more precisely, if $\mathbf{p} = (p, p')^T$, then $\mathbf{p}$ is asymmetrical if $p \neq p'$, or equivalently if $(p, p')^T \neq (p', p)^T$; however, the set $\mathscr{P}$ in (10.3) is symmetrical in the sense that, if $(p, p')^T \in \mathscr{P}$, then $(p', p)^T \in \mathscr{P}$. In words, biases by their nature are asymmetrical, but $\mathscr{P}$ in (10.3) is a symmetrical set of biases. Putting the second and third aspect together, $\mathscr{P}$ in (10.3) limits the magnitude of the departure from uniform assignment, but it does not state a direction for the departure.[2]

10.2.3   Infinite Sets $\mathscr{P}$

Although the example in (10.3) contains only $|\mathscr{P}| = 3$ probability distributions, it is more common to consider a set $\mathscr{P}$ containing infinitely many distributions, including the uniform distribution and asymmetrical distributions that differ from the uniform distribution by a controlled amount, where that amount is suitably defined. Often, $\mathscr{P}$ is a symmetrical set of asymmetrical distributions. For $\Gamma \geq 1$, here is one such infinite symmetrical set of distributions on the two-element set H in (9.2):

$$\mathscr{P}_\Gamma^* = \left\{ \begin{bmatrix} p_{\mathbf{h}_1} \\ p_{\mathbf{h}_2} \end{bmatrix} : p_{\mathbf{h}_1} \geq 0, \, p_{\mathbf{h}_2} \geq 0, \, 1 = p_{\mathbf{h}_1} + p_{\mathbf{h}_2}, \, \frac{1}{\Gamma} \leq \frac{p_{\mathbf{h}_1}}{p_{\mathbf{h}_2}} \leq \Gamma \right\}. \qquad (10.5)$$

For $\Gamma = 2$, the set $\mathscr{P}$ in (10.3) is a subset of $\mathscr{P}_\Gamma^*$ in (10.5), $\mathscr{P} \subset \mathscr{P}_\Gamma^*$, so asserting that the true $\mathbf{p}$ is in $\mathscr{P}$ is asserting much more than asserting $\mathbf{p} \in \mathscr{P}_\Gamma^*$. For $\Gamma = 2$, asserting $\mathbf{p} \in \mathscr{P}_\Gamma^*$ is asserting that the bias is at most 2-to-1 in magnitude, whereas asserting $\mathbf{p} \in \mathscr{P}$ is asserting that there either is no bias or the bias is exactly 2-to-1 in magnitude. For $\Gamma = 3$ in (10.5), there are two inclusions: $\mathscr{P}' \subset \mathscr{P}_\Gamma^*$ in (10.4), but also $\mathscr{P} \subset \mathscr{P}_\Gamma^*$ in (10.3); whereas, $\mathscr{P} \not\subset \mathscr{P}'$. For these reasons, if we want a set of distribution $\mathscr{P}$ that expresses ignorance of the direction of bias, ignorance of the exact magnitude of bias, but a limit on the magnitude of bias, $\mathscr{P}_\Gamma^*$ seems preferable to $\mathscr{P}$ and $\mathscr{P}'$.

---

[2]Sometimes, investigators claim to know the direction of bias, and exploit this claimed knowledge in inference. That is, investigators sometimes claim that the relevant set $\mathscr{P}$ is an asymmetrical set, say including $\mathbf{p} = \left(\frac{2}{3}, \frac{1}{3}\right)^T$ and excluding $\mathbf{p} = \left(\frac{1}{3}, \frac{2}{3}\right)^T$. Bound [26] does this in an interesting study asking whether receipt of Social Security Disability Benefits discourages people who might otherwise return to work. Bound compares two groups: people who had applied for benefits and received them, and people whose applications had been denied. So, the two groups were similar in having applied for disability benefits, but differed in whether they received benefits. Bound argued that the direction of the bias is known: healthier people, those who are better able to work, are more likely to be in the group whose applications were denied. Bound found that, by and large, the denied group did not quickly return to work, despite perhaps being better able to work, arguing that this supports the claim that the disincentive effects of actually receiving benefits are not large. Parsons [170] expressed doubts about Bound's argument, to which Bound replied. For a technical discussion of this example and of biases of known direction, see Ref. [195, §6.5].

10.3 *Some Technical Remarks and Definitions

10.3.1 An Optional Section

A few technical remarks and definitions follow about sets $\mathscr{P}$ of distributions on G. These remarks are helpful at specific moments in certain technical arguments, but they are not at all essential concerns for someone who wishes to see the big picture quickly. So, decide whether to read these remarks now, or whether to move on to the next section.

10.3.2 $\mathscr{P}$ Defines What Is Probable, G Defines What Is Possible

Because each $\mathbf{p} = \left(p_{\mathbf{g}_1}, \ldots, p_{\mathbf{g}_{|G|}} \right)^T \in \mathscr{P}$ is a distribution with each $p_{\mathbf{g}_j} \geq 0$ and $1 = \sum_{j=1}^{|G|} p_{\mathbf{g}_j}$, a set $\mathscr{P}$ of distributions on G is always a bounded set of $|G|$-dimensional vectors. For instance, (10.3)–(10.5) are all contained in the unit square, $[0,1] \times [0,1]$, and so are bounded sets. More precisely, a set $\mathscr{P}$ of distributions on G is always contained in a $(|G| - 1)$-dimensional simplex formed as the convex hull of the $|G|$ degenerate distributions $(1,0,\ldots,0)^T$, $(0,1,\ldots,0)^T$, $\ldots$, $(0,0,\ldots,1)^T$. Let us say that a distribution $\mathbf{p} = \left(p_{\mathbf{g}_1}, \ldots, p_{\mathbf{g}_{|G|}} \right)^T$ on G is interior if $p_{\mathbf{g}_j} > 0$ for $j = 1, \ldots, |G|$; that is, $\mathbf{p}$ is interior if it is an interior point of the simplex viewed as a subset of the $(|G| - 1)$-dimensional flat that contains the simplex. If $p_{\mathbf{g}_j} = 0$ for some j, then by definition $\Pr\left(\mathbf{G} = \mathbf{g}_j\right) = 0$; so, there is a slight inconsistency in saying G is the set of possible treatment assignments if some of the elements of the finite set G are not possible because they have probability zero. So, to remove this inconsistency, without further mention outside §10.3, it is assumed that each probability distribution $\mathbf{p}$ on G is interior.

In brief, elements of G may have arbitrarily small nonzero probability, but it is assumed that no element of G has probability zero.

10.3.3 No $\mathbf{p}$ Is Precluded from $\mathscr{P}_\Gamma$ for Large Enough Γ

For each finite $\Gamma \geq 1$, the set $\mathscr{P}_\Gamma^*$ in (10.4) contains infinitely many distributions, all of them interior. For each interior distribution $\mathbf{p}$ on H in (9.2), there exists a finite $\Gamma \geq 1$ such that $\mathbf{p} \in \mathscr{P}_\Gamma^*$ in (10.4), so as $\Gamma \to \infty$ the sets $\mathscr{P}_\Gamma^*$ in (10.4) gradually encompass all of the interior points. Indeed, this is true of each sensitivity model in §10.4. As this structure is true of each specific model used in this book, it is convenient to assume without further mention that this is true whenever we consider a collection $\mathscr{P}_\Gamma$ of interior distributions $\mathbf{p}$ on G, namely: (I) if $\Gamma \leq \Gamma'$, then $\mathscr{P}_\Gamma \subseteq \mathscr{P}_{\Gamma'}$, and (II) for each interior $\mathbf{p}$ there is some Γ such that $\mathbf{p} \in \mathscr{P}_\Gamma$.

In brief, as Γ increases, the sets of distributions $\mathscr{P}_\Gamma$ become ever more encompassing, so that each interior $\mathbf{p}$ is eventually included. No interior $\mathbf{p}$ is excluded from consideration, but quite a large Γ might be needed to include a particularly extreme $\mathbf{p}$.

10.3.4 Compactness

In sensitivity analyses, we often require a sharp upper bound for a continuous function defined on a set of distributions $\mathscr{P}$. If $\mathscr{P}$ were a compact set, then the upper bound we need would simply be a maximum over $\mathbf{p} \in \mathscr{P}$; otherwise, the bound would be a supremum. As $\mathscr{P}$ is always a bounded set of real vectors, $\mathscr{P}$ would be compact if it was closed, that is, if it contained its limit points. For instance, $\mathscr{P}_\Gamma^*$ in (10.5) is compact; however, if we replaced $\Gamma^{-1} \leq p_{\mathbf{h}_1}/p_{\mathbf{h}_2} \leq \Gamma$ by $\Gamma^{-1} < p_{\mathbf{h}_1}/p_{\mathbf{h}_2} < \Gamma$, then $\mathscr{P}_\Gamma^*$ would no longer be compact. It is difficult to imagine a practical circumstance in which we would wish to use the finite parameter Γ to express our uncertainty about the distribution of treatment assignments in a way that would exclude limit points; that is, it would be odd to say $\Gamma^{-1} < p_{\mathbf{h}_1}/p_{\mathbf{h}_2} < \Gamma$ is possible, but we are certain $p_{\mathbf{h}_1}/p_{\mathbf{h}_2} = \Gamma$ is not possible.

Without further mention, an assumption is added to the collection of sets of distributions $\mathscr{P}_\Gamma$ that appear in sensitivity analyses. This assumption is true of all of the sensitivity models used in this book, true of all of the models in §10.4. Making this into an assumption about $\mathscr{P}_\Gamma$ in general means that there is no need to refer to one of these models or to restrict attention to these models.

Each $\mathscr{P}_\Gamma$ is assumed to be compact, so the supremum of a continuous function on $\mathscr{P}_\Gamma$ is simply a maximum. Because P-values will be sums of some coordinates of $\mathbf{p}$, they will be continuous functions of $\mathbf{p}$; hence, the needed upper bound on the P-values for $\mathbf{p} \in \mathscr{P}_\Gamma$ is a maximum over $\mathscr{P}_\Gamma$, rather than a supremum. This convenience does not affect mathematical arguments, but it permits a simpler translation of the P-value bound into conventional English.

10.4 Sensitivity Analysis

10.4.1 Sensitivity Analysis Viewed Abstractly

In an observational study, the investigator did not assign treatments by coin flips and does not know the true distribution of treatment assignments, say $\mathbf{p}$. Not knowing $\mathbf{p}$, the investigator cannot compute the tail probability (10.2) and the P-value, $P = \Upsilon_{\mathbf{p},\mathsf{G},t}\{t(\mathbf{G})\}$.

Let $\mathscr{P}$ be a set of distributions on G. Typically, $\mathscr{P}$ is a set of possible departures from a uniformly randomized experiment, a neighborhood of $\left(\frac{1}{|\mathsf{G}|}, \ldots, \frac{1}{|\mathsf{G}|}\right)^T$, and the investigator hopes to say that small or moderate departures from the uniform distribution on G would not alter the study's conclusions, for instance, its rejection of H_0 at level α. Define

$$\Upsilon_{\mathscr{P},\mathsf{G},t}(c) = \max_{\mathbf{q} \in \mathscr{P}} \Upsilon_{\mathbf{q},\mathsf{G},t}(c) \quad \text{and} \quad \overline{P} = \Upsilon_{\mathscr{P},\mathsf{G},t}\{t(\mathbf{G})\}, \qquad (10.6)$$

noting that $\overline{P}$ implicitly depends upon $\mathscr{P}$, G and $t(\cdot)$, but the notation for $\overline{P}$ does not indicate this explicitly. If $\overline{P} \leq \alpha$ then H_0 would be rejected at level α for all $\mathbf{p} \in \mathscr{P}$, and in that sense rejection of H_0 is insensitive to departures from uniform assignment that are contained in $\mathscr{P}$. If $\mathbf{p} \in \mathscr{P}$ and H_0 is true, then the probability that $\overline{P} \leq \alpha$ is at most α.[3]

In an observational study, the true distribution of treatment assignments $\mathbf{p}$ is not known, and neither is a set $\mathscr{P}$ that is guaranteed to contain $\mathbf{p}$. There is no basis for computing $\overline{P}$ in (10.6) for one set $\mathscr{P}$, because we do not have a set $\mathscr{P}$ guaranteed to include the true distribution $\mathbf{p}$. So, we need to consider more than one set $\mathscr{P}$. Stated informally, a sensitivity analysis asks: What is the largest set $\mathscr{P}$ that leads to rejection of H_0?

Let us say this precisely. Consider nested sets $\mathscr{P}_\Gamma$, where: (i) the sets are indexed by a real parameter $\Gamma \geq 1$; (ii) $\mathscr{P}_\Gamma \subset \mathscr{P}_{\Gamma'}$ if $\Gamma < \Gamma'$; (iii) the set $\mathscr{P}_1$ contains only the uniform distribution,

$$\mathscr{P}_1 = \left\{ \left(\frac{1}{|G|}, \ldots, \frac{1}{|G|} \right)^T \right\}, \tag{10.7}$$

with $|\mathscr{P}_1| = 1$; and (iv) for each fixed $\mathbf{p}$ with $p_{\mathbf{g}_j} > 0$ for $j = 1, \ldots, |G|$, there exists a $\Gamma \geq 1$ such that $\mathbf{p} \in \mathscr{P}_\Gamma$. For distributions $\mathbf{p}$ on H in (9.2), the sets $\mathscr{P}_\Gamma^*$ in (10.5) fit this description. The sets $\mathscr{P}_\Gamma$ create a yardstick for speaking about the magnitude of bias in treatment assignment, but there is no assumption that the bias is either large or small.

As $\Gamma \to \infty$, the upper bound, $\overline{P}$ in (10.6), on the P-value testing H_0 will tend to 1, $\overline{P} \to 1$, leading to acceptance of the null hypothesis H_0 of no treatment effect.[4] This observation merely reaffirms the familiar fact that association, no matter how strong, does not logically imply causation: sufficiently large biases can explain away as non-causal any observed association. The question answered by a sensitivity analysis is not one of logical implication but of magnitude: What is the magnitude of the bias in treatment assignment that would need to be present to explain away the observed association as something other than an effect caused by the treatment? The sets, $\mathscr{P}_\Gamma$, do not assume anything: they simply create a yardstick, $\mathscr{P}_\Gamma$, and a unit of measure Γ, in terms of which the question may be answered.

---

[3] As in footnote 1, the computation in (10.6) is well-defined; however, G is often a large set, so the computation may not be straightforward. Commonly, $\Upsilon_{\mathscr{P},G,t}(\cdot)$ is either approximated using a large-sample approximation, or in certain cases computed exactly with the aid of the fast Fourier transform. These approximations or computations work well, are described elsewhere [195, 221], and are implemented in various R packages such as senstrat, DOS2, sensitivity2x2xk and sensitivitymult. For present purposes in this book, $\Upsilon_{\mathscr{P},G,t}(\cdot)$ is simply viewed as a function we can compute, as indeed we can.

[4] To prove this, suppose that we test H_0 at some level $\alpha < 1$ and pick a number β with $\alpha < \beta < 1$. Consider the finite set $\mathscr{B}$ containing $|G|$ distributions on G, where the jth distribution in $\mathscr{B}$ has $\Pr(G = \mathbf{g}_j) = \beta$, sharing the remaining probability $1 - \beta$ equally among the remaining $|G| - 1$ elements of G. For sufficiently large Γ, by condition (iv), we have $\mathscr{B} \subset \mathscr{P}_\Gamma$. Therefore, for this Γ,

$$\overline{P} = \Upsilon_{\mathscr{P}_\Gamma,G,t}\{t(G)\} \geq \Upsilon_{\mathscr{B},G,t}\{t(G)\} \geq \beta > \alpha.$$

10.4.2   *Should the Abstract Version of Sensitivity Analysis Be Made More Specific?*

The remainder of §10.4 considers particular forms for the abstract structure of a sensitivity analysis, mentioning particular sets of distributions $\mathscr{P}_\Gamma$ for particular sets G of treatment assignments. Is this a useful thing to do at this moment in this book? Is considering the details of particular cases a useful thing to do, here and now?

Well, it is and it isn't. Fisher's *P*-value in (10.2) is well-defined, as is the sensitivity bound in (10.6). Nothing is missing or vague in (10.2) and (10.6). Various footnotes point to R packages that compute or approximate these quantities; so, in principle, we could leave it at that, and go back to discussing evidence factors. In fact, the main results in Chapter 11 apply very generally, and are best described in the general formulation in (10.2) and (10.6). In that sense, the particulars are a distraction from the task ahead. In that sense, considering the details, here and now, is not a useful thing to do. The details are not needed later.

And yet, (10.2) and (10.6) are fairly abstract. One way we become comfortable with abstractions is by seeing simple cases covered by these abstractions. Another way we become comfortable with abstractions is by recognizing that the abstractions cover several familiar situations. There is quite a bit of published work on sensitivity analysis, and quite a bit of this is covered by (10.2) and (10.6); however, this fact may not be immediately evident. In that sense, considering the details, here and now, is a useful thing to do.

In brief, the particulars that follow are here solely to make (10.2) and (10.6) into a reasonable formulation of sensitivity analysis. A reasonable abstract formulation covers cases we care about. A reasonable abstract formulation removes detail that is not needed and would otherwise be an obstacle to obtaining general results.

As soon as the abstract structure, (10.2) and (10.6), feels tangible and comfortable, perhaps after examining a few but not all of the following particular cases, the reader has the option of moving on to Chapter 11.

10.4.3   *A Specific $\mathscr{P}_\Gamma$ for S Matched Pairs*

In the case of *S* matched treatment/control pairs, the set of treatment assignments G is the set of $|G| = 2^S$ permutation matrices $\mathbf{g}$, each of size $2S \times 2S$, of the form (8.4) with *S* diagonal 2×2 blocks from (8.5). The set $\mathscr{P}_\Gamma$ describes *S* independent flips of *S* biased coins, where coin *s* has probability π_s of picking $\mathbf{a}$ in (8.5) for block *s* of $\mathbf{g}$, and probability $1 - \pi_s$ of instead picking $\mathbf{b}$ in (8.5), where:

$$\frac{1}{1+\Gamma} \leq \pi_s \leq \frac{\Gamma}{1+\Gamma}, \quad s = 1,\ldots,S. \tag{10.8}$$

Writing $z_s(\mathbf{g}) = 1$ if block *s* of $\mathbf{g}$ is $\mathbf{a}$ in (8.5) and $z_s(\mathbf{g}) = 0$ if block *s* of $\mathbf{g}$ is $\mathbf{b}$ in (8.5), a vector $\mathbf{p} = \left(p_{\mathbf{g}_1},\ldots,p_{\mathbf{g}_{|G|}}\right)^T$ is in $\mathscr{P}_\Gamma$ if

$$p_{\mathbf{g}_j} = \Pr\left(G = \mathbf{g}_j\right) = \prod_{s=1}^{S} \pi_s^{z_s(\mathbf{g}_j)} \left\{1 - \pi_s\right\}^{1-z_s(\mathbf{g}_j)} \tag{10.9}$$

$$\text{for some} \quad \begin{bmatrix} \pi_1 \\ \vdots \\ \pi_S \end{bmatrix} \quad \text{satisfying (10.8)}.$$

If $\Gamma = 1$, then $\pi_s = 1/2$ in (10.8), so that (10.9) equals $1/2^S$ where $|G| = 2^S$, yielding the uniform distribution (10.1) on G.

The set $\mathscr{P}_\Gamma$ defined by (10.8)–(10.9) may be interpreted in several ways.[5] Here is one way: Due to biased treatment assignment, two individuals matched for observed covariates may differ in their odds of treatment by at most a factor of Γ; see Refs. [185, 195, §4.2.2]. Here is another equivalent way: A bias of magnitude $\Gamma \geq 1$ may be produced in a matched pair by failing to adjust for an unobserved covariate that increases the odds of treatment by a factor of Λ and increases the odds of a positive pair difference in outcomes by a factor of Δ where $\Gamma = (\Lambda\Delta + 1)/(\Lambda + \Delta)$; see Refs. [231, 234, Table 9.1]. For instance, an unobserved covariate that doubles the odds of treatment, $\Lambda = 2$, and doubles the odds of a positive pair difference in outcomes, $\Delta = 2$, is the same as $\Gamma = (\Lambda\Delta + 1)/(\Lambda + \Delta) = (2 \times 2 + 1)/(2 + 2) = 5/4 = 1.25$, or in (10.8) an interval $(1 + 1.25)^{-1} = 0.4444 \leq \pi_s \leq 0.5556 = 1.25/(1 + 1.25)$.

10.4.4 A Specific $\mathscr{P}_\Gamma$ for Pick Matrices

An (N, m)-pick matrix $\mathbf{g}$ in Definition 4 selects m of the N individuals in $\mathbf{n} = (1, \ldots, N)^T$ for treatment A. If $\mathbf{g}$ picks i for treatment A, write $z_i(\mathbf{g}) = 1$; otherwise, $z_i(\mathbf{g}) = 0$. Also, write $\mathbf{z}(\mathbf{g}) = \{z_1(\mathbf{g}), \ldots, z_N(\mathbf{g})\}^T$. Let $[0,1]^N$ denote the N-dimensional unit cube, so $\mathbf{u} = (u_1, \ldots, u_N)^T \in [0,1]^N$ if $0 \leq u_i \leq 1$ for $i = 1, \ldots, N$. Here, u_i is interpreted to be an unobserved covariate describing individual i. Write $\gamma = \log(\Gamma) \geq 0$. If G is the set of $\binom{N}{m}$ pick matrices $\mathbf{g}$, then for each $\mathbf{u} = (u_1, \ldots, u_N)^T \in [0,1]^N$ the vector $\mathbf{p} = \left(p_{\mathbf{g}_1}, \ldots, p_{\mathbf{g}_{|G|}} \right)^T$ is a probability distribution on G, where

$$p_{\mathbf{g}_j} = \Pr(\mathbf{G} = \mathbf{g}_j) = \frac{\exp\{\gamma \mathbf{u}^T \mathbf{z}(\mathbf{g}_j)\}}{\sum_{\ell=1}^{|G|} \exp\{\gamma \mathbf{u}^T \mathbf{z}(\mathbf{g}_\ell)\}}. \tag{10.10}$$

If $\gamma = 0$ or equivalently if $\Gamma = 1$, then $p_{\mathbf{g}_j} = |G|^{-1}$ in (10.10) is the uniform distribution (10.1) on G. For $\Gamma = e^\gamma$ and $N = 2$, (10.10) reduces to (10.8)–(10.9). Define the set $\mathscr{P}_\Gamma$ of distributions on G to be the set of vectors $\mathbf{p} = \left(p_{\mathbf{g}_1}, \ldots, p_{\mathbf{g}_{|G|}} \right)^T$ given

---

[5] Sensitivity analysis calculations for pairs under model (10.8)–(10.9) are performed by the senWilcox and senU functions in the R package DOS2, and the senm, senmCI, and amplify functions in the package sensitivitymult. These functions also invert tests to obtain sensitivity analyses for confidence intervals and point estimates. In particular, Hodges and Lehmann [104] derive estimates from tests in a manner compatible with confidence intervals derived from tests, and these R functions provide sensitivity analyses for those estimates [188].

by (10.10) as $\mathbf{u}$ ranges over $[0,1]^N$; see Refs. [195, §4.6] and [225].[6] This model may be interpreted as saying that two of the N individuals may differ in their odds of receiving treatment A by at most a factor of Γ; see Ref. [195, §4.2].

10.4.5 A Specific $\mathscr{P}_\Gamma$ for Subpick Matrices

An (N,m,m')-subpick matrix $\mathbf{s}$ in Definition 6 fixes the m individuals previously picked, and selects m' individuals for treatment B from the remaining $N-m$ individuals; it is the direct sum of an $m \times m$ identity matrix and an $(N-m,m')$-pick matrix $\mathbf{g}$ of size $(N-m) \times (N-m)$,

$$\mathbf{s} = \begin{bmatrix} \mathbf{I} & \mathbf{0} \\ \mathbf{0} & \mathbf{g} \end{bmatrix}.$$

Consider taking (10.10) as a model for block $\mathbf{g}$ in $\mathbf{s}$, after making suitable adjustments to reflect the smaller size of the pick matrix $\mathbf{g}$. If S is the set containing the $\binom{N-m}{m'}$-subpick matrices $\mathbf{s}$, then by replacing N by $N-m$, m by m', and $|G| = \binom{N}{m}$ by $|S| = \binom{N-m}{m'}$ in (10.10), a probability distribution $\mathbf{p} = \left(p_{\mathbf{s}_1}, \ldots, p_{\mathbf{s}_{|S|}} \right)^T$ for a random subpick $\mathbf{S}$ drawn from S is

$$p_{\mathbf{s}_j} = \Pr\left(\mathbf{S} = \begin{bmatrix} \mathbf{I} & \mathbf{0} \\ \mathbf{0} & \mathbf{g}_j \end{bmatrix} \right) = \Pr(\mathbf{G} = \mathbf{g}_j),$$

where $\Pr(\mathbf{G} = \mathbf{g}_j)$ has the form (10.10). A set $\mathscr{P}_\Gamma$ of such distributions is obtained as $\mathbf{u}$ ranges over $[0,1]^{N-m}$. Later, this $\mathscr{P}_\Gamma$ will be a set of conditional distributions for an (N,m,m')-subpick conditionally given an (N,m)-pick.[7]

10.4.6 A Specific $\mathscr{P}_\Gamma$ for Stratified Comparisons

A stratified comparison of treated and control groups with S strata involves treatment assignments $\mathbf{k}$ that are the direct sum (8.4) of (n_s, m_s)-pick matrices, $\mathbf{k}_s$, $s = 1, \ldots, S$. If K is the set of these assignments $\mathbf{k}$, then $|K| = \prod_{s=1}^{S} \binom{n_s}{m_s}$. If we sample the S diagonal blocks of $\mathbf{k}$ independently using a model of the form (10.10) for pick matrix $\mathbf{k}_s$, then the probability of $\mathbf{k} \in K$ is the product of S probabilities of the form (10.10). Of course, if $S = 1$ then this reduces to (10.10), whereas if $S \geq 1$ but each $n_s = 2$ and each $m_s = 1$, this reduces to (10.8)–(10.9). As $\mathbf{u}$ varies over the n_s-dimensional unit cube in (10.10), a set of distributions is obtained for each $\mathbf{k}_s$, leading to a corresponding set $\mathscr{P}_\Gamma$ of distributions on K.[8]

The same general approach may be used with stratified comparisons of several treatment groups, formed as the matrix product of direct sums of pick and subpick matrices, as in (8.8).

---

[6]Sensitivity analysis calculations under model (10.10) are performed by the sen2sample function in the R package senstrat.

[7]Sensitivity analysis calculations under this model for a subpick can be performed by the sen2sample function in the R package senstrat, simply by removing the m fixed individuals previously picked for A.

[8]Statified sensitivity analysis can be performed by the senstrat function in the R package senstrat. For analyses of subpicks, one sets aside the units previously picked.

10.5   Summary: Probability on a Set of Treatment Assignments

Chapter 8 represented one treatment assignment for N individuals as one $N \times N$ permutation matrix, $\mathbf{g}$. Chapter 9 considered the set G whose $|G|$ elements $\mathbf{g}$ are the treatment assignments possible in a particular study design. The current chapter has considered probability distributions $\mathbf{p} = \left(p_{\mathbf{g}_1}, \ldots, p_{\mathbf{g}_{|G|}} \right)^T$ on the set G of possible treatment assignments. In a randomized experiment, $\mathbf{p}$ is known, because $\mathbf{p}$ was created by the investigator by assigning treatments at random, most commonly with equal probabilities $p_{\mathbf{g}_j} = |G|^{-1}$ for $j = 1, \ldots, |G|$. In an observational study, treatments are not assigned at random, so $\mathbf{p}$ is unknown. A measured degree of uncertainty about $\mathbf{p}$ is expressed by a set $\mathscr{P}$ containing possible distributions $\mathbf{p}$. A sensitivity analysis considers a nested collection of sets, $\mathscr{P}_\Gamma \subset \mathscr{P}_{\Gamma'}$ for $\Gamma < \Gamma'$. Rejection at level α of the hypothesis H_0 of no effect is insensitive to a bias of Γ if the maximum P-value, $\overline{P}$, is at most α for all $\mathbf{p} \in \mathscr{P}_\Gamma$.

10.6   Complement: Sensitivity Analysis with Doses

In an experiment, N individuals can be assigned to N doses in $N!$ ways. If the odds of receiving one specific dose rather than another were the same for all pairs of two doses and for all individuals, then all $N!$ assignments of doses would have the same probability, $(N!)^{-1}$. An investigator might randomly assign doses picking a random permutation of the doses.

Suppose instead that the odds of receiving one specific dose rather than another might vary from one individual to the next. Suppose that the odds of one specific dose rather than another might differ from one individual to another, but these odds never differ by more than a factor of Γ. You and I might differ in our odds of receiving dose 1 rather than dose 7, but your odds are at most Γ times my odds and at least $1/\Gamma$ times my odds; moreover, this holds not just for you and me, and not just for doses 1 and 7, but for all pairs of individuals and all pairs of doses. For $\Gamma = 1$, this is the uniform distribution on the $N!$ permutations, but, as $\Gamma \to \infty$, this model negligibly constrains the distribution.

Somewhat more precisely, the N doses are independently sampled from N distributions of doses, one distribution for each individual. If these distributions are discrete, they attach probabilities to a discrete set of distributions, and the odds of one dose rather than another is the ratio of the probabilities of these two doses. If these distributions are continuous, then they are assumed to have continuous densities, and the odds of one dose rather than another is the ratio of the densities at these two doses. These odds may vary from individual to individual, but they never differ by more than a factor of $\Gamma \geq 1$. Now, condition on the observed order statistic of the doses, so the conditional distribution is a set of probabilities for the $N!$ permutations of fixed doses. In Ref. [218], this structure leads to a sensitivity analysis for dose-response similar to the analyses described previously. It is straightforward to incorporate stratification for covariates in this analysis.[9]

---

[9]This analysis can be performed using the `crosscut` function in the R package DOS2, or with a little more effort by the `mh` function in the R package `sensitivity2x2xk`.

10.7   Exercises

Exercise 10.1. *This exercise is repeated from Chapter 2. Do a sensitivity analysis using the shinyapp at*

$$\text{https}://\text{rosenbap.shinyapps.io/learnsenShiny/}$$

that runs R in the background, requiring no knowledge of R.

Exercise 10.2. *Install the R packages mentioned in earlier chapters. Copy examples from their help files into your workspace, and perform several sensitivity analyses.*

Chapter 11

Factors

Abstract

Chapter 11 develops the key properties of inference with evidence factors, making use of the structure developed in Chapters 7–10. Chapter 11 also provides the logic underlying the simple analyses presented in Chapter 4. The main result is Theorem 9: under certain conditions, two sensitivity analyses for two factors may be combined by comparing their two upper bounds on P-values to the uniform distribution on the unit square. Theorem 9 is extended to more than two factors in the optional §11.8.

11.1 Marginal and Conditional Distributions

11.1.1 The General Case for Two Factors

Suppose that G, H, and K are sets of $N \times N$ permutation matrices such that $G = HK = \{ \mathbf{hk} : \mathbf{h} \in H, \mathbf{k} \in K \}$, and each $\mathbf{g} \in G$ has one and only one representation as $\mathbf{g} = \mathbf{hk}$, $\mathbf{h} \in H$, $\mathbf{k} \in K$, so that $|G| = |H| \times |K|$; see §9.3. Because this representation is unique, we can replace $\mathbf{g}$ by $\mathbf{hk}$ without ambiguity.

Let

$$\mathbf{p} = \left(p_{\mathbf{g}_1}, \ldots, p_{\mathbf{g}_{|G|}} \right)^T \tag{11.1}$$

be a probability distribution on G, where $p_{\mathbf{g}} = \Pr(\mathbf{G} = \mathbf{g})$ for each $\mathbf{g} \in G$. Then there is a corresponding marginal distribution

$$\mathbf{p}' = \left(p'_{\mathbf{k}_1}, \ldots, p'_{\mathbf{k}_{|K|}} \right)^T \tag{11.2}$$

on K, where

$$p'_{\mathbf{k}} = \sum_{\mathbf{h} \in H} p_{\mathbf{hk}} \quad \text{for } \mathbf{k} \in K. \tag{11.3}$$

Conditionally given $\mathbf{K} = \mathbf{k}$, there is a conditional distribution of $\mathbf{H} \in H$, namely

$$\mathbf{p}''_{\mathbf{k}} = \left(p''_{\mathbf{h}_1 | \mathbf{k}}, \ldots, p''_{\mathbf{h}_{|H|} | \mathbf{k}} \right)^T \tag{11.4}$$

where

$$p''_{\mathbf{h} | \mathbf{k}} = \frac{p_{\mathbf{hk}}}{\sum_{\mathbf{h} \in H} p_{\mathbf{hk}}} = \frac{p_{\mathbf{hk}}}{p'_{\mathbf{k}}}. \tag{11.5}$$

11.1.2 The Special Case of Uniform Randomization

If $\mathbf{p}$ in (11.1) is uniform on G, as in (10.1), with each coordinate equal to $|G|^{-1}$, then $p'_{\mathbf{k}} = |K|^{-1}$ in (11.3) for each $\mathbf{k} \in K$, and $\mathbf{p}' = \left(|K|^{-1}, \ldots, |K|^{-1} \right)^T$ in (11.2) is uniform on K. If $\mathbf{p}$ in (11.1) is uniform on G, as in (10.1), then given $\mathbf{K} = \mathbf{k}$, the conditional distribution $\mathbf{p}''_{\mathbf{k}}$ in (11.4) of $\mathbf{H} \in H$ in (11.5) is uniform on H for every $\mathbf{k} \in K$; that is, $p''_{\mathbf{h}|\mathbf{k}} = |H|^{-1}$ for each $\mathbf{h} \in H$ and $\mathbf{k} \in K$.

Consequently, $\mathbf{H}$ and $\mathbf{K}$ are independent in a uniformly randomized experiment. In contrast, in the general case (11.2)–(11.5), $\mathbf{H}$ and $\mathbf{K}$ may be dependent. In many observational studies, it would be unreasonable to assume that $\mathbf{H}$ and $\mathbf{K}$ are independent.

11.1.3 Joint Distribution from Marginal and Conditional Distributions

It is clear that a joint distribution $\mathbf{p} = \left(p_{\mathbf{g}_1}, \ldots, p_{\mathbf{g}_{|G|}} \right)^T$ on G may be obtained in the usual way from marginal and conditional distributions. If $\mathbf{p}' = \left(p'_{\mathbf{k}_1}, \ldots, p'_{\mathbf{k}_{|K|}} \right)^T$ is a distribution on K, and if $\mathbf{p}''_{\mathbf{k}} = \left(p''_{\mathbf{h}_1|\mathbf{k}}, \ldots, p''_{\mathbf{h}_{|H|}|\mathbf{k}} \right)^T$ is a distribution on H for each $\mathbf{k} \in K$, then $\mathbf{p} = \left(p_{\mathbf{g}_1}, \ldots, p_{\mathbf{g}_{|G|}} \right)^T$ is the corresponding joint distribution on G, where for $\mathbf{g} = \mathbf{hk}$,

$$p_{\mathbf{g}} = p_{\mathbf{hk}} = p''_{\mathbf{h}|\mathbf{k}} \times p'_{\mathbf{k}}. \tag{11.6}$$

For instance, if $\mathbf{K}$ is picked with uniform probabilities from K, and $\mathbf{H}$ is independently picked with uniform probabilities from H, then $\mathbf{G} = \mathbf{HK}$ has a uniform distribution on G.

So far, this is all very familiar. The interesting situation occurs when individual probability distributions on factors are replaced by sets of distributions on factors.

11.2 Joint Distribution of Two Sensitivity Analyses

We are now in a position to consider formally the analyses with evidence factors that were performed in Chapter 5. On what basis are those analyses justified?

Suppose, as before, that G, H, and K are sets of $N \times N$ permutation matrices with $G = HK = \{\mathbf{hk} : \mathbf{h} \in H, \mathbf{k} \in K\}$, and each $\mathbf{g} \in G$ has a unique representation as $\mathbf{g} = \mathbf{hk}, \mathbf{h} \in H, \mathbf{k} \in K$. Perhaps G divides N individuals into three treatment groups, A, B, and C, of sizes m, m', and $N - m - m'$, while K is the set of (N, m)-pick matrices that pick m individuals for group A, and H is the set of (N, m, m')-subpick matrices that pick m' individuals for group B from among the $N - m$ individuals not yet assigned to a treatment group; see, for example, §5.2, §8.4, §8.6, and §9.3 Or perhaps the division into treatment groups A, B, and C occurs separately inside S strata defined by observed covariates; see §5.2 and §8.10. Or perhaps K is the set of 2^S treatment/control assignments within S matched pairs, H is the set of $S!$ permutations of doses among the S pairs, and G is the set of $S! \times 2^S$ treatment assignments for both steps; see §5.3 and §8.8.

Two separate sensitivity analyses have been conducted, one for H, one for K. These analyses ignored each other, and each analysis is valid under certain assumptions. The analysis for $\mathbf{K} \in \mathsf{K}$ paid no attention to $\mathbf{H}$. The analysis for $\mathbf{H} \in \mathsf{H}$ acted as if $\mathbf{K}$ were simply fixed at its observed value, say $\mathbf{K} = \mathbf{k}$, ignoring the fact that the relevant distribution for $\mathbf{H}$ might change if $\mathbf{K}$ were different.

The question is whether these two separate analyses may be combined into a joint analysis, perhaps with a firmer conclusion. At the same time, the joint analysis should add no new assumptions at this stage, no assumptions beyond those required for the separate validity of the two separate sensitivity analyses. Is this possible?

Certainly, we wish to avoid any additional assumption that $\mathbf{H}$ and $\mathbf{K}$ are independent. True, $\mathbf{H}$ and $\mathbf{K}$ would be independent in a uniform randomized experiment, as seen in §11.1; however, this would be a very strong, often unreasonable, additional assumption in many observational studies. In an observational study, the person disinclined to accept treatment A may also try to avoid treatment B, so the two factors may be dependent. In an observational study, the person who elects not to smoke may also be the person who would smoke lightly if she did smoke, so the decision to smoke and how much to smoke may be dependent. If random assignment has made $\mathbf{H}$ and $\mathbf{K}$ independent, then that is one thing; however, in the absence of randomization, there is no basis for assuming that different aspects of treatment assignment are independent, merely because we wish to combine the two sensitivity analyses into one.

The knit product of two sets of probability distributions provides the solution: it creates without additional assumptions the relevant set of joint distributions from sets of marginal and conditional distributions. That is the first task. The second task is to make sense of the informal notions of ignoring $\mathbf{H}$ in factor K and acting as if $\mathbf{K}$ were fixed in factor H. These informal notions will be formalized by using a statistic invariant to $\mathbf{H}$ in factor K and conditioning on $\mathbf{K}$ in factor H. In fact, such an invariant statistic was used in each example in Chapter 5.

11.3   Sets of Marginal and Conditional Distributions

The first sensitivity analysis in §11.2 considered a set of distributions, $\mathscr{P}'_{\Gamma'}$, for $\mathbf{K}$ on K. The second sensitivity analysis in §11.2 considered a set of distributions, $\mathscr{P}''_{\Gamma''}$, for $\mathbf{H}$ on H, acting as if $\mathbf{K}$ were fixed. We want to consider the joint distributions on G compatible with a distribution $\mathbf{p}' \in \mathscr{P}'_{\Gamma'}$ for $\mathbf{K}$ and a distribution $\mathbf{p}'' \in \mathscr{P}''_{\Gamma''}$ for $\mathbf{H}$. A joint distribution on G is essential if there is to be a joint analysis of two evidence factors.

It is a mistake to build a set of joint distributions $\mathbf{p}$ on G in (11.1) for $\mathbf{G} = \mathbf{HK}$ by multiplying, in all possible ways, a distribution $\mathbf{p}' \in \mathscr{P}'_{\Gamma'}$ by a distribution $\mathbf{p}'' \in \mathscr{P}''_{\Gamma''}$. Can you see why?

If we multiply, in all possible ways, a distribution $\mathbf{p}' \in \mathscr{P}'_{\Gamma'}$ by a distribution $\mathbf{p}'' \in \mathscr{P}''_{\Gamma''}$, then we have created joint distributions compatible with $\mathbf{p}' \in \mathscr{P}'_{\Gamma'}$ and $\mathbf{p}'' \in \mathscr{P}''_{\Gamma''}$ while adding the powerful assumption that $\mathbf{H}$ and $\mathbf{K}$ are independent. It was precisely this assumption that we wished to avoid. We wanted to add no new assumptions at this stage, at the moment that we combine the two sensitivity analyses. It is possible that **H** and **K** are dependent, perhaps strongly dependent. The first sensitivity analysis already assumed that some $\mathbf{p}' \in \mathscr{P}'_{\Gamma'}$ was the relevant distribution of **K** on K, and the second sensitivity analysis assumed that some $\mathbf{p}'' \in \mathscr{P}''_{\Gamma''}$ is the relevant distribution for **H** on H. We want to maintain those assumptions, combine the two analyses, adding no additional assumptions at the combination step.

The knit product in Definition 9 is what we need.[1]

Definition 9. *Suppose that* G, H, *and* K *are sets of* $N \times N$ *permutation matrices,* $G = HK$, *where each* $\mathbf{g} \in G$ *has a unique representation as* $\mathbf{g} = \mathbf{hk}$, $\mathbf{h} \in H$, $\mathbf{k} \in K$. *The knit product* $\mathscr{P}'_{\Gamma'} \oslash \mathscr{P}''_{\Gamma''}$ *of a set of distributions* $\mathscr{P}'_{\Gamma'}$ *on* K *and a set of distributions* $\mathscr{P}''_{\Gamma''}$ *on* H *is the set of all joint distributions of* $\mathbf{G} = \mathbf{HK}$ *on* G *formed by selecting a marginal distribution* $\mathbf{p}' \in \mathscr{P}'_{\Gamma'}$ *for* **K**, *and for each* $\mathbf{k} \in K$ *selecting a conditional distribution* $\mathbf{p}'' \in \mathscr{P}''_{\Gamma''}$ *for the distribution of* **H** *given* $\mathbf{K} = \mathbf{k}$.

The set $\mathscr{P}'_{\Gamma'} \oslash \mathscr{P}''_{\Gamma''}$ is composed of the joint distributions of $\mathbf{G} = \mathbf{HK}$ on G compatible with marginal distributions $\mathscr{P}'_{\Gamma'}$ for **K** and conditional distributions $\mathscr{P}''_{\Gamma''}$ for **H**, adding no assumptions at this stage about how **H** and **K** are related.

Why Is the Knit Product Useful? Suppose that we have represented the set G of treatment assignments uniquely as the product $G = HK$, and there is a sensitivity analysis using the marginal distribution of $\mathbf{K} \in K$ alone, and another sensitivity analysis using $\mathbf{H} \in H$ that acts as if **K** were fixed. The knit product makes no new assumptions; yet, as seen later in the chapter, it creates a set of joint distributions such that the two sensitivity analyses done separately are precisely the same as the analogous marginal and conditional analyses that would have been done had they been based on the joint distributions in the knit product.

If $\mathscr{P}'_{\Gamma'}$ contains $\left| \mathscr{P}'_{\Gamma'} \right| = 2$ distributions, if $\mathscr{P}''_{\Gamma''}$ contains $\left| \mathscr{P}''_{\Gamma''} \right| = 3$ distributions, and if $|K| = 5$, then: (i) we can multiply a $\mathbf{p}' \in \mathscr{P}'_{\Gamma'}$ by a $\mathbf{p}'' \in \mathscr{P}''_{\Gamma''}$ in $\left| \mathscr{P}'_{\Gamma'} \right| \times \left| \mathscr{P}''_{\Gamma''} \right| = 2 \times 3 = 6$ ways to obtain independent distributions for **H** and **K**, but (ii) the knit product $\mathscr{P}'_{\Gamma'} \oslash \mathscr{P}''_{\Gamma''}$ contains $\left| \mathscr{P}'_{\Gamma'} \right| \times \left| \mathscr{P}''_{\Gamma''} \right|^{|K|} = 2 \times 3^5 = 486$ distributions. In the knit product, the person most likely to smoke may also be the person most likely to smoke heavily if he smokes.

---

[1] The term "knit product" is used as a weak analogy with the more algebraic description in Ref. [220], where it is connected with the knit product of two groups of permutation matrices. See also §12.4.

11.4 Ignoring a Factor

The sensitivity analysis using distributions $\mathscr{P}'_{\Gamma'}$ for $\mathbf{K} \in \mathsf{K}$ ignored $\mathbf{H} \in \mathsf{H}$. We want to show that the sensitivity analysis we did for $\mathbf{K} \in \mathsf{K}$ ignoring $\mathbf{H} \in \mathsf{H}$ is precisely the same sensitivity analysis that we would have done for $\mathbf{K} \in \mathsf{K}$ had we used the knit product $\mathscr{P}'_{\Gamma'} \oslash \mathscr{P}''_{\Gamma''}$ as the set of joint distributions for the $\mathbf{G} = \mathbf{HK}$ on G. A statistic $t'(\cdot)$ ignores $\mathbf{h} \in \mathsf{H}$ if $t'(\mathbf{hk})$ does not change when $\mathbf{h}$ changes.

Definition 10. *Suppose that* G, H, *and* K *are sets of* $N \times N$ *permutation matrices,* $G = HK$, *where each* $\mathbf{g} \in G$ *has a unique representation as* $\mathbf{g} = \mathbf{hk}$, $\mathbf{h} \in H$, $\mathbf{k} \in K$. *A statistic* $t'(\mathbf{g}) = t'(\mathbf{hk})$ *is invariant to* $\mathbf{h} \in H$ *if* $t'(\mathbf{hk}) = t'(\mathbf{k})$ *for all* $\mathbf{h} \in H$, $\mathbf{k} \in K$.

For instance, when permuting treatment/control within S pairs by K while permuting doses of treatment among pairs by H, Wilcoxon's signed rank statistic $t'(\mathbf{g}) = t'(\mathbf{hk})$ is invariant to permutations of the doses, simply because the statistic does not use the doses in its calculations.

The sets $\mathscr{P}'_{\Gamma'}$ and $\mathscr{P}''_{\Gamma''}$ are indexed by parameters Γ' and Γ'', but to simplify notation, let us fix Γ' and Γ'' and simply write $\mathscr{P}'$ and $\mathscr{P}''$ for $\mathscr{P}'_{\Gamma'}$ and $\mathscr{P}''_{\Gamma''}$.

Suppose $t'(\mathbf{g}) = t'(\mathbf{hk})$ is invariant to $\mathbf{h} \in \mathsf{H}$. All sensitivity analyses are particular instances of (10.6). As in (10.6), a sensitivity analysis using distributions $\mathscr{P}'$ for $\mathbf{K} \in \mathsf{K}$ computes a P-value bound $\overline{P}$ of $\Upsilon_{\mathscr{P}',\mathsf{K},t'}\{t'(\mathbf{K})\}$. As in (10.6), a sensitivity analysis using joint distributions $\mathbf{p} \in \mathscr{P}' \oslash \mathscr{P}''$ for $\mathbf{G} \in \mathsf{G}$ computes a P-value bound of $\Upsilon_{\mathscr{P}' \oslash \mathscr{P}'', \mathsf{G},t'}\{t'(\mathbf{G})\}$. We want to show that these two P-value bounds are equal.

Lemma 7. *If* $t'(\mathbf{g}) = t'(\mathbf{hk})$ *is invariant to* $\mathbf{h} \in \mathsf{H}$, *then the marginal and joint P-value bounds for factor* K *are equal,* $\Upsilon_{\mathscr{P}',\mathsf{K},t'}\{t'(\mathbf{K})\} = \Upsilon_{\mathscr{P}' \oslash \mathscr{P}'', \mathsf{G},t'}\{t'(\mathbf{G})\}$.

Proof. Because $t'(\cdot)$ is invariant, $t'(\mathbf{G}) = t'(\mathbf{HK}) = t'(\mathbf{K})$. Write $\chi(E) = 1$ if event E occurs and $\chi(E) = 0$ otherwise. Then for each fixed c,

$$\Upsilon_{\mathscr{P}' \oslash \mathscr{P}'', \mathsf{G},t'}(c) = \max_{\mathbf{p} \in \mathscr{P}' \oslash \mathscr{P}''} \sum_{\mathbf{g} \in G: t'(\mathbf{g}) \geq c} p_{\mathbf{g}} = \max_{\mathbf{p} \in \mathscr{P}' \oslash \mathscr{P}''} \sum_{\mathbf{k} \in K} \sum_{\mathbf{h} \in H} \chi\{t'(\mathbf{hk}) \geq c\} p_{\mathbf{hk}},$$

which by invariance of $t'(\cdot)$ equals

$$\max_{\mathbf{p} \in \mathscr{P}' \oslash \mathscr{P}''} \sum_{\mathbf{k} \in K} \sum_{\mathbf{h} \in H} \chi\{t'(\mathbf{k}) \geq c\} p_{\mathbf{hk}} = \max_{\mathbf{p} \in \mathscr{P}' \oslash \mathscr{P}''} \sum_{\mathbf{k} \in K} \chi\{t'(\mathbf{k}) \geq c\} \sum_{\mathbf{h} \in H} p_{\mathbf{hk}}$$

$$= \max_{\mathbf{p}' \in \mathscr{P}'} \sum_{\mathbf{k} \in K} \chi\{t'(\mathbf{k}) \geq c\} p'_{\mathbf{k}} = \Upsilon_{\mathscr{P}',\mathsf{K},t'}(c). \tag{11.7}$$

because $p'_{\mathbf{k}} = \sum_{\mathbf{h} \in H} p_{\mathbf{hk}}$ is a marginal distribution $\mathbf{p}'$ in $\mathscr{P}'$. $\qquad\square$

In words, we initially did a sensitivity analysis for each factor separately, for $\mathbf{K} \in \mathsf{K}$ and $\mathbf{H} \in \mathsf{H}$, with no thought about how they might be related. They were two analyses, each dependent on certain assumptions, and we did not want to add any new assumptions. In an effort to relate them, we build the knit product $\mathscr{P}' \oslash \mathscr{P}''$ as a set of all joint distributions on $\mathbf{G} = \mathbf{HK} \in G$ compatible with the assumptions on the separate factors. Lemma 7 says, if $t'(\cdot)$ is invariant, then the sensitivity analysis for $\mathbf{K} \in K$ is the same, whether we view it in isolation, or calculate it from the joint distributions of $\mathbf{G} = \mathbf{HK}$ in the knit product, $\mathbf{p} \in \mathscr{P}' \oslash \mathscr{P}''$.

Ignoring H: Ignoring **H** is the same as using the marginal distribution of **K** in the knit product, providing the test statistic t' is H-invariant.

11.5   Conditioning on a Factor

Consider now a test of H_0 that uses **H** in a test statistic $t''(\mathbf{G}) = t''(\mathbf{HK})$. In general, $t''(\mathbf{hk})$ depends upon both **h** and **k**, unlike the first test statistic $t'(\mathbf{hk}) = t'(\mathbf{k})$ in §11.4. If $\mathbf{G} = \mathbf{HK}$ were distributed on G with a known distribution **p**, as in a randomized experiment, then we could perform a test of H_0 using the conditional distribution of $\mathbf{HK} = \mathbf{Hk}$ given $\mathbf{K} = \mathbf{k}$. Were **p** known, the conditional distribution of **H** given $\mathbf{K} = \mathbf{k}$ would also be known, and it would be given by (11.5).

Suppose, instead, that **p** is not known, as in an observational study, and consider a sensitivity analysis in which **p** is confined to some set $\mathscr{P}_{\Gamma',\Gamma''}$ of distributions on G; however, aside from knowing that $\mathbf{p} \in \mathscr{P}_{\Gamma',\Gamma''}$, the distribution **p** is unknown. The upper bound on the conditional P-value using $t''(\mathbf{HK})$ computes the conditional P-value in the previous paragraph for each $\mathbf{p} \in \mathscr{P}_{\Gamma',\Gamma''}$, and reports as the sensitivity bound, $\overline{P}$, the maximum of these P-values. In other words, we calculate the bound on the conditional tail probability given $\mathbf{K} = \mathbf{k}$,

$$v_{\mathbf{k}}(c) = \max_{\mathbf{p} \in \mathscr{P}_{\Gamma',\Gamma''}} \sum_{\mathbf{h} \in H} \chi\left\{t''(\mathbf{hk}) \geq c\right\} \frac{p_{\mathbf{hk}}}{\sum_{\mathbf{h} \in H} p_{\mathbf{hk}}}, \qquad (11.8)$$

and report the P-value bound $\overline{P} = v_{\mathbf{K}}\{t''(\mathbf{HK})\}$. If $\overline{P} \leq \alpha$, then H_0 is rejected at level α for all $\mathbf{p} \in \mathscr{P}_{\Gamma',\Gamma''}$, and a bias of magnitude (Γ', Γ'') for the joint distribution is too small to explain rejection of H_0 at level α as something other than an effect caused by the treatment. As in §11.4, fix Γ' and Γ'' and write $\mathscr{P}'$ and $\mathscr{P}''$ for $\mathscr{P}'_{\Gamma'}$ and $\mathscr{P}''_{\Gamma''}$.

Commonly, sensitivity bounds are not computed using joint distributions for two factors, as in the previous paragraph. Rather, two unrelated analyses are done. Perhaps the analysis for one factor ignores the other, as in §11.4. Alternatively, perhaps when considering factor, **H**, the other factor is simply regarded as fixed at its observed value, $\mathbf{K} = \mathbf{k}$. The sensitivity analysis that regards $\mathbf{K} = \mathbf{k}$ as fixed uses distributions $\mathscr{P}''$ on H for **H**, meaning that the upper bound on the P-value is quoted as $v_{\mathbf{k}}''\{t''(\mathbf{Hk})\}$, where

$$v_{\mathbf{k}}''(c) = \max_{\mathbf{p}'' \in \mathscr{P}''} \sum_{\mathbf{h} \in H} \chi\left\{t''(\mathbf{hk}) \geq c\right\} p_{\mathbf{h}}''. \qquad (11.9)$$

Lemma 8. *If the set of joint distributions, $\mathscr{P}_{\Gamma',\Gamma''}$, is the knit product, $\mathscr{P}_{\Gamma',\Gamma''} = \mathscr{P}' \oslash \mathscr{P}''$, then $\upsilon_{\mathbf{k}}(c) = \upsilon_{\mathbf{k}}''(c)$ for each c and $\mathbf{k}$.*

Proof. The quantity $\sum_{\mathbf{h}\in\mathsf{H}} \chi\{t''(\mathbf{hk}) \ge c\}\, p_{\mathbf{hk}}/\sum_{\mathbf{h}\in\mathsf{H}} p_{\mathbf{hk}}$ in (11.8) depends on the joint distribution $\mathbf{p} \in \mathscr{P}_{\Gamma',\Gamma''}$ only through its corresponding conditional distribution, $p_{\mathbf{hk}}/\sum_{\mathbf{h}\in\mathsf{H}} p_{\mathbf{hk}}$, of $\mathbf{H}$ given $\mathbf{K} = \mathbf{k}$, and because $\mathscr{P}_{\Gamma',\Gamma''} = \mathscr{P}' \oslash \mathscr{P}''$ is the knit product, the set of possible values for the conditional distribution $p_{\mathbf{hk}}/\sum_{\mathbf{h}\in\mathsf{H}} p_{\mathbf{hk}}$ is precisely the set of $|\mathsf{H}|$-dimensional vectors $\mathbf{p}''$ in $\mathscr{P}''$. It follows that, for each $\mathbf{k} \in \mathsf{K}$, the maxima in (11.8) and (11.9) are equal. $\qquad\square$

Conditioning on $\mathbf{K}$: Acting as if $\mathbf{K}$ were fixed is the same as using the conditional distribution of $\mathbf{H}$ given $\mathbf{K} = \mathbf{k}$ providing the set of joint distributions is the knit product.

In brief, the sensitivity analysis that acts as if $\mathbf{K} = \mathbf{k}$ were fixed by design, namely $\upsilon_{\mathbf{k}}''(\cdot)$, is the same as the sensitivity analysis that conditions on $\mathbf{K} = \mathbf{k}$, providing the set of distributions $\mathscr{P}_{\Gamma',\Gamma''}$ in (11.8) is the knit product, $\mathscr{P}_{\Gamma',\Gamma''} = \mathscr{P}' \oslash \mathscr{P}''$.

11.6 Combining Two Sensitivity Analyses

We have conducted two separate sensitivity analyses testing the null hypothesis of no treatment effect, H_0. Now, we wish to combine them into a single joint sensitivity analysis, adding no new assumptions. This means that the joint analysis assumes what the two separate sensitivity analyses assumed, but nothing else. Let us recall the structure.

1. There are three sets G, H, and K of $N \times N$ permutation matrices, with $\mathsf{G} = \mathsf{HK}$, where each $\mathbf{g} \in \mathsf{G}$ has a unique representation as $\mathbf{g} = \mathbf{hk}$, $\mathbf{h} \in \mathsf{H}$, $\mathbf{k} \in \mathsf{K}$. Each permutation matrix $\mathbf{g} \in \mathsf{G}$ is a possible treatment assignment.

2. One sensitivity analysis used a statistic $t'(\mathbf{g}) = t'(\mathbf{hk})$ that is invariant to $\mathbf{h} \in \mathsf{H}$ in the sense that $t'(\mathbf{hk}) = t'(\mathbf{k})$ for all $\mathbf{h} \in \mathsf{H}$, $\mathbf{k} \in \mathsf{K}$. Because $t'(\mathbf{hk}) = t'(\mathbf{k})$ does not depend upon $\mathbf{h}$, this first sensitivity analysis used a set $\mathscr{P}'$ of marginal distributions for $\mathbf{K} \in \mathsf{K}$, ignoring $\mathbf{H} \in \mathsf{H}$. Specifically, this analysis computed an upper bound $\overline{P}' = \Upsilon_{\mathscr{P}',\mathsf{K},t'}\{t'(\mathbf{K})\}$ in (10.6) on the true P-value, P', that would have been obtained from the true but unknown marginal distribution $\mathbf{p}'\in\mathscr{P}'$. So, we do not know the true P-value, P', but we do know that $P' \le \overline{P}'$, assuming only what the first sensitivity analysis assumed, namely that the true marginal distribution $\mathbf{p}'$ of $\mathbf{K} \in \mathsf{K}$ is in $\mathscr{P}'$.

3. The second sensitivity analysis viewed $\mathbf{K} \in \mathsf{K}$ as fixed, and used a test statistic $t''(\mathbf{hk})$ that depends upon both $\mathbf{h}$ and $\mathbf{k}$. With $\mathbf{K}$ fixed at $\mathbf{k}$, the second sensitivity analysis considered a set of distributions $\mathscr{P}''$ of distributions of $\mathbf{H}$, determining an upper bound $\overline{P}'' = \upsilon_{\mathbf{k}}''\{t''(\mathbf{Hk})\}$ from (11.9) on the true P-value P'' that would have been obtained at the true $\mathbf{p}'' \in \mathscr{P}''$. So we do not know the true P-value, P'', but we do know that $P'' \le \overline{P}''$, assuming only what the second sensitivity analysis

assumed, namely that with $\mathbf{K}$ fixed at $\mathbf{k}$, the true distribution $\mathbf{p}''$ of $\mathbf{H} \in \mathsf{H}$ is in $\mathscr{P}''$.

4. The knit product, $\mathscr{P}' \oslash \mathscr{P}''$, is the set of all joint distributions compatible with a marginal distribution $\mathbf{p}' \in \mathscr{P}'$ for $\mathbf{K} \in \mathsf{K}$, and a conditional distribution $\mathbf{p}'' \in \mathscr{P}''$ for $\mathbf{H}$ given $\mathbf{K} = \mathbf{k}$. No new assumption is introduced by assuming that the joint distribution $\mathbf{p}$ of $\mathbf{G} = \mathbf{HK}$ is in $\mathscr{P}' \oslash \mathscr{P}''$. Lemmas 7 and 8 say that the bounds on P' and P'' obtained from joint distributions in the knit product, $\mathbf{p} \in \mathscr{P}' \oslash \mathscr{P}''$, are identical to the bounds obtained by a different computation from the two separate factors in 2 and 3 above. That is, although we do not know the two P-values, (P', P''), we do know that $(P', P'') \le \left(\overline{P}', \overline{P}'' \right)$ for all $\mathbf{p} \in \mathscr{P}' \oslash \mathscr{P}''$.

Theorem 9. *Assume H_0 is true for the purpose of testing it. If (i) $\mathsf{G} = \mathsf{HK}$, where each $\mathbf{g} \in \mathsf{G}$ has a unique representation as $\mathbf{g} = \mathbf{hk}$, $\mathbf{h} \in \mathsf{H}$, $\mathbf{k} \in \mathsf{K}$, (ii) $t'(\mathbf{g}) = t'(\mathbf{hk})$ is H-invariant, (iii) the distribution $\mathbf{p}'$ of $\mathbf{K}$ is in $\mathscr{P}'$, and (iv) the conditional distribution $\mathbf{p}''$ of $\mathbf{H}$ given $\mathbf{K}$ is in $\mathscr{P}''$, then both the unobserved true P-values, (P', P''), and their observed bounds, $\left(\overline{P}', \overline{P}'' \right)$, are stochastically larger than the uniform distribution on the unit square, $[0, 1]^2$.*

Proof. By (ii) and (iii), the unknown true joint distribution $\mathbf{p}$ of $\mathbf{G} = \mathbf{HK}$ is in the knit product, $\mathbf{p} \in \mathscr{P}' \oslash \mathscr{P}''$. For this true $\mathbf{p}$, the conditions of Proposition 3 in Chapter 7 are satisfied, with $J = 2$, $(V_1, V_2) = (\mathbf{K}, \mathbf{H})$, so that (P', P'') is stochastically larger than uniform. By Lemmas 7 and 8, the joint bounds, $\left(\overline{P}', \overline{P}'' \right)$, obtained from all $\mathbf{p} \in \mathscr{P}' \oslash \mathscr{P}''$ satisfy $(P', P'') \le \left(\overline{P}', \overline{P}'' \right)$, so $\left(\overline{P}', \overline{P}'' \right)$ is also stochastically larger than uniform. $\qquad \square$

Let us put together Theorem 9 and Proposition 4 in Chapter 7. Suppose that we combine the two P-value bounds, $\left(\overline{P}', \overline{P}'' \right)$, using a monotone increasing function $f(\cdot)$, such as the truncated product of P-values (7.7), rejecting the hypothesis of no effect, H_0, when the combined P-value in Proposition 4, namely $P_{\{1,2\}}$, is at most α. If the hypothesis H_0 of no effect is true, and if $\mathbf{p}' \in \mathscr{P}'$, $\mathbf{p}'' \in \mathscr{P}''$, then the probability that $P_{\{1,2\}} \le \alpha$ is at most α. In other words, if $P_{\{1,2\}} \le \alpha$ then the biased treatment assignments in $\mathscr{P}'$ and $\mathscr{P}''$ are insufficient to explain rejection of H_0 at level α.

The conclusion of Theorem 9 is that two P-values, (P', P''), and two P-value bounds, $\left(\overline{P}', \overline{P}'' \right)$, are stochastically larger than independent uniform random variables. However, the premises of Theorem 9 did not assume that $\mathbf{H}$ and $\mathbf{K}$ are independent. Quite the contrary, the premises of Theorem 9 allow the joint distribution of $\mathbf{H}$ and $\mathbf{K}$ to exhibit any dependence compatible with $\mathbf{p}' \in \mathscr{P}'$ and $\mathbf{p}'' \in \mathscr{P}''$. The dependence of $\mathbf{H}$ and $\mathbf{K}$ for $\mathbf{p} \in \mathscr{P}' \oslash \mathscr{P}''$ can be quite strong.

11.7   Summary: Combining Two Sensitivity Analyses

A central result, Theorem 9, has shown how to combine two sensitivity analyses without adding new assumptions, that is, with no assumptions beyond those already present in the two separate sensitivity analyses. Theorem 9 created the set—the knit product—containing all of the joint distributions compatible with the assumptions of the separate sensitivity analyses, and did a joint sensitivity analysis using that set of joint distributions. Perhaps surprisingly, the joint upper bound $\left(\overline{P}', \overline{P}''\right)$ on the pair of P-values testing no effect is identical to the pair of bounds from the two separate sensitivity analyses, and $\left(\overline{P}', \overline{P}''\right)$ may be handled as if they were two independent P-values testing H_0, despite allowing for strong dependence between the two factors.

11.8   Complement: More than Two Factors

11.8.1   All L Factors

For more than two factors, recall Definition 8 in §9.3. Theorem 9 is the special case of Proposition 10 in which there are $L = 2$ factors.

Proposition 10. *Assume H_0 is true for the purpose of testing it. Suppose that (i) $\mathsf{G} = \mathsf{A}_1 \mathsf{A}_2 \cdots \mathsf{A}_L$, where each $\mathbf{g} \in \mathsf{G}$ has a unique representation as $\mathbf{g} = \mathbf{a}_1 \cdots \mathbf{a}_L$, $\mathbf{a}_\ell \in \mathsf{A}_\ell$, $\ell = 1, \ldots, L$, (ii) $t_\ell(\mathbf{g}) = t_\ell(\mathbf{a}_1 \cdots \mathbf{a}_L)$ is $\mathsf{A}_1 \mathsf{A}_2 \cdots \mathsf{A}_{\ell-1}$-invariant, in the sense that $t_\ell(\mathbf{a}_1 \cdots \mathbf{a}_L) = t_\ell(\mathbf{a}_\ell \cdots \mathbf{a}_L)$, for $\ell = 2, \ldots, L$, (iii) the marginal distribution $\mathbf{p}_L$ of $\mathbf{A}_L \in \mathsf{A}_L$ is in $\mathscr{P}_L$, and (iv) the distribution $\mathbf{p}_\ell$ of $\mathbf{A}_\ell \in \mathsf{A}_\ell$ with fixed $(\mathbf{A}_{\ell+1}, \ldots, \mathbf{A}_L) = (\mathbf{a}_{\ell+1}, \ldots, \mathbf{a}_L)$ is in $\mathscr{P}_\ell$ for $\ell = 1, \ldots, L-1$. Let P_L be the unknown true P-value testing H_0 using $t_L(\mathbf{A}_L)$, and let $\overline{P}_L$ be its upper bound over marginal distributions $\mathbf{p}_L \in \mathscr{P}_L$. For $\ell = 1, \ldots, L-1$, let P_ℓ be the unknown true P-value testing H_0 using $t_\ell(\mathbf{A}_\ell \mathbf{a}_{\ell+1} \cdots \mathbf{a}_L)$, and let $\overline{P}_\ell$ be its upper bound over distributions $\mathbf{p}_\ell \in \mathscr{P}_\ell$. Then the joint distribution of both the unobserved true P-values, $(P_1, \ldots, P_L)^T$, and their observed bounds, $(\overline{P}_1, \ldots, \overline{P}_L)^T$, are stochastically larger than the uniform distribution on $[0,1]^L$.*

11.8.2   Some of the L Factors

Let $\mathscr{J} \subseteq \{1, \ldots, L\}$ pick out some but not necessarily all of the L factors. As in Proposition 3, it is often important in practice to consider the behavior of some of the factors, $\ell \in \mathscr{J}$, without assuming that $\mathbf{p}_\ell \in \mathscr{P}_\ell$ for all of the factors, $\ell = 1, \ldots, L$. Nonetheless, as in Proposition 3, the test using factor ℓ fixes all of $(\mathbf{A}_{\ell+1}, \ldots, \mathbf{A}_L) = (\mathbf{a}_{\ell+1}, \ldots, \mathbf{a}_L)$. To simplify the statement of Proposition 11, avoiding special discussion of P_1 and P_L, understand P_L as having no conditioning and P_1 as having no invariance.

Proposition 11. *Suppose that (i) $\mathsf{G} = \mathsf{A}_1 \mathsf{A}_2 \cdots \mathsf{A}_L$, where each $\mathbf{g} \in \mathsf{G}$ has a unique representation as $\mathbf{g} = \mathbf{a}_1 \cdots \mathbf{a}_L$, $\mathbf{a}_\ell \in \mathsf{A}_\ell$, $\ell = 1, \ldots, L$, (ii) for $\ell \in \mathscr{J}$, the statistic $t_\ell(\mathbf{g}) = t_\ell(\mathbf{a}_1 \cdots \mathbf{a}_L)$ is $\mathsf{A}_1 \mathsf{A}_2 \cdots \mathsf{A}_{\ell-1}$-invariant, (iii) $\mathbf{p}_\ell \in \mathscr{P}_\ell$ for $\ell \in \mathscr{J}$, where $\mathbf{p}_\ell$ is* *the distribution of $\mathbf{A}_\ell \in A_\ell$ with fixed $(\mathbf{A}_{\ell+1}, \ldots, \mathbf{A}_L) = (\mathbf{a}_{\ell+1}, \ldots, \mathbf{a}_L)$. For $\ell \in \mathscr{J}$, let P_ℓ be the unknown true P-value testing H_0 using $t_\ell(\mathbf{A}_\ell \mathbf{a}_{\ell+1} \cdots \mathbf{a}_L)$, and let $\overline{P}_\ell$ be its upper bound over distributions $\mathbf{p}_\ell \in \mathscr{P}_\ell$. Then the joint distribution of both the unobserved true P-values, P_ℓ, $\ell \in \mathscr{J}$, and their observed bounds, $\overline{P}_\ell$, $\ell \in \mathscr{J}$, are stochastically larger than the uniform distribution on $[0,1]^{|\mathscr{J}|}$.*

11.9   Exercises

Exercise 11.1. *Review Exercises 5.1–5.3 in Chapter 5. Verify the conditions of Theorem 9, thereby showing that the analyses you did in Exercises 5.1–5.3 are appropriate. By verifying these conditions, you demonstrate that the pair of P-value bounds are jointly stochastically larger than the uniform distribution on the unit square when Fisher's hypothesis of no effect is true and the biases in the two factors are at most Γ and Γ'. (Hint: This example is essentially a one-way comparison of three groups, but the outcome is binary rather than continuous. The pick and subpick matrices provide the needed factorization of the set of treatment assignments, as in §9.3. The analysis of Table 4.2 is invariant to the choice of subpick matrix.)*

Exercise 11.2. *This exercise continues Exercise 5.5 concerning DNA damage from chromium exposure at a tannery [306]. Verify the conditions of Theorem 9, thereby showing that the analysis you did in Exercise 5.5 is appropriate. (Hint: The relevant factorization of the treatment assignments involves stratified pick and subpick matrices acting within each of 30 blocks. That is, the permutation matrices are 90×90 block diagonal matrices with 30 blocks of size 3×3, and each block involves a pick and a subpick matrix.)*

Exercise 11.3. *Consider again the proof of Lemma 7. In that proof, the quantity $\sum_{\mathbf{k} \in K} \sum_{\mathbf{h} \in H} \chi\{t'(\mathbf{hk}) \geq c\} p_{\mathbf{hk}}$ is seen to depend upon the joint distribution $p_{\mathbf{hk}}$ of $(\mathbf{H}, \mathbf{K})$ only indirectly through its corresponding marginal distribution $p'_{\mathbf{k}} = \sum_{\mathbf{h} \in H} p_{\mathbf{hk}}$ of $\mathbf{K}$. Would this still be true if $t'(\cdot)$ were not invariant to $\mathbf{h} \in H$? Why or why not?*

Exercise 11.4. *Consider again the proof of Lemma 8. For a set $\mathscr{P}_{\Gamma',\Gamma''}$ of joint distributions of $(\mathbf{H}, \mathbf{K})$, write $\mathscr{P}_{\Gamma',\Gamma'',\mathbf{k}}$ for the corresponding set of conditional distributions $p_{\mathbf{hk}} / \sum_{\mathbf{h} \in H} p_{\mathbf{hk}}$ of $\mathbf{H}$ given $\mathbf{K} = \mathbf{k}$, so each such conditional distribution is a distribution on H. If $\mathscr{P}_{\Gamma',\Gamma''} = \mathscr{P}' \oslash \mathscr{P}''$, as in Lemma 8, then $\mathscr{P}_{\Gamma',\Gamma'',\mathbf{k}} = \mathscr{P}''$ for every $\mathbf{k} \in K$. If $\mathscr{P}_{\Gamma',\Gamma''}$ was not the knit product in such a way that $\mathscr{P}_{\Gamma',\Gamma'',\mathbf{k}}$ changed with $\mathbf{k} \in K$, then would it still be true that $\upsilon_{\mathbf{k}}(c) = \upsilon''_{\mathbf{k}}(c)$? Why or why not?*

Chapter 12

*Groups of Permutation Matrices

Abstract

This optional chapter explores the connection between evidence factors and algebraic groups of permutation matrices. The main results of Chapter 11, namely Theorem 9 and Proposition 10, required the unique representation of a set G of permutation matrices as the product of other sets of permutation matrices. These unique representations take natural forms when G is a group of permutation matrices.

12.1 Why Groups?

The main results of Chapter 11, namely Theorem 9 and Proposition 10, required the unique representation of a set G of permutation matrices as the product of other sets of permutation matrices. Additionally, one test statistic had to be invariant under the action of the permutation matrices in one of these sets of permutation matrices. These topics may be discussed without reference to group theory, but they have a natural home in group theory. If there is a group of permutation matrices and a subgroup of that group, then the needed factorization arises from one of the most basic constructions in group theory, namely the representation of the group in terms of the cosets of the subgroup. The formal structure needed for three evidence factors appears if the subgroup itself has a subgroup. Various group products—the direct product, the semidirect product, the wreath product—produce the required factorization in a natural way. These products may be iterated to produce several evidence factors satisfying the conditions of Proposition 10.

In brief, if you wanted to construct new evidence factors satisfying the conditions of Theorem 9 and Proposition 10, then the perspective provided by group theory is helpful.

12.2 Groups

12.2.1 Definition of a Group

Section 12.2 contains a few definitions and facts about groups of $N \times N$ permutation matrices. These definitions and facts are found in the first chapter of most books about groups; e.g., Refs. [92, 134, 236].

Let G be a nonempty set of $N \times N$ permutation matrices. By definition, the set G is a group if it has two properties: (I) the product of any two elements of G is also in G, and (II) the inverse of any element of G is also in G. That is, property (I) says: $\mathbf{a} \in$ G and $\mathbf{b} \in$ G implies $\mathbf{ab} \in$ G. Similarly, property (II) says: $\mathbf{a} \in$ G implies $\mathbf{a}^{-1} \in$ G.

For example, H in (9.2) is a group: $\mathbf{h}_1\mathbf{h}_1 = \mathbf{h}_1 \in$ H, $\mathbf{h}_2\mathbf{h}_2 = \mathbf{h}_1 \in$ H, $\mathbf{h}_1\mathbf{h}_2 = \mathbf{h}_2\mathbf{h}_1 = \mathbf{h}_2 \in$ H, and $\mathbf{h}_1^{-1} = \mathbf{h}_1 \in$ H, $\mathbf{h}_2^{-1} = \mathbf{h}_2 \in$ H. In the same way, K in (9.1) is a group. The subset $\{\mathbf{k}_1, \mathbf{k}_2, \mathbf{k}_3\} \subset$ K in (9.1) is not a group because $\mathbf{k}_2\mathbf{k}_3 = \mathbf{k}_4 \notin \{\mathbf{k}_1, \mathbf{k}_2, \mathbf{k}_3\}$ so (I) does not hold; however, $\{\mathbf{k}_1, \mathbf{k}_2, \mathbf{k}_3\}^{-1} = \{\mathbf{k}_1, \mathbf{k}_2, \mathbf{k}_3\}$, so (II) does hold.

The definition of a group implies that the $N \times N$ identity matrix $\mathbf{I}$ is in G: (a) because G is not empty, it contains at least one $N \times N$ permutation matrix $\mathbf{g}$, (b) by property (II), $\mathbf{g}^{-1} \in$ G, (c) by property (I), $\mathbf{I} = \mathbf{gg}^{-1} \in$ G.

The definition of a group may be restated using the notion of closure from §9.4: G is a group of $N \times N$ permutation matrices if $GG \subseteq G$ and $G^{-1} \subseteq G$.

12.2.2 Subgroups

If G is a group of $N \times N$ permutation matrices, then a subset $S \subseteq$ G is a subgroup of G if S is a group. For instance, K in (9.1) is a subgroup of the group of all 4×4 permutation matrices, and so is H in (9.2); moreover, H and K are subgroups of the group HK, which in turn is a subgroup of the group of all 4×4 permutation matrices. Also, in (9.1), $\{\mathbf{k}_1, \mathbf{k}_2\} \subset$ K is a subgroup of K, but $\{\mathbf{k}_2, \mathbf{k}_3\} \subset$ K is not a subgroup.

Trivially, G is a subgroup of G and $\{\mathbf{I}\}$ is a subgroup of G. Moreover, $\mathbf{I} \in$ S for every subgroup S of G.

12.2.3 Cosets

Let S be a subgroup of a group G of $N \times N$ permutation matrices, and let $\mathbf{g}$ be an element of G. Then $S\mathbf{g} = \{\mathbf{sg} : \mathbf{s} \in S\}$ is a subset of G, because G is a group, so G satisfies property (I). The set $S\mathbf{g}$ is called a right coset of S. For example, in (9.1) and (9.2), H is a subgroup of the group HK, and the coset $H\mathbf{k}_4 = \{\mathbf{h}_1, \mathbf{h}_2\}\mathbf{k}_4 = \{\mathbf{h}_1\mathbf{k}_4, \mathbf{h}_2\mathbf{k}_4\}$ is

$$H\mathbf{k}_4 = \left\{ \begin{bmatrix} 0 & 1 & 0 & 0 \\ 1 & 0 & 0 & 0 \\ 0 & 0 & 0 & 1 \\ 0 & 0 & 1 & 0 \end{bmatrix}, \begin{bmatrix} 0 & 0 & 0 & 1 \\ 0 & 0 & 1 & 0 \\ 0 & 1 & 0 & 0 \\ 1 & 0 & 0 & 0 \end{bmatrix} \right\}. \tag{12.1}$$

Of course, in (9.1) and (9.2), $H\mathbf{k}_1 = H\mathbf{I} = H$.

It is easy to see that $S\mathbf{g}$ and S contain the same number of permutation matrices. Specifically, there are $|S|$ products of the form $\mathbf{a} = \mathbf{gs}$, $\mathbf{s} \in S$, so $|S\mathbf{g}| \le |S|$; however, these $|S|$ products $\mathbf{a} = \mathbf{gs}$ are all distinct permutation matrices, because $\mathbf{g}^{-1}\mathbf{a} = \mathbf{s}$, so $|S\mathbf{g}| = |S|$.

Cosets of a Subgroup The cosets of a subgroup partition a finite group into mutually exclusive and exhaustive sets of the same size.

If $\mathbf{g} \in S$, then $S\mathbf{g} = S$ by property (I). If $\mathbf{g} \notin S$, then $S\mathbf{g} \neq S$, because $\mathbf{I} \in S$, so $\mathbf{Ig} = \mathbf{g} \in S\mathbf{g}$.

Two cosets, $S\mathbf{a}$ and $S\mathbf{b}$, may or may not be the same. When does $S\mathbf{a} = S\mathbf{b}$? Clearly, $S\mathbf{a} = S\mathbf{b}$ if and only if $S\mathbf{a}\mathbf{b}^{-1} = S$ if and only if $\mathbf{a}\mathbf{b}^{-1} \in S$.

If $\mathbf{a} \in G$ and $\mathbf{b} \in G$, then say $\mathbf{a}$ is related to $\mathbf{b}$ if $\mathbf{a}\mathbf{b}^{-1} \in S$. The relation just defined is an equivalence relation, as will now be demonstrated. First, $\mathbf{a}$ is related to itself, because $\mathbf{a}\mathbf{a}^{-1} = \mathbf{I} \in S$, because S is a subgroup. Second, if $\mathbf{a}$ is related to $\mathbf{b}$ then $\mathbf{b}$ is related to $\mathbf{a}$, because $\mathbf{a}\mathbf{b}^{-1} \in S$ implies $\left(\mathbf{a}\mathbf{b}^{-1}\right)^{-1} \in S$ by property (II), and $\left(\mathbf{a}\mathbf{b}^{-1}\right)^{-1} = \mathbf{b}\mathbf{a}^{-1}$; so, $\mathbf{b}\mathbf{a}^{-1} \in S$. Finally, if $\mathbf{a}$ is related to $\mathbf{b}$ and $\mathbf{b}$ is related to $\mathbf{c}$, then $\mathbf{a}$ is related to $\mathbf{c}$, because $\mathbf{a}\mathbf{b}^{-1} \in S$ and $\mathbf{b}\mathbf{c}^{-1} \in S$ imply, by property (I), that $\mathbf{a}\mathbf{b}^{-1}\mathbf{b}\mathbf{c}^{-1} = \mathbf{a}\mathbf{c}^{-1} \in S$. So, the relationship just defined is an equivalence relationship on G, so G partitions into mutually exclusive and exhaustive equivalence classes, with $\mathbf{a}$ and $\mathbf{b}$ in the same class if and only if $\mathbf{a}\mathbf{b}^{-1} \in S$. By the previous paragraph, these equivalence classes are precisely the right cosets.

In brief, the right cosets $S\mathbf{g}$ of S partition G into $|G|/|S|$ mutually exclusive and exhaustive sets, each containing $|S|$ permutation matrices.

In parallel, the set $\mathbf{g}S$ is called a left coset of S, with similar properties.

12.2.4 Representatives of the Cosets

Let S be a subgroup of a group G of $N \times N$ permutation matrices. There are $|G|/|S|$ distinct right cosets of S, but there are $|G|$ names, $S\mathbf{g}$, $\mathbf{g} \in G$, for these cosets; so, there are too many names. As the cosets are nonoverlapping, it is easy to assign each coset a unique name: (i) visit each of the $|G|/|S|$ cosets of S, (ii) pick one arbitrary element $\mathbf{t}$, from each coset, giving the unique name $S\mathbf{t}$ to that coset, and (iii) collect the names $\mathbf{t}$ in a set T with $|G|/|S|$ elements, each of which is a permutation matrix. The set T is called a system of distinct representatives of the cosets.

For example, $G = HK$ in (9.1) and (9.2) contains $|G| = 8$ permutation matrices, and its subgroup H contains $|H| = 2$ permutation matrices, so H has $|G|/|H| = 4$ cosets, each of size $|H\mathbf{g}| = 2$, one of which is in (12.1). The set K is a system of $|G|/|H| = 4$ distinct representatives from the cosets. In this rather special case, it is also true that H is a system of $|G|/|K| = 2$ representatives from the four cosets of the subgroup K of $G = HK$. Unlike this special example, if T is a system of distinct representatives from the cosets of a subgroup S, then T need not be a subgroup.

Taken together, the subgroup S and the system of distinct representatives T yield a unique representation of each $\mathbf{g} \in G$ as $\mathbf{g} = \mathbf{s}\mathbf{t}$ with $\mathbf{s} \in S$ and $\mathbf{t} \in T$. Every $\mathbf{g}$ has such a representation because the cosets $S\mathbf{t}$, $\mathbf{t} \in T$, exhaustively cover G. The representation is unique because the cosets, $S\mathbf{t}$, $\mathbf{t} \in T$, are mutually exclusive, so each $\mathbf{g} \in G$ is in only one coset, say $S\mathbf{t}$, and if $\mathbf{g} = \mathbf{s}\mathbf{t}$ and $\mathbf{g} = \mathbf{a}\mathbf{t}$ with $\mathbf{s} \in S$ and $\mathbf{a} \in S$, then $\mathbf{s} = \mathbf{g}\mathbf{t}^{-1} = \mathbf{a}$.

Unique Representation as a Product If S is a subgroup of a group G of $N \times N$ permutation matrices, then every element of G can be written in precisely one way as the product of an element of S and an element of a system T of distinct representatives of the cosets of S.

12.3   Groups in Evidence Factors: Some Examples

In Theorem 9, it was important to write the elements of a set of permutation matrices in a unique way as the product of elements drawn from two subsets, and we now have a general way to do this. Specifically, if S is a subgroup of a group G of $N \times N$ permutation matrices, then we may always construct a system T of distinct representatives from the cosets of a subgroup S; then, each $\mathbf{g} \in G$ has one and only one representation as $\mathbf{g} = \mathbf{st}$ with $\mathbf{s} \in S$ and $\mathbf{t} \in T$.

Let us reexamine Chapters 8–9 in light of §12.2.

Example 1. *Pick Matrices*

Let G be the group of all $N \times N$ permutation matrices, so $|G| = N!$, and let S be the subgroup containing the $m! \times (N-m)!$ block diagonal permutation matrices of the form (8.3); that is, each $\mathbf{s} \in S$ is the direct sum of an $m \times m$ permutation matrix and an $(N-m) \times (N-m)$ permutation matrix. Then the $\binom{N}{m}$ pick matrices in Definition 8.4 are a system T of distinct representatives of the right cosets of S, with $G = ST$, so there are two factors for use in Theorem 9. Of course, $|S| \times |T| = m! \times (N-m)! \times \binom{N}{m} = N! = |G|$.

Section 8.7 considers two treatments, each with doses. There, T picks individuals for one treatment or the other, and S assigns doses within each treatment.

As discussed below in §12.4, the direct sum S may itself be written as two factors, so $G = ST$ yields three factors for use in Proposition 10. One factor of S permutes doses of treatment 1, while the other factor permutes doses of treatment 2.

Example 2. *Subpick Matrices*

Let G, S, and T be defined as in Example 1. Let A be the subgroup of both G and S containing the $m! \times m'! \times (N-m-m')!$ block diagonal permutation matrices of the form (8.4) with $L = 3$ blocks; that is, each $\mathbf{a} \in A$ is the direct sum of an $m \times m$ permutation matrix, an $m' \times m'$ permutation matrix, and an $(N-m-m') \times (N-m-m')$ permutation matrix. Denote by B the set of (N, m, m')-subpick matrices, so B contains $\binom{N-m}{m'}$ permutation matrices of the form in Definition 6. As discussed in §9.3, the assignments of N individuals to treatment groups of sizes m, m' and $N-m-m'$ are uniquely represented in the factorization BT as the product of a subpick matrix and a pick matrix. Additionally, B is a system of distinct representatives of the right cosets of A in S, with $S = AB$. Also, BT is a system of distinct representatives of the right cosets of A in G, with $G = ABT = ST$, where

$$|A| \times |B| \times |T| = m! \times m'! \times (N-m-m')! \times \binom{N-m}{m'} \times \binom{N}{m} = N! = |G|.$$

So, $G = ABT$ yields three factors for use in Proposition 10. As discussed below in §12.4, the subgroup A may itself be written as three factors, so that $G = ABT$ yields five factors for use in Proposition 10.

Split matrices in §8.12 behave in a parallel way.

Section 8.10 considered the same situation repeated in S strata of varying sizes n_s, $s = 1, \ldots S$, with m_s individuals receiving the first treatment, m'_s receiving the second treatment, and $n_s - m_s - m'_s$ receiving the third treatment. In this case, the group G contains $\prod n_s!$ block-diagonal permutation matrices of the form (8.4). Here, G factors in a manner analogous to the case without strata (or equivalently with $S = 1$ stratum).

Example 3. *Within and Between Blocks*

In §8.8, the N units are divided into S strata, each stratum containing $N/S = n$ units. Units within strata are permuted into treatment positions, and strata are also permuted into treatment positions. In (8.12), the subgroup S contains the $S!$ permutation matrices of size $N \times N$ formed as Kronecker products $\mathbf{a} \otimes \mathbf{I}$ as $\mathbf{a}$ ranges over the $S!$ permutation matrices of size $S \times S$. The system of distinct representatives T consists of direct sums of S permutation matrices of size $n \times n$, so T contains $|T| = (n!)^S$ permutation matrices. In this special case, T is also a subgroup. The group G is $G = ST$ with $S! \times (n!)^S$ permutation matrices.

Section §8.8 also considered an alternative subgroup S with fewer than $S!$ permutation matrices, $|S| \leq S!$, with $N \times N$ permutation matrices $\mathbf{s} = \mathbf{a} \otimes \mathbf{I}$ as $\mathbf{a}$ ranges over a subgroup A of the $S \times S$ permutation matrices. This alternative subgroup S permitted only permutations of strata that resembled each other, say strata containing people of the same gender and age. In parallel, the S blocks of $\mathbf{t} \in T$ might all be drawn from one subgroup of the group B of the $n \times n$ permutation matrices, $|B| \leq n!$. In this case, $G = ST$ contains $|G| = |S| \times |B|^S$ permutation matrices (8.12), rather than $S! \times (n!)^S$ matrices. As $G = ST$ has the two properties required of a group, properties (I) and (II), $G = ST$ is a group, called the wreath product [236, p. 175] of B by A, with subgroups S and T.

12.4 Group Products

12.4.1 Normal Subgroups

Let S be a subgroup of a group G of $N \times N$ permutation matrices. Then S is said to be a normal subgroup if $\mathbf{g}^{-1}\mathbf{sg} \in S$ for every $\mathbf{g} \in G$ and $\mathbf{s} \in S$. Here are several equivalent ways to say this: (i) $\mathbf{g}^{-1}Sg \subseteq S$ for every $\mathbf{g} \in G$, (ii) $\mathbf{g}^{-1}Sg = S$ for every $\mathbf{g} \in G$, and (iii) left and right cosets are equal, $Sg = gS$.

In (9.1) and (9.2), H and K are both subgroups of the group $G = HK$. The subgroup H is not a normal subgroup: for instance, $\mathbf{k}_2^{-1}\mathbf{h}_2\mathbf{k}_2 \notin H$. In contrast, the subgroup K is a normal subgroup, as is checked in two steps. First, as $\mathbf{h}_1 = \mathbf{I}$, it follows trivially that $\mathbf{h}_1^{-1}\mathbf{kh}_1 = \mathbf{k} \in K$ for each $\mathbf{k} \in K$. So, consider $\mathbf{h}_2 \in H$. Now, $\mathbf{h}_2 = \mathbf{h}_2^{-1}$ swaps the two pairs, while each $\mathbf{k} \in K$ swaps treatments inside the two pairs, leaving the pairs in their original order. So $\mathbf{h}_2^{-1}\mathbf{kh}_2 = \mathbf{h}_2\mathbf{kh}_2$ first swaps the two pairs, then changes treatment assignments within pairs, then swaps the two pairs back into their original order. The claim that $\mathbf{h}_2^{-1}\mathbf{k}\mathbf{h}_2 \in K$ is the claim that it was silly to swap the pairs if you were going to swap them back: the pairs are now back in their original order, and you could have produced the same effect by using a different element of K to produce the same permutation of individuals into treatment positions. For instance, $\mathbf{h}_2^{-1}\mathbf{k}_2\mathbf{h}_2 = \mathbf{k}_3$.

The group $G = HK$ built from (9.1) and (9.2), and larger versions of this group, is the group of invariances of the joint distribution of an iid sample from a distribution symmetric about zero, and it is widely discussed in the statistical literature; e.g., Ref. [15]. This group is isomorphic to the reflection group generated by coordinate sign changes and coordinate permutations for a real vector [90, 117], leading to various probability inequalities [44, 61, 62] that are useful in obtaining the bounds that appear in sensitivity analyses [185]. The stratified analysis in Table 5.7 refers to a subgroup of this group, where the subgroup is also a reflection group, a so-called parabolic subgroup [73, 117, §1.10].

The subgroups H and K in (9.1) and (9.2) are a very special case of (8.12) in §8.9, and of the wreath product $G = ST$ in Example 3. Instead of permuting within and between two pairs, the $N \times N$ matrices in (8.12) permute S strata of the same size, n, and permute within each stratum, where $N = Sn$. In the wreath product $G = ST$ in Example 3, T is a normal subgroup, but S is not generally a normal subgroup [236, p. 175].

Let A be a group of $m \times m$ permutation matrices, let B be a group of $(N-m) \times (N-m)$ permutation matrices, and let G be the set of $N \times N$ permutation matrices formed as the direct sum of an $\mathbf{a} \in A$ and a $\mathbf{b} \in B$,

$$G = \left\{ \begin{bmatrix} \mathbf{a} & \mathbf{0} \\ \mathbf{0} & \mathbf{b} \end{bmatrix} : \mathbf{a} \in A, \mathbf{b} \in B \right\}. \qquad (12.2)$$

Then G in (12.2) is a group because it has the defining properties (I) and (II). Two subgroups of G are:

$$S = \left\{ \begin{bmatrix} \mathbf{a} & \mathbf{0} \\ \mathbf{0} & \mathbf{I} \end{bmatrix} : \mathbf{a} \in A \right\} \text{ and } T = \left\{ \begin{bmatrix} \mathbf{I} & \mathbf{0} \\ \mathbf{0} & \mathbf{b} \end{bmatrix} : \mathbf{b} \in B \right\}. \qquad (12.3)$$

Indeed, both S and T in (12.3) are normal subgroups of G in (12.2); for instance,

$$\begin{bmatrix} \mathbf{a} & \mathbf{0} \\ \mathbf{0} & \mathbf{b} \end{bmatrix}^{-1} \begin{bmatrix} \mathbf{c} & \mathbf{0} \\ \mathbf{0} & \mathbf{I} \end{bmatrix} \begin{bmatrix} \mathbf{a} & \mathbf{0} \\ \mathbf{0} & \mathbf{b} \end{bmatrix} = \begin{bmatrix} \mathbf{a}^{-1}\mathbf{c}\mathbf{a} & \mathbf{0} \\ \mathbf{0} & \mathbf{I} \end{bmatrix} \in S \text{ for all } \mathbf{a}, \mathbf{c} \in A, \mathbf{b} \in B,$$

because $\mathbf{a}^{-1}\mathbf{c}\mathbf{a} \in A$ by property (I). The group G in (12.2) is called the direct product of S and T in (12.3), or the direct product of A and B. In words, an experiment or group G of treatment assignments has two normal subgroups whenever the N individuals in the experiment may be divided into two nonoverlapping parts, one of size m, the other of size $N-m$, where the assignment of treatments in the first part has nothing to do with the assignment of treatments in the second part.

12.4.2 Several Group Products

Suppose that a group G of $N \times N$ permutation matrices has subgroups S and T. When can G be represented uniquely as the product of S and T? If each element $\mathbf{g} \in G$ has one and only one representation as $g = st$, $s \in S$, $t \in T$, then G is called one of several names: the Zapa-Szep product of S and T [28, 269], the essentially disjoint product [183, p. 33, p. 151], or the knit product [6]. Consequences of the definition include the following. If G is the knit product of its subgroups S and T, then (i) $G = ST$, (ii) $|G| = |S| \times |T|$, (iii) $S \cap T = \{I\}$, and (iv) $ST = TS$, even if the group elements do not commute [134, p. 6, §1.1.5].[1]

Suppose that G is the knit product of its subgroups S and T. Several special cases of the knit product are familiar. If either S or T is a normal subgroup, then G is called the semidirect product of S and T. If both S and T are normal subgroups, then G is called the direct product of S and T. For instance, G in (12.2) is the direct product of S or T in (12.3), so G is also the semidirect and knit product of S and T. The wreath product in Example 3 is a knit product, a semidirect product, but not a direct product. Suppose that G has a subgroup S, so that $G = ST$, where T is a system of distinct representatives of the right cosets of S; so, if T is a subgroup, then G is the knit product of S and T.

In brief, group products are a rich source of the unique representations used in Theorem 9 and Proposition 10 of Chapter 11.

12.4.3 Some Useful Semidirect Products

The wreath product in Example 3 is a particularly tidy semidirect product: all S strata have the same size, n, and the same internal structure expressed by the group B. Statistical practice is often less tidy than this. In the simplest case, suppose that there are L_2 matched pairs of a smoker and a nonsmoker, and L_3 matched triples of a smoker and two nonsmokers, so $N = 2L_2 + 3L_3$. Generally, the structure of the matched sets contains information. In the United States today, smoking is uncommon among educated and wealthier individuals, but it is not uncommon among individuals with less education and income. Run an optimal matching algorithm with income and education among the covariates, producing a mixture of pairs and triples, and the result is likely to contain pairs of individuals with less education and income, and triples with more education and income, because educated, wealthy nonsmokers are in abundant supply. More generally, Pimentel, Yoon, and Keele [174] observe that, in large samples, the number of controls available at a given value of observed covariates is predicted by the reciprocal of the odds of the propensity score (their entire number); so, the structure of matched sets is informative, reflecting the propensity score. Therefore, it makes sense to restrict treatment assignments to sets of permutation matrices that preserve the structure of the matched sets. We would like to permute the pairs separately from the triples. If we let G be a direct sum of a wreath

---

[1]Technically, there are two ways to describe a group product. An internal definition starts with a group, G, and two of its subgroups, S and T, and the definition of a particular group product states a condition such that G is the product of S and T. The definition just given is the internal definition of the knit product. An external definition starts with two groups, S and T, and builds a third group, G, from them. See, for example, the construction of G in (12.2) from A and B. There is then a theorem which says that these two structures refer to isomorphic groups. For instance, A and S in (12.3) are distinct groups—the matrices are of different sizes—but they are isomorphic, so it is rather fussy to distinguish them. This level of detail is not needed here, so I move between internal and external definitions without comment.

product for the L_2 pairs and another wreath product for the L_3 triples, then G is a semidirect product that is not a wreath product. In the notation of Example 3, the wreath product for the pairs has a group A_2 of $L_2 \times L_2$ permutation matrices that permute pairs and the group B_2 comprised of the two 2×2 matrices in (8.5) that permute treatments inside pairs. The wreath product for the triples has a group A_3 of $L_3 \times L_3$ permutation matrices that permute the triples, and a group B_3 that permutes one individual into the first position, the smoker position, in a matched triple:

$$B_3 = \left\{ \begin{bmatrix} 1 & 0 & 0 \\ 0 & 1 & 0 \\ 0 & 0 & 1 \end{bmatrix}, \begin{bmatrix} 0 & 1 & 0 \\ 0 & 0 & 1 \\ 1 & 0 & 0 \end{bmatrix}, \begin{bmatrix} 0 & 0 & 1 \\ 1 & 0 & 0 \\ 0 & 1 & 0 \end{bmatrix} \right\}. \tag{12.4}$$

Because nothing distinguishes the two nonsmoking positions in a matched triple, the test statistic for smoker-versus-control would be selected to be invariant to the positioning of the two nonsmokers in a triple.

Suppose that, instead of smokers and nonsmokers, the matched pairs compared treatment 1 and treatment 2, while the triples compared treatments 1, 2, and 3. The relevant semidirect product would be as above, except the group B_3 would contain all $3! = 6$ permutation matrices of size 3×3.

In a full matching [95, 97, 124, 187, 266], a matched set contains either one treated individual and one or more controls, or one control and one or more treated individuals.[2] Full matching is often possible when pair matching is not possible, and it produces closer matches on covariates. Again, the structure of a full match is informative, reflecting the distribution of propensity scores [174]. In the simplest case, there are L_2 pairs, L_3 triples with two controls, and L_3' triples with two treated individuals. The semidirect product is similar to the one described above, except that it permutes the two types of triples within types, yielding a direct sum of three wreath products.

In brief, Theorem 9 is applicable in settings in which strata sizes or structures vary, yet doses or other treatments are permuted among strata.

12.5   Summary: Groups Provide the Needed Factors

Theorem 9 may be understood and used without reference to group theory. Nonetheless, Theorem 9 makes reference to the unique representation of a set of treatment assignments, or a set of permutation matrices, as the products of two subsets. The relevant factorization exists whenever there is a group G of $N \times N$ permutation matrices and a subgroup S; see §12.3. The group products in §12.4 provide a variety of useful factorizations.

Exercises

Exercise 12.1. *Verify that B_3 in (12.4) is a group. How does multiplication of its three elements change the vector $\mathbf{n} = (1, 2, 3)^T$?*

---

[2]Hansen's R package optmatch performs optimal full matching.

Exercise 12.2. *Consider $N \times N$ permutation matrices of the form*

$$\begin{bmatrix} 1 & 0 \\ 0 & \mathbf{p} \end{bmatrix}, \tag{12.5}$$

where $\mathbf{p}$ is an $(N-1) \times (N-1)$ permutation matrix. Let F be the set of all permutation matrices of the form (12.5). What is $|\mathsf{F}|$? Show that F is a group. Show that F is a subgroup of the group G of all $N!$ permutation matrices of size $N \times N$. How many cosets does F have in G? Give a system of distinct representatives for the right cosets of F. How does multiplication by elements of F act on the vector $\mathbf{n} = (1, \ldots, N)^T$? (Hint: Reexamine Example 1.)

Exercise 12.3. *Which of the elements of B_3 in (12.4) are $(3, 1)$-pick matrices? In B_3, replace*

$$\begin{bmatrix} 0 & 1 & 0 \\ 0 & 0 & 1 \\ 1 & 0 & 0 \end{bmatrix} \quad by \quad \begin{bmatrix} 0 & 1 & 0 \\ 1 & 0 & 0 \\ 0 & 0 & 1 \end{bmatrix},$$

and call the result B_3'. Which elements of B_3' are $(3, 1)$-pick matrices? Is B_3' a group? Consider the subgroup

$$\mathsf{F}_3 = \left\{ \begin{bmatrix} 1 & 0 & 0 \\ 0 & 1 & 0 \\ 0 & 0 & 1 \end{bmatrix}, \begin{bmatrix} 1 & 0 & 0 \\ 0 & 0 & 1 \\ 0 & 1 & 0 \end{bmatrix} \right\}$$

of the group G of all 3×3 permutation matrices. How many cosets does F_3 have in G? How large is each coset? Is B_3 in (12.4) a system of distinct representatives for the right cosets of F_3 in G? Is B_3' a system of distinct representatives for the right cosets of F_3 in G?

Part IV

Aspects of Design

Chapter 13

Constructing Matched Samples with Evidence Factors

Abstract

How should we match for observed covariates in a study that contains evidence factors? The literature discusses a few options, including complete blocks with several treatment groups, incomplete blocks, and certain more focused strategies. These options are described in conceptual terms. A variety of computational issues arise, as some problems have polynomial-time solutions, and others do not. Some designs permit essentially independent comparisons despite reuse of same data, while other designs secure independent comparisons by splitting the data. The loss of sample size for each factor from splitting can be substantial, and it may be avoidable in a carefully planned study. Parallel issues arise when stratification and covariance adjustment are used in place of matching.

13.1 Aspects of Design

13.1.1 Importance of Design

Evidence factors are planned aspects of an observational study; they need to be built into the study design. Evidence factors require additional data that would not be needed for a simple treatment/control comparison. The structure of the additional data needs to be compatible with an analysis that yields two essentially independent factors; see Chapter 11. To be convincing, evidence must be conceived before examining outcomes. The design incorporates a plan for a primary analysis.

The importance of design in confirmatory studies is often stressed. For instance, Tukey wrote [274, p. 22]:

> Preplan the main analysis. ... I see no real alternative, in most truly confirmatory studies, to having a single main question—in which a question is specified by all of design, collection, monitoring, and analysis.

Rubin [241, pp. 20, 25, 26] wrote:

> Observational studies can and should be designed to approximate randomized experiments as closely as possible. In particular, observational studies should be designed using only background information to create subgroups of similar

treated and control units, where 'similar' here refers to their distributions of background variables. Of great importance, this activity should be conducted without any access to any outcome data, thereby assuring the objectivity of the design. ... [I]n randomized experiments the design phase takes place prior to seeing any outcome data. And this critical feature of randomized experiments can be duplicated in observational studies ... [O]objectivity is not the same as finding truth, but I believe that it is generally a necessary ingredient if we are to find truth. The key idea is to conduct the design before ever seeing any outcome data ... The design should include the specification of the analysis that is to be carried out. [pp. 20, 25, 26]

13.1.2   Algorithmic Aspects of Design with Evidence Factors

The current chapter is concerned with the algorithmic aspects of forming matched comparisons with evidence factors. For instance, in §4.4, matched triples of restaurants created two evidence factors in Card and Krueger's [34] study of the minimum wage. The first factor was a comparison of Pennsylvania and New Jersey, where New Jersey had raised its minimum wage and Pennsylvania had not. The second factor was a comparison inside New Jersey of restaurants with starting wages near the old minimum wage or well above it. A New Jersey restaurant with a starting wage at or near the old minimum wage had to make substantial adjustments to accommodate the new minimum wage. How does one match to compare three treatment groups?

The algorithmic aspects of design with evidence factors are not well developed. One reason for this is that, by the usual standard, the computational task in matching three groups is much harder than in forming matched pairs for two groups. This is surprising, at first, because the tasks sound similar. So, let us develop a clear way of speaking about this.

13.1.3   How Fast Is an Algorithm?

In algorithm design, the usual standard for appraising an algorithm counts the number of steps required to produce a solution. Obviously, the number of steps will depend upon the size of the problem, and also on the particulars of the input. Suppose there are N numbers and we want to sort them into increasing order. Obviously, we expect to work harder when N is larger. Also, if the numbers were already in increasing order, then we would simply have to verify this, but if they were very much out of order, then we would have to work harder to bring them into order. So the usual standard is adjusted to be the maximum number of steps required to produce a solution for any input of size N. Let $d(N)$ be that number.

Even this is problematic, because the notion of "one step" is vague. One person might write C code that swaps two numbers that are out of order using two lines of code, while another might do the same thing with three lines of codes. Is this one step? Is it two steps for the first person and three steps for the second? Perhaps it would take four lines of Fortran code to do what could be done in two lines of C code. Perhaps four lines of Fortran code execute as fast as two lines of C code, or perhaps that is true on one computer and not on another. All of this seems tedious and beside the point, which is: Can we solve large problems quickly? To some extent, the four answers we have—$d(N)$ steps for one swap, $2d(N)$ steps for two lines of C code, $3d(N)$ steps for three lines of C code, and $4d(N)$ steps for four lines of Fortran code—feel like the same answer. The usual solution is to leave vague what is vague.[1] Instead of focusing on $d(N)$, we drop a constant of proportionality, and focus on $O\{d(N)\}$ as $N \to \infty$. For instance, no matter how disorganized N numbers are, it is possible to sort them into increasing order in $O\{N\log(N)\}$ steps [248, Chapter 1]. An algorithm runs in polynomial time if $d(N) \leq \varsigma N^\lambda$ for all N for some fixed numbers $\varsigma > 0$ and $\lambda > 0$, in which case $d(N) = O(N^\lambda)$. For instance, sorting N numbers can be done in $O\{N\log(N)\}$ steps, so it can be done in polynomial time. In brief, we can sort large files relatively quickly.

Suppose that we have N individuals, some of whom are treated, the rest controls, and between each treated individual and each control there is a nonnegative distance. This distance indicates how similar these two individuals are in terms of measured covariates. There are more controls than treated individuals, and as $N \to \infty$ the ratio of control to treated individuals remains nearly constant. We wish to pair each treated individual with a different control such that the total of the distances for paired individuals is as small as possible. This problem can be solved in $O(N^3)$ steps [132, Theorem 11.2]. This time bound assumes any treated individual can be paired with any control (with all $O(N)$ controls); however, we often impose restrictions, such as a caliper of the propensity score [230, 303], so that each treated individual can only be paired with a subset of the controls. If each treated individual must be assigned to one of $O\{\log(N)\}$ controls, then the time bound is improved from $O(N^3)$ to $O\{N^2\log(N)\}$; see Ref. [132, Theorem 11.2].

Calculations of this sort are definitely useful as a guide to statistical practice, but they have limitations and must be informed by practical experience. An algorithm with a less satisfying time bound[2] may perform as well or better in typical problems than the algorithm with the best time bound, in part because the worst problem that provides the bound may not resemble a typical problem. In particular, an algorithm and code for optimal matching [21, 22] that is widely used in R has a less satisfying time bound; however, experience shows that it solves large statistical problems quickly.[3] Statisticians face various risks in their professional work, for instance, being part of a research team that recommends an ineffective or harmful drug. In this context, the risk associated with calling a computer program and having to kill the job because it takes too long is a rather small risk. Worrying that an algorithm may be slow for a worst-case problem unlikely to arise in practice may constitute worrying about a detail when larger issues are at stake. Certain statistical problems

---

[1] Wittgenstein [294, p. 45]: "What is ragged should be left ragged."

[2] A less satisfying time bound may be less satisfying in various ways. It may simply be a larger bound, $O(N^\omega)$ with $\omega > \lambda$. Alternatively, the bound may not depend solely on N, but may involve other features of the input besides its size. For an optimization problem, the solution may be guaranteed to be within ε of the optimum, for any specified $\varepsilon > 0$, rather than achieving the optimum, but the time bound may depend on ε. There are many variations on these themes.

[3] The Fortran code for this algorithm may be used within R by installing and loading the optmatch and rcbalance packages, and applying the callrelax function in the rcbalance package.

that lack worst-case time bounds are often solved quickly without them [309]. In certain statistical problems, we seek to optimize a function, but in truth any solution guaranteed to be close to the optimum would suffice.[4]

Consider, now, the problem of forming matched triples from three treatment groups, A, B, and C, as in §4.4 for the minimum wage data. Suppose that we want to form matched triples, (A, B, C), so that the sum of the three distances, AB, AC, BC, is minimized. This problem sounds similar to the minimum distance pair match problems, with its $O(N^3)$ time bound. In fact, for minimum distance matching of three groups, no polynomial time algorithm is known, and it is believed that none exists, no matter how large one sets λ.[5] What can be done?

13.1.4   Outline

In light of these computational issues, two ways to match with three treatment groups, A, B, and C are considered in §13.2 and §13.3. The methods are described in concise, conceptual terms, with reference to published articles for specifics. With additional specifics, each of these methods extends to more than three groups, as discussed in the articles.

The first approach in §13.2 solves the original problem approximately in polynomial time [126]. The time bound is still $O(N^3)$, but an optimal solution need not be produced; rather, the solution is at a measured distance from the optimum.

The second approach in §13.3 changes the problem, solving the new problem optimally in $O(N^3)$ steps [147]. Instead of forming matched triples, the three treatments, A, B, and C are compared in matched pairs, perhaps balanced to create a balanced incomplete block design. This design has both advantages and disadvantages.

Section 13.4 discusses a study design that makes comparisons within and between institutions that provide treatments. Sometimes two very different processes are at work: one leads a person to an institution, the other assigns treatments within that institution. These two processes can produce two evidence factors.

Study designs are compared in §13.5. Some study designs secure independent evidence factors by splitting the sample into nonoverlapping parts, but §13.5 emphasizes that the resulting loss of sample size for each factor can often be avoided by careful design.

Matching often provides a simple design, together with fine control of imbalances in covariates. An alternative proceeds without matching, perhaps combining stratification and covariance adjustment, as illustrated in §2.3. This presents no special issues, providing: (i) the same strata are used for both evidence factors, and (ii) as in §2.3 and Ref. [194], the covariance adjustment does not include the treatment group as a predictor. In particular, finding evidence factors without splitting the sample arises in the same way, whether or not matching is used in design; see §13.5 and Ref. [127].

---

[4]For instance, Wald [280, Theorem 2] proved the consistency of the maximum likelihood estimate by showing that any estimate is consistent if its likelihood ratio exceeds a positive constant, even if it does not maximize the likelihood.

[5]More precisely, Crama and Spieksma [52, Theorem 1] show that the problem is NP-hard.

13.2 Nearly Optimal Complete Blocks

13.2.1 Approximation Algorithms

Approximation algorithms provide, in polynomial time, near-optimal solutions to optimization problems that are computationally intractable [278, 290]. For example, an $O\left(N^3\right)$ time 2-approximation algorithm for a minimization problem provides, in $O\left(N^3\right)$ steps, a solution that is at most twice the true minimum [290, Definition 1.1]. An approximation algorithm makes two promises about the worst case: (i) in the worst case, the time is at most $O\left(N^3\right)$, (ii) in the worst case, the solution is at most twice the true minimum.

In matching three groups of equal size, Crama and Spieksma [52] developed a matching algorithm for approximately minimizing the total distance within matched triples. Their method and results are not quite applicable for statistical matching problems, for several reasons. First, in statistical matching problems, the groups are not initially the same size. In §4.4, there are 66 restaurants in Pennsylvania, 150 low-wage restaurants in New Jersey and 135 high-wage restaurants in New Jersey. The statistical problem must start with the smallest group, here Pennsylvania, and lacks certain symmetries of the original problem. Equally important, statistical matching problems often impose additional constraints to balance covariates, such as fine and near-fine balance constraints. Karmakar and colleagues [126] modified the argument of Crama and Spieksma [52] to provide an $O\left(N^3\right)$ time 2-approximation algorithm for the statistical problem with groups of unequal size and near-fine balance constraints. Only a few aspects of these algorithms are sketched here. See also Ref. [162].

13.2.2 What Is a Fine Balance Constraint?

Fine balance means that the marginal distribution of a nominal covariate is exactly the same in the treated group and the matched control group [226]. The covariate may have thousands or tens of thousands of levels. This definition makes no reference to who is matched to whom. Pairs may not be matched for a finely balanced nominal covariate: the promise is simply that the distribution of the covariate is the same in the treated and matched control groups viewed as groups. For instance, in health outcomes research, one may wish to finely balance hundreds of ICD-10 Principal Diagnosis Codes or Surgical Procedure Codes [303]. Alternatively, one nominal covariate with many levels may be formed from the interaction of several nominal covariates [313].

Fine balance is not always feasible. There may be no matched control group that exhibits fine balance. Near-fine balance means that the marginal distributions of a nominal covariate in treated and matched-control groups differ to the smallest extent possible [299]. By definition, near-fine balance equals fine balance whenever fine balance is feasible. By definition, near-fine balance is always feasible.

Refined balance creates a hierarchical or tree structure for violations of fine balance, so that gaps in fine balance are filled by neighboring categories in the tree. Pimentel and colleagues [172, Table 1] used refined balance to balance a tree-structured nominal covariate with more that 2.8 million categories as its leaves.

Fine, near-fine, and refined balance are constraints on an optimization problem. The total within-pair covariate distance is minimized subject to constraints. For two groups, treatment and control, this constrained optimization problem may be formulated as finding a minimum cost flow in a suitable network. For two treatment groups, the constrained optimization problem may be solved in $O(N^3)$ steps.

What can be done with three treatment groups?

13.2.3   An Approximation Algorithm with Near-fine Balance

The algorithm requires a distance that satisfies the triangle inequality. The triangle inequality says that the distance between x and z is at most the distance between x and y plus the distance between y and z, for any y. In words, a detour to y cannot shorten the trip from x to z. For instance, the Euclidean norm and the Mahalanobis norm satisfy the triangle inequality, as do various distances formed by suitably combining such distances with weights to emphasize certain covariates [126, §4].

The algorithm proceeds in two steps. First, it finds a minimum distance pair match subject to near-fine constraints of the 66 Pennsylvania restaurants and the 135 high-wage New Jersey restaurants, making 66 matched pairs. It then computes a distance between each of the 66 pairs and each of the 150 low-wage restaurants in New Jersey. That distance is the sum of three distances for the two restaurants in the pair and the one low-wage restaurant. In the second step, the algorithm finds a minimum distance pair match subject to near-fine constraints of the 66 pairs and the 150 low-wage restaurants in New Jersey. Each of the two steps is an optimal pair match, so each step takes $O\left(N^3\right)$ time, and the entire algorithm runs in $O\left(N^3\right)$ time.

The algorithm need not find the set of 66 triples that minimizes the total distance within triples. The pairing chosen in the first step may seem regrettable when we examine the restricted choices it has left for us in the second step. Some tinkering with the triangle inequality shows our regret cannot be very large, with the consequence that the algorithm returns a total distance that is at most twice the true minimum.

This method created the match in §4.4. See §13.7 for the R code.

13.2.4   One Comparison Takes Precedence

Depending upon the scientific context, one of the comparisons of three treatment groups may take precedence over the others. With treatment groups A, B and C, the comparison of A and B may be of overriding importance. For instance, it may be that comparisons involving group C are useful as checks for bias, but the main interest entails comparing A and B; e.g., Ref. [264]. When matching creates the treatment groups, it may be important that the existence of group C not alter the composition of A and B, as in Refs. [173, §5.3] and [232].

If the comparison of A and B is of overriding importance, it is natural to match A and B to minimize the distance within pairs, perhaps subject to a fine balance constraint. Having done that, one seeks to bring C into the match, minimizing its distance to the AB pairs, perhaps subject to a fine balance constraint. Notably, this is precisely what Karmakar's algorithm does. So, that algorithm is an approximation algorithm if one wishes to minimize the within-block distances among the three treatment groups, but it is the optimal solution to a matching problem that gives total priority to the comparison of groups A and B.

13.3 Optimal Incomplete Block Designs

13.3.1 Incomplete Blocks

In an incomplete block design, the block size is smaller than the number of treatments. For instance, with three treatments, A, B, and C, an incomplete block design consists of matched pairs of two individuals receiving different treatments. An incomplete block design is balanced if every pair of two treatments occurs together in a block with equal frequency. With three treatments in pairs, the design is balanced if the number of AB pairs equals the number of AC pairs, which in turn equals the number of BC pairs. Incomplete block designs play an important role in the theory of experimental design [40, 50, 297].

13.3.2 Nonbipartite Matching

Consider an even number, Q, of objects together with a nonnegative, possibly infinite distance between each pair of two objects. The problem is to divide the Q objects into $Q/2$ disjoint pairs to minimize the total of the $Q/2$ within-pair distances [63, 145].

This is called weighted "nonbipartite matching," for "not-two-parts." An infinite distance may be viewed as an attempt to forbid certain pairings, but that may or may not be possible: there may or may not be a pairing with finite total distance. The problem can be solved in $O(Q^3)$ steps [132, Corollary 11.12].[6] Nonbipartite matching has a variety of statistical applications [146].

If the number, N, of individuals to be matched is odd, then add a phantom individual at zero distance from everyone else, making $Q = N + 1$ objects. Nonbipartite matching forms $Q/2$ pairs, so that discarding the one individual paired with the phantom leaves $(N - 1)/2$ pairs. The discarded individual is the one who was most difficult to match, in the sense that discarding this individual led to the smallest total distance for the $(N - 1)/2$ pairs. By introducing additional phantoms at zero distance from some individuals and at infinite distance from others, a wide variety of problems may be solved [146]. The $O(Q^3)$ time bound is lost if general integer programming methods are used; however, additional matching techniques become available [314].

---

[6]In R, the nbpMatching package [146] provides access to the Fortran code of Derigs [54]. See also the nmatch function in the designmatch package.

13.3.3 *Minimum Distance Incomplete Block Designs*

In Card and Krueger's [34] study of the minimum wage in §4.4, there were initially $q_A = 66$ restaurants in Pennsylvania, $q_B = 150$ low-wage restaurants in New Jersey and $q_C = 135$ high-wage restaurants in New Jersey with complete data on employment and starting wages, or $66 + 150 + 135 = 351$ restaurants in total.[7] Between any two restaurants in different treatment groups, there is a distance measuring how similar these restaurants are in terms of observed covariates. The distance between two restaurants in the same treatment group is set to ∞ to prevent the pairing of two restaurants in the same group. Nonbipartite matching may be used in several ways to produce an incomplete block design that minimizes the total within-block distance subject to various specifications [147].

In any design, let v_{AB} be the number of AB pairs, v_{AC} be the number of AC pairs, and v_{BC} be the number of BC pairs. A balanced incomplete block design has $v_{AB} = v_{AC} = v_{BC}$, but we need not use a balanced design. In this same design, let w_A be the number of blocks that include treatment A, w_B be the number of blocks that include treatment B, and w_C be the number of blocks that include treatment C. Of course, these quantities are related; for instance, $w_A = v_{AB} + v_{AC}$ and $w_A \leq q_A$. Specifically,

$$
\begin{bmatrix} w_A \\ w_B \\ w_C \end{bmatrix} = \begin{bmatrix} 1 & 1 & 0 \\ 1 & 0 & 1 \\ 0 & 1 & 1 \end{bmatrix} \begin{bmatrix} v_{AB} \\ v_{AC} \\ v_{BC} \end{bmatrix} \tag{13.1}
$$

and

$$
\begin{bmatrix} v_{AB} \\ v_{AC} \\ v_{BC} \end{bmatrix} = \frac{1}{2} \begin{bmatrix} 1 & 1 & -1 \\ 1 & -1 & 1 \\ -1 & 1 & 1 \end{bmatrix} \begin{bmatrix} w_A \\ w_B \\ w_C \end{bmatrix}. \tag{13.2}
$$

Consider the largest possible incomplete block design. It is not balanced. As $66 + 150 + 135 = 351$ is odd, we must add one phantom to the distance matrix. Group B is the largest, with $q_B = 150$ low-wage restaurants in New Jersey. So we pair the phantom with a restaurant in group B by adding a row and column to the distance matrix at 0 distance from each member of group B and at infinite distance from all other restaurants. Without the restaurant in group B that was paired to the phantom, $w_A = 66$, $w_B = 149$, $w_C = 135$, and (13.2) yields $v_{AB} = 40$, $v_{AC} = 26$, and $v_{BC} = 109$, for $175 = 40 + 26 + 109$ pairs comprised of $350 = 2 \times 175$ restaurants. The restaurant in group B that is most difficult to match is excluded by this process.

Figure 13.1 shows the matched pair differences in the after-minus-before changes in full-time equivalent employment. The covariates and outcomes are as in §4.4; however, there are now matched pairs rather than matched triples. In parallel with §4.4, Figure 13.2 merges the two comparisons of New Jersey and Pennsylvania. The two boxplots in Figures 13.1 and 13.2 are independent simply because no restaurant appears in more than one boxplot.

---

[7]In the evident package in R, this is the ckA data frame with 351 rows. The match in Figure 13.1 was built by applying the nbpMatching package to ckA; however, this requires a few clerical steps in R to create the distance matrix and then reorganize the output into a matched data set, so these details are not included in the text of this book.

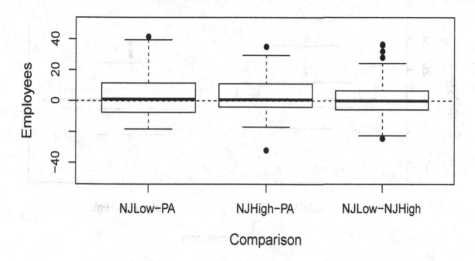

Figure 13.1 *Matched pair differences in the after-minus-before changes in the numbers of full-time equivalent employees in the largest incomplete block design, with 350 restaurants in 175 matched pairs. The three boxplots contain 40, 26, and 109 pairs. The dashed horizontal line is at zero.*

Consider a balanced incomplete block design. As $v_{AB} + v_{AC} = w_A \leq q_A = 66$ and $v_{AB} = v_{AC}$, it follows that the largest possible balanced design has $v_{AB} = v_{AC} = v_{BC} = 33$, or $3 \times 33 = 99$ pairs, comprised of $2 \times 99 = 198$ restaurants of the 351 restaurants. Each treatment group is represented in $w_A = w_B = w_C = 66$ pairs of the 99 pairs. Additional phantoms are added to the distance matrix to remove the appropriate numbers of pairs from groups B and C. For instance, we need $w_B - w_A = 150 - 66 = 84$ phantoms at zero distance from group B and at infinite distance from other groups to remove 84 restaurants from group B. A balanced incomplete block design for the minimum wage data is given in Ref. [147].

13.4   Variation in Treatment within and Between Institutions

Treatments are often provided by institutions, be they hospitals, schools, prisons, or psychiatric clinics. People find themselves at one institution rather than another, and inside that institution are given one treatment rather than another. So, two selection processes are at work, one that brings a person to a particular institution, the other that selects a treatment for that person within that institution. Either or both steps may depart from random assignment, but the two processes are often very different, perhaps subject to different selection biases. Perhaps people find themselves

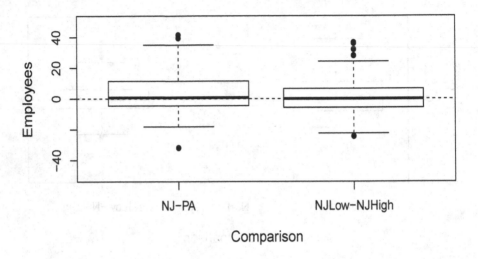

Figure 13.2 *Matched pair differences in the after-minus-before changes in the numbers of full-time equivalent employees in the largest incomplete block design, with 350 restaurants in 175 matched pairs. The two comparisons involving Pennsylvania have been combined. The two boxplots contain 66 and 109 pairs. The dashed horizontal line is at zero.*

at the local institution, the neighborhood school, the local hospital. Perhaps the local school regards evolution and divine creation as two equally valid theories, but perhaps in that school, students studying for the national Advanced Placement Examination in Biology are taught evolution exclusively. Institutions may have general preferences, yet make exceptions; different institutions may do this differently. Is it possible to use this structure to produce two evidence factors?

Institutions may vary in their typical practice, employing one treatment far more often than another. Institutions may also vary in how they select some people for one treatment, other people for another treatment. Perhaps people are offered a choice inside one institution, but experts allocate treatments at another institution. Perhaps experts at different institutions hold different opinions about the best treatment. Perhaps different experts within a single institution hold different opinions or preferences.

Knee surgery may be performed using either general or regional anesthesia. With regional anesthesia, pain may be blocked by injection of a local anesthetic at specific sites within the spinal column, but the patient may be awake, perhaps sedated. With general anesthesia, the patient is unconscious. Opinions vary about whether general or regional anesthesia is better for patients, and whether the decision is more important for some patients than for others, say for elderly patients. Some hospitals typically use one form of anesthesia for knee surgery, while other hospitals typically use the other, and still other hospitals commonly use both forms. Inside an institution, one anesthesiologist may prefer regional anesthesia, a second anesthesiologist may prefer general anesthesia, and a third may prefer that the patient make an informed choice. Hospitals and their patient populations differ in many ways other than the type of anesthesia they commonly use, so one might wish to control for the hospital. Then again, the allocation of patients to hospitals may be more haphazard than decisions inside the hospital about which patient should be given which type of anesthesia; so, one might like to compare patients who received a particular anesthetic just because that anesthetic is the usual practice in the local hospital. Can we see it both ways?

Zubizarreta and colleagues [311] examined Medicare data and chart reviews for knee surgery performed at 47 hospitals in New York, Texas and Illinois. They built two nonoverlapping matched comparisons. In the first comparison, each hospital contributes the same number of patients to the general and regional anesthesia groups. In this comparison, there is a nominal covariate with 47 categories representing the hospital, and that covariate is finely balanced. In the second comparison, the "usual practice comparison," each hospital contributes patients to one treatment group or the other, but never to both. Table 13.1 shows the patient counts for five of the 47 hospitals, specifically hospitals 24 through 28, where all the possible patterns occur.

Table 13.1 *Counts of patients receiving general or regional anesthesia for hospitals 24 through 28 of 47 hospitals. The table distinguishes the "finely balanced match" and the "usual practice" match*

Hospital ID	Finely Balanced		Usual Practice	
	General	Regional	General	Regional
	⋮	⋮	⋮	⋮
24	29	29	0	14
25	14	14	0	41
26	17	17	71	0
27	35	35	168	0
28	92	92	0	0
	⋮	⋮	⋮	⋮

In Table 13.1, hospitals 26 and 27 have a decided preference for general anesthesia, while hospital 25 has a preference for regional anesthesia. These hospitals contribute most of their patients to the usual practice match, and in such hospitals, a patient is likely to receive the type of anesthesia commonly used in that hospital. In hospitals 24 and 28, the division into general and regional anesthesia is more evenly divided, and these hospitals contribute most of their patients to the finely balanced match. Both comparisons may be biased, but the biases are likely to be different. In the finely balanced match, the predominant selection takes place inside the hospital, as one patient receives general anesthesia and another receives regional anesthesia.

In the usual practice match, the predominant selection takes place between hospitals that may differ in other ways. The match controlled for numerous covariates, some from chart abstraction, such as age, gender, diabetes and other comorbid conditions, obesity, the American Society of Anesthesiologists' physical status classification, the APACHE score, and others [311, Table 2 and Figure 1]. The finely balanced match consisted of 1354 pairs of two patients, and the usual practice match consisted of 944 pairs. In a trivial way, not unlike Figure 13.2, the two comparisons or factors have outcomes that are conditionally independent given covariates, simply because the two comparisons do not share patients. See Ref. [311, §4] for discussion of the optimal matching algorithm.

The main outcome was a binary indicator of success thirty days after surgery. Success entailed: (i) being alive at 30 days, (ii) without a deep vein thrombosis during those 30 days, and (iii) without readmission to the hospital during those 30 days. As in the benzene example in §4.5, the two factors do not concur in this example. In the finely balanced match, regional anesthesia was associated with a substantially higher rate of success, with an odds ratio of 1.52 (95% CI: [1.16, 2.01]) and two-sided P-value 0.003. In the usual practice match, there was little sign of a difference, with odds ratio 1.06 (95% CI: [0.76, 1.47]), and P-value 0.80. In words, inside hospitals, patients selected for regional anesthesia appear to have better outcomes, but patients at hospitals that routinely use regional anesthesia do not appear to have better outcomes. This conflict is certainly a reason to hesitate before claiming that the associations reflect effects actually caused by the type of anesthesia.

The direction of the effect, if any, was always in doubt, so the combined test should be two-sided, in the sense of §6.2. That is, two one-sided truncated products are computed, truncating at 0.1, and the smaller of the two resulting, one-sided P-values is doubled. In other words, as in §6.2, the two tests support each other only if they point in the same direction. Here, this two-sided, combined P-value is 0.014 at $\Gamma = 1$ but is 0.05 at $\Gamma = 1.082$.

13.5   Comparing Study Designs: Which Design Is Best?

13.5.1   Incomplete Block Designs: Balanced or Unbalanced?

Consider, first, incomplete block designs, balanced or not. An incomplete block design that discards some restaurants produces a closer pairing for the restaurants it does pair. Optimal nonbipartite matching pairs phantoms with the least matchable restaurants. So, there is a trade-off between sample size and a compelling comparison. The minimum wage study is not extremely large, so sample size remains relevant.

13.5.2   Block Designs: Complete or Incomplete?

Now, compare complete and incomplete block designs. Which is better? For complete blocks, the match in §4.4 and §13.2 formed 66 matched triples, so 66 Pennsylvania restaurants were compared to 132 New Jersey restaurants. For incomplete blocks, the first boxplot in Figure 13.2 compared 66 Pennsylvania restaurants to 66

New Jersey restaurants. So, that favors the complete block design: its Pennsylvania versus New Jersey comparison used twice as many restaurants in New Jersey. In contrast, in the complete block design, the matched triples compare 66 low-wage New Jersey restaurants to 66 high-wage New Jersey restaurants, while in the incomplete block design, the second boxplot in Figure 13.2 compares 109 low-wage New Jersey restaurants to 109 high-wage restaurants; however, this is not an entirely fair comparison, and therefore it does not really favor incomplete block designs in general. The incomplete block design in §13.3 used the maximum number of pairs, but the complete block design in §4.4 made no attempt to do this. For complete blocks, the sample sizes are sufficient to match 1-to-2-to-2, making 66 blocks each with one Pennsylvania restaurant, two low-wage New Jersey restaurants and two high-wage New Jersey restaurants. If sample size were the only consideration—it is not—but if it were, then that complete block design would win in terms of sample size. That complete block design would compare 66 Pennsylvania restaurants—all of them—to $66 \times 4 = 264$ New Jersey restaurants, and then would compare 132 low-wage New Jersey restaurants to 132 high-wage New Jersey restaurants. Even though the incomplete block design used 350/351 restaurants, while that complete block design used $66 + 264 = 330$ restaurants, the complete block design had a larger sample size in each evidence factor because it used the same restaurants twice, whereas Figure 13.2 uses each restaurant once. If sample size is a concern, there can be a big gain in effective sample size from using the same data twice in a manner compatible with Theorem 9 of Chapter 11.

Avoid Splitting the Data When Obtaining Independent Factors Splitting data to produce two independent evidence factors does yield independent factors; however, it reduces the effective sample size in each factor, often substantially. When possible, use Theorem 9 in Chapter 11 to obtain essentially independent evidence factors using the same data twice, without split samples. When Theorem 9 is applicable, the combined meta-analysis of two essentially independent factors can have an effective sample size that is twice the actual sample size. Moreover, to the extent that the two factors are affected by different unmeasured biases, the evidence in favor of a causal effect, and against a bias, may be strengthened to a measurable degree indicated by a joint sensitivity analysis. Use the data twice; do not cut the data in half.

The issues are the same, whether or not matching is used. Suppose strata and covariance adjustment were used in place of matching, as in §2.3. If two independent evidence factors were produced by splitting the data set, then the factors would indeed be independent, but the sample size in each factor would be reduced. If instead the same data were used twice, say with the stratified picks and subpicks in §8.10, then there would be no reduction in sample size. Despite using the data twice, the two factors formed from picks and subpicks are essentially independent, in the sense of Theorem 9 of Chapter 11, so the evidence they provide may be combined as if it came from two independent studies. See Ref. [127] for an example using covariance adjustment with strata to obtain three evidence factors.

13.5.3   Complete or Incomplete Blocks: Design Sensitivity

Sample size is one consideration, but there are others. The design sensitivity strongly affects the power of a sensitivity analysis, becoming the decisive consideration as the sample size increases; see §2.4 and Refs. [198, 215]. Consider one factor in §13.2 and §13.3, namely the comparison of New Jersey and Pennsylvania, with the change in full-time equivalent employment as the outcome. Even as $N \to \infty$, the design sensitivity for matched triples in §13.2 is larger than the design sensitivity for matched pairs in §13.3; see Refs. [212, Table 4] and [214, Table 3]. So, complete blocks are favored by two considerations that each increase the power of a sensitivity analysis: (i) design sensitivity and (ii) the ability to reuse rather than split the sample. In a certain sense, consideration (i) is more important than consideration (ii), because (i) continues to affect the power of a sensitivity analysis as $N \to \infty$. It is appropriate to consider the impact of study design on the design sensitivity for each evidence factor [125]. For detailed discussion of issues that affect design sensitivity, see Ref. [223, Part III].

13.5.4   Complete or Incomplete Blocks: What if Some Individuals Cannot Tolerate Some Treatments?

A curious, if limited, fact does favor incomplete block designs. Sometimes the world itself resembles an incomplete block design, so that similar people can have either of two treatments, but rarely can have all three treatments. The best incomplete block design in a world that resembles an incomplete block design may permit closer pairs than would be possible with a complete block design. Consider the following toy example. Suppose that we have two Pennsylvania restaurants, two low-wage New Jersey restaurants, and two high-wage New Jersey restaurants, in that order, as restaurants 1, 2, ..., 6, with the following 6×6 covariate distance matrix. As is true throughout §13.3, there are infinite distances between restaurants in the same treatment group—Pennsylvania, low-wage New Jersey, high-wage New Jersey—to prevent the pairing of restaurants in the same treatment group. Here is the symmetric 6×6 distance matrix for the 6 restaurants:

$$\begin{bmatrix} \infty & \infty & 0 & 0 & 100 & 100 \\ \infty & \infty & 100 & 100 & 0 & 0 \\ 0 & 100 & \infty & \infty & 0 & 0 \\ 0 & 100 & \infty & \infty & 0 & 0 \\ 100 & 0 & 0 & 0 & \infty & \infty \\ 100 & 0 & 0 & 0 & \infty & \infty \end{bmatrix}.$$

A balanced incomplete block design would form three pairs, say $(1,3)$, $(2,5)$, $(4,6)$ for a total distance of $0 = 0+0+0$. A complete block design would form two triples, each containing one restaurant from each treatment group. There are four possible triples that contain restaurant 1, namely $(1,3,5)$, $(1,3,6)$, $(1,4,5)$, and $(1,4,6)$, and each of these contributes a distance of $0 + 100 + 0 = 100$. The same pattern occurs with the complete block containing restaurant 2. By replacing the 100s by larger numbers, we see that the total distance for a complete block design can be vastly larger than for an incomplete block design.

This sort of pattern occurs with certain medications [133]: each patient has several options, but few patients have all the options.

13.6 Summary: Build Evidence Factors into the Design

This chapter has considered matching to control observed covariates in studies with evidence factors. The statistical literature has focused on matching two groups, treated and control, but designs with evidence factors are more complex, and a variety of new issues arise. Complete and incomplete block designs were compared in terms of: (i) their abilities to make full use of the available data, (ii) their abilities to pair closely, (iii) design sensitivity, and (iv) computational considerations in matching. In §13.4, two evidence factors came into existence by matching.

Section 13.5 compared competing designs with two evidence factors. Although no one design is best in all respects, complete blocks that use all of the data twice—aided by Theorem 9 in Chapter 11—had advantages in terms of sample size, power, and design sensitivity.

Two essentially independent comparisons—two evidence factors—can be obtained in either of two ways: (i) by splitting the data into non-overlapping pieces or (ii) by using all of the data twice when Theorem 9 in Chapter 11 is applicable. The effective sample size in each factor is often much larger if all the data are used twice, and splitting is avoided; see §13.5. A larger effective sample size in each factor becomes an even larger effective sample size in the combined meta-analysis of the two factors working in unison. In appropriate circumstances when Theorem 9 is applicable, the combined meta-analysis of two essentially independent factors can have an effective sample size that is twice the actual sample size.

13.7 Using R

The balanced complete blocks match in §13.2 for Card and Krueger's [34] data was built using Karmakar's `approxmatch` package. To use the `approxmatch` package, you must separately load Hansen's `optmatch` package, which uses Fortran code from Bersekas and Tseng [21, 22]. The data are in the `evident` package as ckA. The matched data are also in the `evident` package as ck. In effect, the following code constructs ck from ckA.

```
library(evident)
data(ckA)
library(optmatch)
library(approxmatch)
attach(ckA)

dist=multigrp_dist_struc(ckA,as.character(grp),
```

```
    list(mahal=c("chain1","chain2","chain3",
    "HRSOPEN")),wgts=1)

mtch=tripletmatching(dist,as.character(grp),
    indexgroup="PA",ckA,"CHAIN",design=c(1,1,1))
```

Chapter 14

Design Elements for Evidence Factors

Abstract

This chapter is a brief look backwards. Section 14.1 recalls some common design elements that produce evidence factors, and situates these design elements both in examples and in the technical discussion of previous chapters. Section 14.2 restates the mathematical argument in English.

14.1 Some Common Design Elements

14.1.1 Why Look Back?

The properties of evidence factors are consequences of Theorem 9 and Propositions 10 and 11 of Chapter 11. The premises of these results are the conditions that design elements must satisfy if several analyses are to be combined as if they came from independent studies. In this section, particular design elements are reconnected to Theorem 9, recalling the relevant examples and factorizations of sets of treatment assignments expressed as permutation matrices.

14.1.2 Enhancement or Mitigation of Treatment

A treatment may exist in an enhanced or a mitigated form, so treated versus control becomes one evidence factor, and enhanced treatment versus mitigated treatment becomes a second factor. This situation arose in §4.2, §4.4 and in Exercises 4.1 and 4.2. The enhanced form of treatment may itself have an enhanced form, leading to additional factors. For instance, in §4.3, a high occupational exposure to lead might be further enhanced by poor hygiene when leaving work. Any treatment group may be subdivided; see §8.12.

If there are no matched sets, or strata, then this situation falls under the scope of Theorem 9 of Chapter 11 through pick matrices and subpick matrices. If there are matched sets or strata, then the situation falls under the scope of Theorem 9 through matrices formed as direct sums of pick matrices or of subpick matrices. See Chapters 8 and 9.

Suppose that the study consists of pairs and triples, where the triples contain enhanced treatment, mitigated treatment, and control, but the pairs contain only enhanced treatment and control. This situation falls under the scope of Theorem 9 as a direct sum of a design for pairs and a design for triples, similar to (8.15) in §8.10. There are many variations on this theme: several designs with slightly different structures are pasted together into one design by taking the direct sum of the treatment assignments for the different designs.

14.1.3   Doses

In place of, or in addition to, enhanced or mitigated treatment as two groups, there may be a continuous dose of treatment, as in §4.5, §5.4, and §8.7. So, one factor compares treated and control, while the other factor looks for a dose-response relationship in the treated group. For instance, in §5.4, exposure to benzene appeared harmful, but the duration of exposure to benzene did not predict the frequency of chromosome aberrations. Each of several treatment groups may have doses, say pack-years of smoking for current smokers, pack-years for former smokers, compared to never-smoking controls who lack doses. The doses in distinct treatment groups need not be commensurate; e.g., the dose of one drug may not be commensurate with the dose of a different drug. Distinct treatment groups with doses fall under the scope of Theorem 9 by combining pick or subpick matrices with matrices that permute doses within treatment groups, as discussed in §8.7.

14.1.4   Treatments that Vary Within and Between Matched Sets

One factor may consist of a treatment-versus-control comparison within matched pairs, or matched sets, or blocks, and this may be the first factor. The treatment may vary in intensity between pairs, sets or blocks, perhaps because the dose of treatment varies from one treated person to another, and this may form a second factor. See the examples in §4.1 and §4.3.

This situation falls under the scope of Theorem 9 of Chapter 11 by way of permutations of the blocks of block-diagonal permutation matrices, as discussed in §8.9. As illustrated in §5.3 and discussed in §8.9, the permutation of doses among matched sets may be restricted: it may swap doses only among matched sets with similar covariates, thereby adjusting twice for the observed covariates. This may be done to appropriate residuals from a robust covariance adjustment, as illustrated in §2.3, making a third adjustment for the observed covariates.

The matched sets or blocks need not have the same size or structure, providing the permutation of doses is restricted to permute a dose from one set to another of the same size and structure, in parallel with (8.15) in §8.10.

14.1.5   Instruments

A valid instrument is a randomized treatment that encourages a change in behavior, in which encouragement affects the outcome only if it alters behavior. A valid instrument affords an estimate of the effect of the change in behavior on those people who would change their behavior if encouraged to do so [4]. A basic example of an instrument occurs in a randomized trial with noncompliance with the assigned treatment [88]. Instruments were discussed in §3.4.

If encouragement is not randomized, or if the encouragement has effects of its own, then the instrument is not valid; so, it may fail to provide an estimate of the effect of a change in behavior. In practice, most purported instruments were not assigned by randomization, so their validity is a matter of speculation. Sensitivity analyses for potentially biased encouragement closely parallel sensitivity analyses for any other treatment, and much is known about what makes some instruments sensitive to small biases and other instruments insensitive to large biases [223, §5.3]. Evidence factor analyses apply directly to instruments, that is, to treatments that encourage but do not fully control a change in behavior. One evidence factor may use one instrument, a second evidence factor may condition on the first factor as if it were a covariate, examining what is added by a second instrument, and a third factor may condition on both instruments yielding a direct comparison of treated and control groups [127].

14.1.6 Several Evidence Factors

The various design elements may be superimposed upon one another to produce more than two evidence factors. A few of the many ways of doing this were illustrated in §8.10.

14.2 *Symmetric Sets of Biases

This section restates the technical argument in English.

A treatment assignment is a random permutation: it permutes people into treatment positions. In a randomized experiment, the permutation is picked by random numbers generated by the computer. Beginning in §1.1, treatment assignment was seen to be equitable if the probability distribution of the treatment assignment possessed certain symmetries. Symmetry referred to both the support of the distribution and the probabilities on this support. Beginning in the subsection "Randomized Trials Contain Simpler Randomized Trials" of §1.1, symmetries of treatment assignments were seen to possess subsymmetries, perhaps marginal symmetries, perhaps conditional symmetries.

In observational studies, treatment assignment may be inequitable: the distribution of the treatment assignment may not be symmetric, so that it favors some people over others. A bias in treatment assignment is an asymmetry in its distribution. As a matter of routine, biases from measured covariates are removed by adjustments, such as combinations of matching, stratification, and covariance adjustment; see §2.3. Removing biases from measured covariates is important, but it leaves untouched the central problem in causal inference, namely unmeasured biases.

Biases from unmeasured covariates are typically unknown. After adjustment for observed covariates, we think that treatment assignment may still have a distribution that is inequitable or asymmetric, favoring some individuals over others. However, we do not know that asymmetric distribution. So, we consider a set of distributions of treatment assignment as the basis for sensitivity analyses describing the range of possible inferences about treatment effects for a certain magnitude of bias in treatment assignment. We do not know the magnitude of bias either, so we consider several magnitudes, determining the smallest magnitude of bias that would alter the qualitative conclusions about treatment effects. That is, we consider a nested sequence of such sets of distributions, indexed by one or more parameters, say Γ, where later sets in the sequence, with larger Γ's, contain more distributions and permit larger biases or larger asymmetries in the distribution of treatment assignments. In any one such set of distributions of treatment assignment, most distributions are biased and asymmetric; however, given that we do not know the unmeasured bias, we considered a symmetric set of biases, a symmetric set of asymmetries.[1] Theorem 9 of Chapter 11 indicated that symmetric sets of biases yield evidence factors. Whatever bias occurs in the first or marginal factor, the set of biases that may affect the second or conditional factor remains the same. The set of distributions of dose assignments in Figure 4.2(b) is the same no matter what is observed in treatment-control assignments in Figure 4.2(a). The set of conditional distributions of dose assignments in Figure 4.2(b) is unaffected by the treatment-control assignments in Figure 4.2(a): both the support of these conditional distributions and the set of distributions on that support remain the same. This is true despite the fact that individual joint distributions of dose-assignments and treatment-control assignments may exhibit dependence.

---

[1]Symmetric sets of asymmetric objects are familiar. Consider the function $f(x,y) = (x-y)^2$ defined on the unit square, $0 \leq x \leq 1, 0 \leq y \leq 1$, so $f(x,y)$ is a symmetric function defined on a symmetric domain. The minimum value of $f(x,y)$ is zero, attained whenever $x = y$, so the set of minimal solutions is the set $\{(x,y) : x = y\}$; that is, both the individual solutions and the set of individual solutions exhibit a symmetry. In contrast, the maximum value of $f(x,y)$ on its domain is 1, attained at two points, $(x,y) = (1,0)$ and $(x,y) = (0,1)$, so the set of solutions $\{(1,0), (0,1)\}$ is a symmetric set of individually asymmetric objects.

Bibliography

[1] J. M. Abowd, F. Kramarz, D. N. Margolis, and T. Philippon. The tail of two countries: Minimum wages and employment in France and the United States. *IZA Discussion Series*, 203, 2000.

[2] J. L. Ackrill. *A New Aristotle Reader*. Princeton University Press, Princeton, NJ, 1987.

[3] K. Alam. Some nonparametric tests of randomness. *Journal of the American Statistical Association*, 69(347):738–739, 1974.

[4] J. D. Angrist, G. W. Imbens, and D. B. Rubin. Identification of causal effects using instrumental variables. *Journal of the American statistical Association*, 91(434):444–455, 1996.

[5] C. S. Armstrong, A. D. Jagolinzer, and D. F. Larcker. Chief executive officer equity incentives and accounting irregularities. *Journal of Accounting Research*, 48(2):225–271, 2010.

[6] F. Ates and A. S. Çevik. Knit products of some groups and their applications. *Rendiconti del Seminario Matematico della Università di Padova*, 121:1–11, 2009.

[7] S. Athey, G. W. Imbens, and S. Wager. Approximate residual balancing: Debiased inference of average treatment effects in high dimensions. *Journal of the Royal Statistical Society*, B 80(4):597–623, 2018.

[8] O. Auerbach, A. P. Stout, E. C. Hammond, and L. Garfinkel. Changes in bronchial epithelium in relation to cigarette smoking and in relation to lung cancer. *New England Journal of Medicine*, 265(6):253–267, 1961.

[9] R. R. Bahadur. Stochastic comparison of tests. *Annals of Mathematical Statistics*, 31(2):276–295, 1960.

[10] J. C. Bailar and H. L. Gornik. Cancer undefeated. *New England Journal of Medicine*, 336(22):1569–1574, 1997.

[11] G. W. Basse, A. Feller, and P. Toulis. Randomization tests of causal effects under interference. *Biometrika*, 106(2):487–494, 2019.

[12] P. Bauer. Multiple testing in clinical trials. *Statistics in Medicine*, 10(6):871–890, 1991.

[13] P. Bauer and M. Kieser. A unifying approach for confidence intervals and testing of equivalence and difference. *Biometrika*, 83(4):934–937, 1996.

[14] L. A. Bazzano, J. He, P. Muntner, S. Vupputuri, and P. K. Whelton. Relationship between cigarette smoking and novel risk factors for cardiovascular disease in the United States. *Annals of Internal Medicine*, 138(11):891–897, 2003.

[15] C. B. Bell and H. S. Haller. Bivariate symmetry tests: Parametric and nonparametric. *Annals of Mathematical Statistics*, 40:259–269, 1969.

[16] R. L. Berger. Multiparameter hypothesis testing and acceptance sampling. *Technometrics*, 24(4):295–300, 1982.

[17] R. L Berger and J. C. Hsu. Bioequivalence trials, intersection-union tests and equivalence confidence sets. *Statistical Science*, 11(4):283–319, 1996.

[18] B. Bergmann and G. Hommel. Improvements of general multiple test procedures for redundant systems of hypotheses. In *Multiple Hypothesenprüfung/Multiple Hypotheses Testing*, pages 100–115. Springer, 1988.

[19] R. H. Berk and A. Cohen. Asymptotically optimal methods of combining tests. *Journal of the American Statistical Association*, 74(368):812–814, 1979.

[20] R. H. Berk and D. H. Jones. Relatively optimal combinations of test statistics. *Scandinavian Journal of Statistics*, pages 158–162, 1978.

[21] D. P. Bertsekas. A new algorithm for the assignment problem. *Mathematical Programming*, 21(1):152–171, 1981.

[22] D. P. Bertsekas and P. Tseng. The relax codes for linear minimum cost network flow problems. *Annals of Operations Research*, 13(1):125–190, 1988.

[23] M. W. Birch. The detection of partial association, I: The 2×2 case. *Journal of the Royal Statistical Society B*, 26(2):313–324, 1964.

[24] M. Bogomolov and R. Heller. Discovering findings that replicate from a primary study of high dimension to a follow-up study. *Journal of the American Statistical Association*, 108(504):1480–1492, 2013.

[25] R. C. Bose and S. S. Shrikhande. On the falsity of Euler's conjecture about the non-existence of two orthogonal Latin squares of order 4t + 2. *Proceedings of the National Academy of Sciences of the United States of America*, 45(5):734, 1959.

[26] J. Bound. The health and earnings of rejected disability insurance applicants. *American Economic Review*, 79(3):482–503, 1989.

[27] W. Brannath, M. Posch, and P. Bauer. Recursive combination tests. *Journal of the American Statistical Association*, 97(457):236–244, 2002.

[28] M. G. Brin. On the Zappa-Szép product. *Communications in Algebra*, 33(2):393–424, 2005.

[29] B. M. Brown. Symmetric quantile averages and related estimators. *Biometrika*, 68(1):235–242, 1981.

[30] C. F. Burman, C. Sonesson, and O. Guilbaud. A recycling framework for the construction of Bonferroni-based multiple tests. *Statistics in Medicine*, 28(5):739–761, 2009.

[31] A. L. Byrd and J. A. Segre. Adapting Koch's postulates. *Science*, 351(6270):224–226, 2016.

[32] P. Cahuc and A. Zylberberg. *The Natural Survival of Work: Job Creation and Job Destruction in a Growing Economy*. MIT Press, 2006.

[33] D. T. Campbell and R. F. Boruch. Making the case for randomized assignment to treatments by considering the alternatives: Six ways in which quasi-experimental evaluations in compensatory education tend to underestimate effects. In *Evaluation and Experiment*, pages 195–296. Academic Press, 1975.

[34] D. Card and A. B. Krueger. Minimum wages and employment: A case study of the fast food industry in New Jersey and Pennsylvania. *American Economic Review*, 84(4):772–793, 1994.

[35] D. Card and A. B. Krueger. Minimum wages and employment: A case study of the fast-food industry in New Jersey and Pennsylvania: Reply. *American Economic Review*, 90(5):1397–1420, 2000.

[36] D. Choi. Estimation of monotone treatment effects in network experiments. *Journal of the American Statistical Association*, 112(519):1147–1155, 2017.

[37] W. S. Cleveland. *The Elements of Graphing Data*. Murray Hill, NJ, 2nd edition, 1994.

[38] W. G. Cochran. The planning of observational studies of human populations (with discussion). *Journal of the Royal Statistical Society*, A 128(2):234–266, 1965.

[39] W. G. Cochran. The effectiveness of adjustment by subclassification in removing bias in observational studies. *Biometrics*, pages 295–313, 1968.

[40] W. G. Cochran and G. M. Cox. *Experimental Designs*. John Wiley, 1957.

[41] W. G. Cochran and D. B. Rubin. Controlling bias in observational studies: A review. *Sankhyā*, A 35:417–446, 1973.

[42] A. Cohen and H. B. Sackrowitz. On stochastic ordering of random vectors. *Journal of Applied Probability*, 32(4):960–965, 1995.

[43] A. R. Collins. The comet assay for DNA damage and repair. *Molecular Biotechnology*, 26(3):249, 2004.

[44] J. C. Conlon, R. Leon, F. Proschan, and J. Sethuraman. G-ordered functions, with applications in statistics. Technical report, Florida State University, Department of Statistics, Technical Report, 1977.

[45] W. J. Conover and D. S. Salsburg. Locally most powerful tests for detecting treatment effects when only a subset of patients can be expected to respond to treatment. *Biometrics*, pages 189–196, 1988.

[46] J. Cornfield, W. Haenszel, E. C. Hammond, A. M. Lilienfeld, M. B. Shimkin, and E. L. Wynder. Smoking and lung cancer: Recent evidence and a discussion of some questions. *Journal of the National Cancer institute*, 22(1):173–203, 1959.

[47] J. Cornfield, W. Haenszel, E. C. Hammond, A. M. Lilienfeld, M. B Shimkin, and E. L. Wynder. Smoking and lung cancer: Recent evidence and a discus-

sion of some questions (Reprinted with new Discussion by D. R. Cox, J. B. greenhouse, J. P. Vandenbroucke, M. Zwahlen. *International Journal of Epidemiology*, 38(5):1175–1191, 2009.

[48] D. R. Cox. The interpretation of the effects of non-additivity in the Latin square. *Biometrika*, 45(1):69–73, 1958.

[49] D. R. Cox. The role of significance tests [with discussion]. *Scandinavian Journal of Statistics*, 4(2):49–70, 1977.

[50] D. R. Cox and N. Reid. *The Theory of the Design of Experiments*. CRC Press, 2000.

[51] D.R. Cox. *Planning of Experiments*. John Wiley, 1958.

[52] Y. Crama and F. C. R. Spieksma. Approximation algorithms for three-dimensional assignment problems with triangle inequalities. *European Journal of Operational Research*, 60(3):273–279, 1992.

[53] B. R. Davis, J. A. Cutler, D. J. Gordon, et al. Rationale and design for the antihypertensive and lipid lowering treatment to prevent heart attack trial (ALLHAT). *American Journal of Hypertension*, 9(4):342–360, 1996.

[54] U. Derigs. Solving non-bipartite matching problems via shortest path techniques. *Annals of Operations Research*, 13(1):225–261, 1988.

[55] J. Dewey. *The Sources of a Science of Education*. Horace Liveright, 1987.

[56] A. Dmitrienko and A. C. Tamhane. Gatekeeping procedures in clinical trials. In A. Dmitrienko, A. C. Tamhane, and F. Bretz, editors, *Multiple Testing Problems in Pharmaceutical Statistics*, pages 165–192. Chapman and Hall/CRC, 2009.

[57] R. Doll and A. B. Hill. The mortality of doctors in relation to their smoking habits. *British Medical Journal*, 1(4877):1451, 1954.

[58] F. I. Dretske. Reasons and falsification. *Philosophical Quarterly*, 15(58):20–34, 1965.

[59] F. Dudbridge and B. P. C. Koeleman. Rank truncated product of p-values, with application to genomewide association scans. *Genetic Epidemiology*, 25(4):360–366, 2003.

[60] M. Dwass. Some k-sample rank-order tests. In I. Olkin, editor, *Contributions to Probability and Statistics: Essays in Honor of Harold Hotelling*. Stanford University Press, 1960.

[61] M. L. Eaton. A review of selected topics in multivariate probability inequalities. *Annals of Statistics*, 10:11–43, 1982.

[62] M. L. Eaton and M. D. Perlman. Reflection groups, generalized Schur functions, and the geometry of majorization. *Annals of Probability*, 5:829–860, 1977.

[63] J. Edmonds. Maximum matching and a polyhedron with 0, 1-vertices. *Journal of Research of the National Bureau of Standards B*, 69(125-130):55–56, 1965.

[64] A. S. Evans. Causation and disease: The Henle-Koch postulates revisited. *The Yale Journal of Biology and Medicine*, 49(2):175, 1976.

[65] A. S. Evans. *Causation and Disease: A Chronological Journey*. Plenum, 1993.

[66] H. Finner. Two-sided tests and one-sided confidence bounds. *Annals of Statistics*, 22(3):1502–1516, 1994.

[67] R.A. Fisher. *Statistical Methods for Research Workers*. Oliver and Boyd, Edinburgh, 1925.

[68] R.A. Fisher. *Design of Experiments*. Oliver and Boyd, Edinburgh, 1935.

[69] M. A. Fligner and D. A. Wolfe. Nonparametric prediction intervals for a future sample median. *Journal of the American Statistical Association*, 74(366a):453–456, 1979.

[70] C. B. Fogarty. Studentized sensitivity analysis for the sample average treatment effect in paired observational studies. *Journal of the American Statistical Association*, 2020.

[71] C. B. Fogarty and D. S. Small. Sensitivity analysis for multiple comparisons in matched observational studies through quadratically constrained linear programming. *Journal of the American Statistical Association*, 111(516):1820–1830, 2016.

[72] D. P. Foster and R. A. Stine. α-investing: A procedure for sequential control of expected false discoveries. *Journal of the Royal Statistical Society B*, 70(2):429–444, 2008.

[73] A. R. Francis and H. P. Wynn. Subgroup majorization. *Linear Algebra and Its Applications*, 444:53–66, 2014.

[74] N. D. Freedman, Y. Park, C. C. Abnet, A. R. Hollenbeck, and R. Sinha. Association of coffee drinking with total and cause-specific mortality. *The New England Journal of Medicine*, 366:1891–1904, 2012.

[75] C. D. Furberg, J. T. Wright, B. R. Davis, et al. Major outcomes in high-risk hypertensive patients randomized to angiotensin-converting enzyme inhibitor or calcium channel blocker vs diuretic: The antihypertensive and lipid-lowering treatment to prevent heart attack trial (ALLHAT). *Journal of the American Medical Association*, 288(23):2981–2997, 2002.

[76] M. Gardner. Mathematical games: How three mathematicians disproved a celebrated conjecture of Leonard Euler. *Scientific American*, 201(5):181–188, 1959.

[77] J. J. Gart. A median test with sequential application. *Biometrika*, 50(1/2):55–62, 1963.

[78] J. L. Gastwirth. On robust procedures. *Journal of the American Statistical Association*, 61(316):929–948, 1966.

[79] J. L. Gastwirth. The first-median test: A two-sided version of the control median test. *Journal of the American Statistical Association*, 63(322):692–706, 1968.

[80] J. L. Gastwirth. Methods for assessing the sensitivity of statistical comparisons used in title vii cases to omitted variables. *Jurimetrics J.*, 33:19, 1992.

[81] J. L. Gastwirth, A. M. Krieger, and P. R. Rosenbaum. Cornfield's inequality. *Wiley StatsRef: Statistics Reference Online*, 2014.

[82] A. Gelman and J. Hill. *Data Analysis Using Regression and Multilevel/Hierarchical Models*. Cambridge University Press, 2006.

[83] A. Glazer. Advertising, information, and prices—A case study. *Economic Inquiry*, 19(4):661, 1981.

[84] J. J. Goeman and A. Solari. The sequential rejection principle of familywise error control. *Annals of Statistics*, 38:3782–3810, 2010.

[85] J. J. Goeman, A. Solari, and T. Stijnen. Three-sided hypothesis testing: Simultaneous testing of superiority, equivalence and inferiority. *Statistics in Medicine*, 29(20):2117–2125, 2010.

[86] K. M. Grassel, G. J. Wintemute, M. A. Wright, and M. P. Romero. Association between handgun purchase and mortality from firearm injury. *Injury Prevention*, 9(1):48–52, 2003.

[87] S. W. Greenhouse. Jerome Cornfield's contributions to epidemiology. *Biometrics*, 38(Supplement):33–45, 1982.

[88] R. Greevy, J. H. Silber, A. Cnaan, and P. R. Rosenbaum. Randomization inference with imperfect compliance in the ACE-inhibitor after anthracycline randomized trial. *Journal of the American Statistical Association*, 99(465):7–15, 2004.

[89] R. A. Groeneveld. Asymptotically optimal group rank tests for location. *Journal of the American Statistical Association*, 67(340):847–849, 1972.

[90] L. C. Grove and C. T. Benson. *Finite Reflection Groups*. Springer, 1985.

[91] S. Haack. *Evidence and Inquiry*. Oxford: Blackwell, 1995.

[92] M. Hall. *The Theory of Groups*. Chelsea Publishing, 1976.

[93] M. A. Hamilton. Choosing the parameter for a 2×2 table or a $2 \times 2 \times 2$ table analysis. *American Journal of Epidemiology*, 109(3):362–375, 1979.

[94] E. C. Hammond. Smoking in relation to mortality and morbidity: Findings in first thirty-four months of follow-up in a prospective study started in 1959. *Journal of the National Cancer Institute*, 32(5):1161–1188, 1964.

[95] B. B. Hansen. Full matching in an observational study of coaching for the SAT. *Journal of the American Statistical Association*, 99(467):609–618, 2004.

[96] B. B. Hansen. Optmatch: Flexible, optimal matching for observational studies. *New Functions for Multivariate Analysis*, 7(2):18–24, 2007.

[97] B. B. Hansen and S. O. Klopfer. Optimal full matching and related designs via network flows. *Journal of computational and Graphical Statistics*, 15(3):609–627, 2006.

[98] R. Heller, M. Bogomolov, and Y. Benjamini. Deciding whether follow-up studies have replicated findings in a preliminary large-scale omics study.

Proceedings of the National Academy of Sciences, 111(46):16262–16267, 2014.

[99] R. Heller, P. R. Rosenbaum, and D. S. Small. Split samples and design sensitivity in observational studies. *Journal of the American Statistical Association*, 104(487):1090–1101, 2009.

[100] S. Heng, D. S. Small, and P. R. Rosenbaum. Finding the strength in a weak instrument in a study of cognitive outcomes produced by Catholic high schools. *Journal of the Royal Statistical Society A*, 2020.

[101] A. L. Herbst, H. Ulfelder, and D. C. Poskanzer. Adenocarcinoma of the vagina: Association of maternal stilbestrol therapy with tumor appearance in young women. *New England Journal of Medicine*, 284(16):878–881, 1971.

[102] M. A. Hernan and J. M. Robins. *Causal Inference*. Chapman and Hall/CRC, 2011.

[103] J. L. Hodges and E. L. Lehmann. Rank methods for combination of independent experiments in analysis of variance. *Annals of Mathematical Statistics*, pages 482–497, 1962.

[104] J. L. Hodges and E. L. Lehmann. Estimates of location based on rank tests. *The Annals of Mathematical Statistics*, 34(2):598–611, 1963.

[105] W. Hoeffding. A class of statistics with asymptotically normal distribution. *Annals of Mathematical Statistics*, 19(3):293–325, 1948.

[106] R. V. Hogg. On conditional expectations of location statistics. *Journal of the American Statistical Association*, 55(292):714–717, 1960.

[107] R. V. Hogg. On the resolution of statistical hypotheses. *Journal of the American Statistical Association*, 56(296):978–989, 1961.

[108] R. V. Hogg. Iterated tests of the equality of several distributions. *Journal of the American Statistical Association*, 57(299):579–585, 1962.

[109] M. Hollander. Certain uncorrelated nonparametric test statistics. *Journal of the American Statistical Association*, 63(322):707–714, 1968.

[110] M. Hollander, D. A. Wolfe, and E. Chicken. *Nonparametric Statistical Methods*. John Wiley & Sons, 2013.

[111] S. Holm. A simple sequentially rejective multiple test procedure. *Scandinavian Journal of Statistics*, 6(2):65–70, 1979.

[112] J. Y. Hsu, D. S. Small, and P. R. Rosenbaum. Effect modification and design sensitivity in observational studies. *Journal of the American Statistical Association*, 108(501):135–148, 2013.

[113] J. Y. Hsu, J. R. Zubizarreta, D. S. Small, and P. R Rosenbaum. Strong control of the familywise error rate in observational studies that discover effect modification by exploratory methods. *Biometrika*, 102(4):767–782, 2015.

[114] R. L. Hubbard, S. G. Craddock, P. M. Flynn, J. Anderson, and R. M. Etheridge. Overview of 1-year follow-up outcomes in the Drug Abuse Treatment Outcome Study (DATOS). *Psychology of Addictive Behaviors*, 11(4):261, 1997.

[115] P. J. Huber. *Robust Statistics*. John Wiley & Sons, 1981.

[116] M. G. Hudgens and M. E. Halloran. Toward causal inference with interference. *Journal of the American Statistical Association*, 103(482):832–842, 2008.

[117] J. E. Humphreys. *Reflection Groups and Coxeter Groups*. Cambridge University Press, 1990.

[118] G. W. Imbens and P. R. Rosenbaum. Robust, accurate confidence intervals with a weak instrument: Quarter of birth and education. *Journal of the Royal Statistical Society, A*, 168(1):109–126, 2005.

[119] J. P. A. Ioannidis, P. Boffetta, J. Little, T. R. O'Brien, A. G. Uitterlinden, P. Vineis, D. J. Balding, A. Chokkalingam, S. M. Dolan, W. D. Flanders, and J. P. Higgins. Assessment of cumulative evidence on genetic associations. *International Journal of Epidemiology*, 37(1):120–132, 2008.

[120] T. Irwin. Ways to first principles: Aristotle's methods of discovery. *Philosophical Topics*, 15(2):109–134, 1987.

[121] T. Irwin. *Aristotle's Nicomachean Athics*. Hackett Publishing, 2019.

[122] H. Jick, O. S. Miettinen, R. K. Neff, S. Shapiro, O. P. Heinonen, D. Slone, and Boston Collaborative Drug Surveillance Program. Coffee and myocardial infarction. *New England Journal of Medicine*, 289(2):63–67, 1973.

[123] Kumar Jogdeo. Association and probability inequalities. *Annals of Statistics*, pages 495–504, 1977.

[124] H. Kang, B. Kreuels, J. May, and D. S. Small. Full matching approach to instrumental variables estimation with application to the effect of malaria on stunting. *The Annals of Applied Statistics*, 10(1):335–364, 2016.

[125] B. Karmakar, B. French, and D. S. Small. Integrating the evidence from evidence factors in observational studies. *Biometrika*, 106(2):353–367, 2019.

[126] B. Karmakar, D. S. Small, and P. R. Rosenbaum. Using approximation algorithms to build evidence factors and related designs for observational studies. *Journal of Computational and Graphical Statistics*, 28(3):698–709, 2019.

[127] B. Karmakar, D. S. Small, and P. R. Rosenbaum. Reinforced designs: Multiple instruments plus control groups as evidence factors in an observational study of the effectiveness of Catholic schools. *Journal of the American Statistical Association*, 115(to appear):1–33, 2020.

[128] B. Karmakar, D. S. Small, and P. R. Rosenbaum. Using evidence factors to clarify exposure biomarkers. *American Journal of Epidemiology*, 189(3):243–249, 2020.

[129] O. Kempthorne. *The Design and Analysis of Experiments*. Wiley, 1952.

[130] G. G. Koch and S. A. Gansky. Statistical considerations for multiplicity in confirmatory protocols. *Drug Information Journal*, 30(2):523–534, 1996.

[131] N. Kopjar and V. Garaj-Vrhovac. Application of the alkaline comet assay in human biomonitoring for genotoxicity: A study on Croatian medical personnel handling antineoplastic drugs. *Mutagenesis*, 16(1):71–78, 2001.

[132] B. Korte and J. Vygen. *Combinatorial Optimization: Theory and Algorithms.* Springer, 5th edition, 2012.

[133] N. Koyawala, J. H. Silber, P. R. Rosenbaum, W. Wang, A. S. Hill, J. G. Reiter, B. A. Niknam, O. Even-Shoshan, R. D. Bloom, D. Sawinski, S. Nazarian, J. Trofe-Clark, M. A. Lim, J. D. Schold, and P. P. Reese. Comparing outcomes between antibody induction therapies in kidney transplantation. *Journal of the American Society of Nephrology*, 28(7):2188–2200, 2017.

[134] H. Kurzweil and B. Stellmacher. *The Theory of Finite Groups: An Introduction.* Springer, 2006.

[135] D. A. Lawlor, K. Tilling, and G. Davey Smith. Triangulation in aetiological epidemiology. *International Journal of Epidemiology*, 45(6):1866–1886, 2016.

[136] K. Lee, D. S. Small, J. Y. Hsu, J. H. Silber, and P. R. Rosenbaum. Discovering effect modification in an observational study of surgical mortality at hospitals with superior nursing. *Journal of the Royal Statistical Society A*, 181(2):535–546, 2018.

[137] K. Lee, D. S. Small, and P. R. Rosenbaum. A new, powerful approach to the study of effect modification in observational studies. *Biometrics*, 74(4):1161–1170, 2018.

[138] E. L. Lehmann. Testing multiparameter hypotheses. *Annals of Mathematical Statistics*, 23(4):541–552, 1952.

[139] E. L. Lehmann. Nonparametric confidence intervals for a shift parameter. *Annals of Mathematical Statistics*, 34(4):1507–1512, 1963.

[140] E. L. Lehmann. *Nonparametrics: Statistical Methods Based on Ranks.* Holden-Day, 1975.

[141] E. L. Lehmann and J. P. Romano. *Testing Statistical Hypotheses.* Springer, 3rd Edition, 2006.

[142] E. L. Lehmann and C. Stein. On the theory of some non-parametric hypotheses. *The Annals of Mathematical Statistics*, 20(1):28–45, 1949.

[143] Y. Lepage. A combination of Wilcoxon's and Ansari-Bradley's statistics. *Biometrika*, 58(1):213–217, 1971.

[144] A. M. Lilienfeld. "On the methodology of investigations of etiologic factors in chronic diseases"—Some comments. *Journal of Chronic Diseases*, 10(1):41–46, 1959.

[145] L. Lovász and M. D. Plummer. *Matching Theory*, volume 367. American Mathematical Society/Chelsea, 1986.

[146] B. Lu, R. Greevy, X. Xu, and C. Beck. Optimal nonbipartite matching and its statistical applications. *American Statistician*, 65(1):21–30, 2011.

[147] B. Lu and P. R. Rosenbaum. Optimal pair matching with two control groups. *Journal of Computational and Graphical Statistics*, 13(2):422–434, 2004.

[148] H. B. Mann and D. R. Whitney. On a test of whether one of two random variables is stochastically larger than the other. *The Annals of Mathematical Statistics*, pages 50–60, 1947.

[149] C. F. Manski, J. V. Pepper, Y. F. Thomas, the Committee on Data, and Research for Policy on Illegal Drugs. *Assessment of Two Cost-Effectiveness Studies on Cocaine Control Policy*. Washington, DC: National Academies Press, 1999.

[150] N. Mantel and W. Haenszel. Statistical aspects of the analysis of data from retrospective studies of disease. *Journal of the National Cancer Institute*, 22(4):719–748, 1959.

[151] R. Marcus, E. Peritz, and K. R. Gabriel. On closed testing procedures with special reference to ordered analysis of variance. *Biometrika*, 63(3):655–660, 1976.

[152] J. I. Marden. Use of nested orthogonal contrasts in analyzing rank data. *Journal of the American Statistical Association*, 87(418):307–318, 1992.

[153] J. S. Maritz. A note on exact robust confidence intervals for location. *Biometrika*, 66(1):163–170, 1979.

[154] E. P. Markowski and T. P. Hettmansperger. Inference based on simple rank step score statistics for the location model. *Journal of the American Statistical Association*, 77(380):901–907, 1982.

[155] A. W. Marshall, I. Olkin, and B. C. Arnold. *Inequalities: Theory of Majorization and its Applications*. Springer, 1979.

[156] L. C. McCandless, P. Gustafson, and A. Levy. Bayesian sensitivity analysis for unmeasured confounding in observational studies. *Statistics in Medicine*, 26(11):2331–2347, 2007.

[157] D. Mehrotra, Xi. Lu, and X. Li. Rank-based analyses of stratified experiments. *American Statistician*, 64(2):121–130, 2010.

[158] J. Milyo and J. Waldfogel. The effect of price advertising on prices: Evidence in the wake of 44 Liquormart. *American Economic Review*, 89(5):1081–1096, 1999.

[159] D. E. Morton, A. J. Saah, S. L. Silberg, W. L. Owens, M. A. Roberts, and M. D. Saah. Lead absorption in children of employees in a lead-related industry. *American Journal of Epidemiology*, 115(4):549–555, 1982.

[160] R. Mukerjee and C. F. J. Wu. *A Modern Theory of Factorial Design*. Springer, 2007.

[161] M. R. Munafò and G. Davey Smith. Repeating experiments is not enough. *Nature*, 553(7689):399–401, 2018.

[162] G. Nattino, B. Lu, J. Shi, S. Lemeshow, and H. Xiang. Triplet matching for estimating causal effects with three treatment arms: A comparative study of mortality by trauma center level. *Journal of the American Statistical Association*, pages 1–10, 2020.

[163] D. Neumark and W. L. Wascher. *Minimum Wages*. MIT Press, 2008.

[164] J. Neyman. On the application of probability theory to agricultural experiments: Essay on principles. Section 9. (English translation of Neyman (1923)). *Statistical Science*, 5(4):465–472, 1990.

[165] G. E. Noether. Efficiency of the Wilcoxon two-sample statistic for randomized blocks. *Journal of the American Statistical Association*, 58(304):894–898, 1963.

[166] G. E. Noether. Some simple distribution-free confidence intervals for the center of a symmetric distribution. *Journal of the American Statistical Association*, 68(343):716–719, 1973.

[167] P. S. Olmstead and J. W. Tukey. A corner test for association. *Annals of Mathematical Statistics*, 18(4):495–513, 1947.

[168] C. L. Park. What is the value of replicating other studies? *Research Evaluation*, 13(3):189–195, 2004.

[169] E. T. Parker. Orthogonal Latin squares. *Proceedings of the National Academy of Sciences of the United States of America*, 45(6):859, 1959.

[170] D. O. Parsons. The health and earnings of rejected disability insurance applicants: comment. *American Economic Review*, 81(5):1419–1426, 1991.

[171] C.S. Peirce. *The Essential Peirce, Volume 1: Selected Philosophical Writings (1867–1893)*. Indiana University Press, 1992.

[172] S. D. Pimentel, R. R. Kelz, J. H. Silber, and P. R. Rosenbaum. Large, sparse optimal matching with refined covariate balance in an observational study of the health outcomes produced by new surgeons. *Journal of the American Statistical Association*, 110(510):515–527, 2015.

[173] S. D. Pimentel, D. S. Small, and P. R Rosenbaum. Constructed second control groups and attenuation of unmeasured biases. *Journal of the American Statistical Association*, 111(515):1157–1167, 2016.

[174] S. D. Pimentel, F. Yoon, and L. Keele. Variable-ratio matching with fine balance in a study of the peer health exchange. *Statistics in Medicine*, 34(30):4070–4082, 2015.

[175] E. J. G. Pitman. Significance tests which may be applied to samples from any populations. *Supplement to the Journal of the Royal Statistical Society*, 4(1):119–130, 1937.

[176] G. Polya. Heuristic reasoning and the theory of probability. *American Mathematical Monthly*, 48(7):450–465, 1941.

[177] G. Polya. *Mathematics and Plausible Reasoning, Volume II: Patterns of Plausible Inference*. Princeton University Press, 2nd edition, 1968.

[178] J. W. Pratt. Length of confidence intervals. *Journal of the American Statistical Association*, 56(295):549–567, 1961.

[179] R. H. Randles and R. V. Hogg. Certain uncorrelated and independent rank statistics. *Journal of the American Statistical Association*, 66(335):569–574, 1971.

[180] N. Rescher. *Cognitive Harmony: The Role of Systemic Harmony in the Constitution of Knowledge*. University of Pittsburgh Press, Pittsburgh, PA, 2005.

[181] S. I. Resnick. *A Probability Path*. Springer, 2003.

[182] T. M. Rivers. Viruses and Koch's postulates. *Journal of Bacteriology*, 33(1):1, 1937.

[183] S. Roman. *Fundamentals of Group Theory*. Springer, 2011.

[184] P. R. Rosenbaum. From association to causation in observational studies: The role of tests of strongly ignorable treatment assignment. *Journal of the American Statistical Association*, 79(385):41–48, 1984.

[185] P. R. Rosenbaum. Sensitivity analysis for certain permutation inferences in matched observational studies. *Biometrika*, 74(1):13–26, 1987.

[186] P. R. Rosenbaum. On permutation tests for hidden biases in observational studies: An application of Holley's inequality to the Savage lattice. *Annals of Statistics*, pages 643–653, 1989.

[187] P. R. Rosenbaum. A characterization of optimal designs for observational studies. *Journal of the Royal Statistical Society B*, 53(3):597–610, 1991.

[188] P. R. Rosenbaum. Hodges-Lehmann point estimates of treatment effect in observational studies. *Journal of the American Statistical Association*, 88(424):1250–1253, 1993.

[189] P. R. Rosenbaum. Quantiles in nonrandom samples and observational studies. *Journal of the American Statistical Association*, 90(432):1424–1431, 1995.

[190] P. R. Rosenbaum. Signed rank statistics for coherent predictions. *Biometrics*, 556–566, 1997.

[191] P. R. Rosenbaum. Reduced sensitivity to hidden bias at upper quantiles in observational studies with dilated treatment effects. *Biometrics*, 55(2):560–564, 1999.

[192] P. R. Rosenbaum. Effects attributable to treatment: Inference in experiments and observational studies with a discrete pivot. *Biometrika*, 88(1):219–231, 2001.

[193] P. R. Rosenbaum. Replicating effects and biases. *The American Statistician*, 55(3):223–227, 2001.

[194] P. R. Rosenbaum. Covariance adjustment in randomized experiments and observational studies (with discussion). *Statistical Science*, 17(3):286–327, 2002.

[195] P. R. Rosenbaum. *Observational Studies*. Springer, 2nd edition, 2002.

[196] P. R. Rosenbaum. Does a dose–response relationship reduce sensitivity to hidden bias? *Biostatistics*, 4(1):1–10, 2003.

[197] P. R. Rosenbaum. Exact confidence intervals for nonconstant effects by inverting the signed rank test. *American Statistician*, 57(2):132–138, 2003.

[198] P. R. Rosenbaum. Design sensitivity in observational studies. *Biometrika*, 91(1):153–164, 2004.

[199] P. R. Rosenbaum. Attributable effects in case^2 studies. *Biometrics*, 61(1):246–253, 2005.

[200] P. R. Rosenbaum. Heterogeneity and causality: Unit heterogeneity and design sensitivity in observational studies. *American Statistician*, 59(2):147–152, 2005.

[201] P. R. Rosenbaum. Reasons for effects. *Chance*, 18(1):5–10, 2005.

[202] P. R. Rosenbaum. Confidence intervals for uncommon but dramatic responses to treatment. *Biometrics*, 63(4):1164–1171, 2007.

[203] P. R. Rosenbaum. Interference between units in randomized experiments. *Journal of the American Statistical Association*, 102(477):191–200, 2007.

[204] P. R. Rosenbaum. Sensitivity analysis for m-estimates, tests, and confidence intervals in matched observational studies. *Biometrics*, 63(2):456–464, 2007.

[205] P. R. Rosenbaum. Testing hypotheses in order. *Biometrika*, 95(1):248–252, 2008.

[206] P. R. Rosenbaum. Design sensitivity and efficiency in observational studies. *Journal of the American Statistical Association*, 105(490):692–702, 2010.

[207] P. R. Rosenbaum. Evidence factors in observational studies. *Biometrika*, 97(2):333–345, 2010.

[208] P. R. Rosenbaum. A new U-statistic with superior design sensitivity in matched observational studies. *Biometrics*, 67(3):1017–1027, 2011.

[209] P. R. Rosenbaum. Some approximate evidence factors in observational studies. *Journal of the American Statistical Association*, 106(493):285–295, 2011.

[210] P. R. Rosenbaum. An exact adaptive test with superior design sensitivity in an observational study of treatments for ovarian cancer. *The Annals of Applied Statistics*, 6(1):83–105, 2012.

[211] P. R. Rosenbaum. Testing one hypothesis twice in observational studies. *Biometrika*, 99(4):763–774, 2012.

[212] P. R. Rosenbaum. Impact of multiple matched controls on design sensitivity in observational studies. *Biometrics*, 69(1):118–127, 2013.

[213] P. R. Rosenbaum. Using differential comparisons in observational studies. *Chance*, 26(3):18–25, 2013.

[214] P. R. Rosenbaum. Weighted m-statistics with superior design sensitivity in matched observational studies with multiple controls. *Journal of the American Statistical Association*, 109(507):1145–1158, 2014.

[215] P. R. Rosenbaum. Bahadur efficiency of sensitivity analyses in observational studies. *Journal of the American Statistical Association*, 110(509):205–217, 2015.

[216] P. R. Rosenbaum. Cochran's causal crossword. *Observational Studies*, 1:205–211, 2015.

[217] P. R. Rosenbaum. Two R packages for sensitivity analysis in observational studies. *Observational Studies*, 1(1):1–17, 2015.

[218] P. R. Rosenbaum. The cross-cut statistic and its sensitivity to bias in observational studies with ordered doses of treatment. *Biometrics*, 72(1):175–183, 2016.

[219] P. R. Rosenbaum. Using Scheffé projections for multiple outcomes in an observational study of smoking and periodontal disease. *The Annals of Applied Statistics*, 10(3):1447–1471, 2016.

[220] P. R. Rosenbaum. The general structure of evidence factors in observational studies. *Statistical Science*, 32(4):514–530, 2017.

[221] P. R. Rosenbaum. Sensitivity analysis for stratified comparisons in an observational study of the effect of smoking on homocysteine levels. *Annals of Applied Statistics*, 12(4):2312–2334, 2018.

[222] P. R. Rosenbaum. A conditional test with demonstrated insensitivity to unmeasured bias in matched observational studies. *Biometrika*, doi:10.1093/biomet/asaa032, 2020.

[223] P. R. Rosenbaum. *Design of Observational Studies*. Springer, 2nd edition, 2020.

[224] P. R. Rosenbaum. Modern algorithms for matching in observational studies. *Annual Review of Statistics and Its Application*, 7:143–176, 2020.

[225] P. R. Rosenbaum and A. M. Krieger. Sensitivity of two-sample permutation inferences in observational studies. *Journal of the American Statistical Association*, 85(410):493–498, 1990.

[226] P. R. Rosenbaum, R. N. Ross, and J. H. Silber. Minimum distance matched sampling with fine balance in an observational study of treatment for ovarian cancer. *Journal of the American Statistical Association*, 102(477):75–83, 2007.

[227] P. R. Rosenbaum and D. B. Rubin. Assessing sensitivity to an unobserved binary covariate in an observational study with binary outcome. *Journal of the Royal Statistical Society B*, 45(2):212–218, 1983.

[228] P. R. Rosenbaum and D. B. Rubin. The central role of the propensity score in observational studies for causal effects. *Biometrika*, 70(1):41–55, 1983.

[229] P. R. Rosenbaum and D. B. Rubin. Reducing bias in observational studies using subclassification on the propensity score. *Journal of the American Statistical Association*, 79(387):516–524, 1984.

[230] P. R. Rosenbaum and D. B. Rubin. Constructing a control group using multivariate matched sampling methods that incorporate the propensity score. *American Statistician*, 39(1):33–38, 1985.

[231] P. R. Rosenbaum and J. H. Silber. Amplification of sensitivity analysis in matched observational studies. *Journal of the American Statistical Association*, 104(488):1398–1405, 2009.

[232] P. R. Rosenbaum and J. H. Silber. Using the exterior match to compare two entwined matched control groups. *The American Statistician*, 67(2):67–75, 2013.

[233] P. R. Rosenbaum and D. S. Small. An adaptive Mantel–Haenszel test for sensitivity analysis in observational studies. *Biometrics*, 73(2):422–430, 2017.

[234] P.R. Rosenbaum. *Observation and Experiment: An Introduction to Causal Inference*. Harvard University Press, Cambridge, MA, USA, 2017.

[235] W. F. Rosenberger and J. M. Lachin. *Randomization in Clinical Trials: Theory and Practice*. John Wiley & Sons, 2015.

[236] J. J. Rotman. *An Introduction to the Theory of Groups*. Springer, 1995.

[237] D. B. Rubin. Estimating causal effects of treatments in randomized and non-randomized studies. *Journal of Educational Psychology*, 66(5):688, 1974.

[238] D. B. Rubin. Assignment to treatment group on the basis of a covariate. *Journal of Educational Statistics*, 2(1):1–26, 1977.

[239] D. B. Rubin. Using multivariate matched sampling and regression adjustment to control bias in observational studies. *Journal of the American Statistical Association*, 74(366a):318–328, 1979.

[240] D. B. Rubin. Comment: Which ifs have causal answers? *Journal of the American Statistical Association*, 81(396):961–962, 1986.

[241] D. B. Rubin. The design versus the analysis of observational studies for causal effects: Parallels with the design of randomized trials. *Statistics in Medicine*, 26(1):20–36, 2007.

[242] K. E. Rudolph and E. A. Stuart. Using sensitivity analyses for unobserved confounding to address covariate measurement error in propensity score methods. *American Journal of Epidemiology*, 187(3):604–613, 2018.

[243] D. Salsburg. Alternative hypotheses for the effects of drugs in small-scale clinical studies. *Biometrics*, pages 671–674, 1986.

[244] I. R. Savage. On the independence of tests of randomness and other hypotheses. *Journal of the American Statistical Association*, 52(277):53–57, 1957.

[245] H. Scheffe. *The Analysis of Variance*. John Wiley & Sons, 1959.

[246] S. Schwartz, F. Li, and J. P. Reiter. Sensitivity analysis for unmeasured confounding in principal stratification settings with binary variables. *Statistics in Medicine*, 31(10):949–962, 2012.

[247] B. Schweizer and E. F. Wolff. On nonparametric measures of dependence for random variables. *Annals of Statistics*, 9(4):879–885, 1981.

[248] R. Sedgewick and P. Flajolet. *An Introduction to the Analysis of Algorithms*. Addison-Wesley, 1996.

[249] US Public Health Service. *Smoking and Health: Report of the Advisory Committee to the Surgeon General*. US Department of Health and Human Services, 1964.

[250] US Public Health Service. *The Health Consequences of Involuntary Exposure to Tobacco Smoke: A Report of the Surgeon General*. US Department of Health and Human Services, 2006.

[251] US Public Health Service. *The Health Consequences of Smoking—50 Years of Progress: A Report of the Surgeon General.* US Department of Health and Human Services, 2014.

[252] J. P. Shaffer. Bidirectional unbiased procedures. *Journal of the American Statistical Association*, 69(346):437–439, 1974.

[253] J. P. Shaffer. Modified sequentially rejective multiple test procedures. *Journal of the American Statistical Association*, 81(395):826–831, 1986.

[254] M. Shaked and J. G. Shanthikumar. *Stochastic Orders.* Springer, 2007.

[255] S. S. Shapiro and M. B. Wilk. An analysis of variance test for normality. *Biometrika*, 52(3/4):591–611, 1965.

[256] J. H. Silber, A. Cnaan, B. J. Clark, S. M. Paridon, A. J. Chin, J. Rychik, A. N. Hogarty, M. I. Cohen, G. Barber, M. Rutkowski, and T. R. Kimball. Enalapril to prevent cardiac function decline in long-term survivors of pediatric cancer exposed to anthracyclines. *Journal of Clinical Oncology*, 22(5):820–828, 2004.

[257] J. H. Silber, P. R. Rosenbaum, M. D. McHugh, J. M. Ludwig, H. L. Smith, B. A. Niknam, O. Even-Shoshan, L. A. Fleisher, R. R. Kelz, and L. H. Aiken. Comparison of the value of nursing work environments in hospitals across different levels of patient risk. *JAMA Surgery*, 151(6):527–536, 2016.

[258] R. J. Simes. An improved Bonferroni procedure for multiple tests of significance. *Biometrika*, 73(3):751–754, 1986.

[259] N. P. Singh, M. T. McCoy, R. R. Tice, and E. L. Schneider. A simple technique for quantitation of low levels of DNA damage in individual cells. *Experimental Cell Research*, 175(1):184–191, 1988.

[260] M. E. Sobel. What do randomized studies of housing mobility demonstrate? causal inference in the face of interference. *Journal of the American Statistical Association*, 101(476):1398–1407, 2006.

[261] K. W. Staley. Robust evidence and secure evidence claims. *Philosophy of Science*, 71(4):467–488, 2004.

[262] W. R. Stephenson. A general class of one-sample nonparametric test statistics based on subsamples. *Journal of the American Statistical Association*, 76(376):960–966, 1981.

[263] G. J. Stigler. The economics of minimum wage legislation. *American Economic Review*, 36(3):358–365, 1946.

[264] B. L. Strom, R. Schinnar, J. Karlawish, S. Hennessy, V. Teal, and W. B. Bilker. Statin therapy and risk of acute memory impairment. *JAMA Internal Medicine*, 175(8):1399–1405, 2015.

[265] E. A. Stuart. Matching methods for causal inference: A review and a look forward. *Statistical Science*, 25(1):1, 2010.

[266] E. A. Stuart and K. M. Green. Using full matching to estimate causal effects in nonexperimental studies: Examining the relationship between adolescent

marijuana use and adult outcomes. *Developmental Psychology*, 44(2):395, 2008.

[267] M. Susser. *Causal Thinking in the Health Sciences*. Oxford University Press, New York, 1973.

[268] M. Susser. *Epidemiology, Health and Society: Selected Papers*. Oxford University Press, New York, 1987.

[269] J. Szép. On the structure of groups which can be represented as the product of two subgroups. *Acta Scientiarum Mathematicarum (Szeged)*, 12:57–61, 1950.

[270] E. J. Tchetgen Tchetgen and T. J. VanderWeele. On causal inference in the presence of interference. *Statistical Methods in Medical Research*, 21(1):55–75, 2012.

[271] S. L. Tomar and S. Asma. Smoking-attributable periodontitis in the United States: Findings from NHANES III. *Journal of Periodontology*, 71(5):743–751, 2000.

[272] D. F. Tough and J. Sprent. Lifespan of lymphocytes. *Immunologic Research*, 14(1):1–12, 1995.

[273] N. Y. Tretyakova, A. Groehler IV, and S. Ji. DNA–protein cross-links: Formation, structural identities, and biological outcomes. *Accounts of Chemical Research*, 48(6):1631–1644, 2015.

[274] J. W. Tukey. We need both exploratory and confirmatory. *American Statistician*, 34(1):23–25, 1980.

[275] B. T. Tunca and U. Egeli. Cytogenetic findings on shoe workers exposed long-term to benzene. *Environmental Health Perspectives*, 104(suppl 6):1313–1317, 1996.

[276] M. J. Van der Laan and S. Rose. *Targeted Learning: Causal Inference for Observational and Experimental Data*. Springer, 2011.

[277] C. van Eeden. An analogue, for signed rank statistics, of Jureckova's asymptotic linearity theorem for rank statistics. *Annals of Mathematical Statistics*, 43(3):791–802, 1972.

[278] V. V. Vazirani. *Approximation Algorithms*. Springer, 2013.

[279] S. Wager and S. Athey. Estimation and inference of heterogeneous treatment effects using random forests. *Journal of the American Statistical Association*, 113(523):1228–1242, 2018.

[280] A. Wald. Note on the consistency of the maximum likelihood estimate. *Annals of Mathematical Statistics*, 20(4):595–601, 1949.

[281] L. Walker, H. LeVine, and M. Jucker. Koch's postulates and infectious proteins. *Acta Neuropathologica*, 112(1):1, 2006.

[282] J. Waller. *The Discovery of the Germ: Twenty Years that Transformed the Way We Think About Disease*. Columbia University Press, New York, 2002.

[283] G. Wassmer and W. Brannath. *Group Sequential and Confirmatory Adaptive Designs in Clinical Trials*. Springer, 2016.

[284] L. Weiss. A note on confidence sets for random variables. *The Annals of Mathematical Statistics*, 26(1):142–144, 1955.

[285] B. L. Welch. On the z-test in randomized blocks and Latin squares. *Biometrika*, 29(1/2):21–52, 1937.

[286] B. L. Wiens. A fixed sequence Bonferroni procedure for testing multiple endpoints. *Pharmaceutical Statistics*, 2(3):211–215, 2003.

[287] B. L. Wiens and A. Dmitrienko. The fallback procedure for evaluating a single family of hypotheses. *Journal of Biopharmaceutical Statistics*, 15(6):929–942, 2005.

[288] F. Wilcoxon. Individual comparisons by ranking methods. *Biometrics*, 1(6):80–83, 1945.

[289] M. B. Wilk. The randomization analysis of a generalized randomized block design. *Biometrika*, 42(1/2):70–79, 1955.

[290] D. P. Williamson and D. B. Shmoys. *The Design of Approximation Algorithms*. Cambridge university press, 2011.

[291] S. G. Winter and G. Szulanski. Replication as strategy. *Organization Science*, 12(6):730–743, 2001.

[292] L. Wittgenstein. *Philosophical Investigations*. Macmillan, 1954.

[293] L. Wittgenstein. *On Certainty*. Harper and Row, 1969.

[294] L. Wittgenstein. *Culture and Value*. University of Chicago Press, 1984.

[295] D. A. Wolfe. Some general results about uncorrelated statistics. *Journal of the American Statistical Association*, 68(344):1013–1018, 1973.

[296] D. A. Wolfe and R. V. Hogg. On constructing statistics and reporting data. *The American Statistician*, 25(4):27–30, 1971.

[297] C. F. J. Wu and M. S. Hamada. *Experiments: Planning, Analysis, and Optimization*, volume 552. John Wiley & Sons, 2011.

[298] Fang-Yang Wu, Pao-Wen Chang, Chin-Ching Wu, and Hsien-Wen Kuo. Correlations of blood lead with DNA-protein cross-links and sister chromatid exchanges in lead workers. *Cancer Epidemiology and Prevention Biomarkers*, 11(3):287–290, 2002.

[299] D. Yang, D. S. Small, J. H. Silber, and P. R. Rosenbaum. Optimal matching with minimal deviation from fine balance in a study of obesity and surgical outcomes. *Biometrics*, 68(2):628–636, 2012.

[300] F. Yang, J. R. Zubizarreta, D. S. Small, S. Lorch, and P. R. Rosenbaum. Dissonant conclusions when testing the validity of an instrumental variable. *American Statistician*, 68(4):253–263, 2014.

[301] K. Yano, G. G. Rhoads, and A. Kagan. Coffee, alcohol and risk of coronary heart disease among Japanese men living in Hawaii. *New England Journal of Medicine*, 297(8):405–409, 1977.

[302] J. Yerushalmy and C. E. Palmer. On the methodology of investigations of etiologic factors in chronic diseases. *Journal of Chronic Diseases*, 10(1):27–40, 1959.

[303] R. Yu, J. H. Silber, and P. R. Rosenbaum. Matching methods for observational studies derived from large administrative databases (with discussion). *Statistical Science*, 2020.

[304] S. Zaheer, S. D. Pimentel, K. D. Simmons, L. E. Kuo, J. Datta, N. Williams, D. L. Fraker, and R. R. Kelz. Comparing international and United States undergraduate medical education and surgical outcomes using a refined balance matching methodology. *Annals of Surgery*, 265(5):916–922, 2017.

[305] D. V. Zaykin, L. A. Zhivotovsky, P. H. Westfall, and B. S. Weir. Truncated product method for combining p-values. *Genetic Epidemiology*, 22(2):170–185, 2002.

[306] M. Zhang, Z. Chen, Q. Chen, H. Zou, J. Lou, and J. He. Investigating DNA damage in tannery workers occupationally exposed to trivalent chromium using comet assay. *Mutation Research/Genetic Toxicology and Environmental Mutagenesis*, 654(1):45–51, 2008.

[307] Q. Zhao. On sensitivity value of pair-matched observational studies. *Journal of the American Statistical Association*, 2018.

[308] Q. Zhao. Covariate balancing propensity score by tailored loss functions. *The Annals of Statistics*, 47(2):965–993, 2019.

[309] J. R. Zubizarreta. Using mixed integer programming for matching in an observational study of kidney failure after surgery. *Journal of the American Statistical Association*, 107(500):1360–1371, 2012.

[310] J. R. Zubizarreta, M. Cerdá, and P. R. Rosenbaum. Effect of the 2010 Chilean earthquake on posttraumatic stress reducing sensitivity to unmeasured bias through study design. *Epidemiology*, 24(1):79, 2013.

[311] J. R. Zubizarreta, M. Neuman, J. H. Silber, and P. R. Rosenbaum. Contrasting evidence within and between institutions that provide treatment in an observational study of alternate forms of anesthesia. *Journal of the American Statistical Association*, 107(499):901–915, 2012.

[312] J. R. Zubizarreta, R. D. Paredes, and P. R. Rosenbaum. Matching for balance, pairing for heterogeneity in an observational study of the effectiveness of for-profit and not-for-profit high schools in Chile. *Annals of Applied Statistics*, 8(1):204–231, 2014.

[313] J. R. Zubizarreta, C. E. Reinke, R. R. Kelz, J. H. Silber, and P. R. Rosenbaum. Matching for several sparse nominal variables in a case-control study of readmission following surgery. *American Statistician*, 65(4):229–238, 2011.

[314] J. R. Zubizarreta, D. S. Small, N. K. Goyal, S. Lorch, and P. R. Rosenbaum. Stronger instruments via integer programming in an observational study of late preterm birth outcomes. *Annals of Applied Statistics*, 7(1):25–50, 2013.

Index

Printed in the United States
by Baker & Taylor Publisher Services

Printed in the United States
by Baker & Taylor Publisher Services